Geographic Health Data

Fundamental Techniques for Analysis

FSC
www.fsc.org
MIX
Paper from responsible sources
FSC® C013604

Geographic Health Data

Fundamental Techniques for Analysis

Edited by

Francis P. Boscoe

Department of Epidemiology and Statistics,
University at Albany, New York, USA

www.cabi.org

CABI is a trading name of CAB International

CABI
Nosworthy Way
Wallingford
Oxfordshire OX10 8DE
UK

Tel: +44 (0)1491 832111
Fax: +44 (0)1491 833508
E-mail: info@cabi.org
Website: www.cabi.org

CABI
38 Chauncey Street
Suite 1002
Boston, MA 02111
USA

Tel: +1 800 552 3083 (toll free)
Tel: +1 (0)617 395 4051
E-mail: cabi-nao@cabi.org

A catalogue record for this book is available from the British Library, London, UK.

Library of Congress Cataloging-in-Publication Data

Geographic health data : fundamental techniques for analysis / Francis P. Boscoe, editor.
p. ; cm.
Includes bibliographical references and index.
ISBN 978-1-78064-089-1 (alk. paper)
I. Boscoe, Francis P.
[DNLM: 1. Geographic Information Systems. 2. Geographic Mapping. 3. Health Information Systems. W 26.55.I4]

R859.7.E43
610.285--dc23

2013010067

ISBN-13: 978 1 78064 089 1

Commissioning editor: Rachel Cutts
Editorial assistant: Alexandra Lainsbury
Production editor: Lauren Povey

Typeset by SPi, Pondicherry, India.
Printed and bound in the UK by CPI Group (UK) Ltd, Croydon, CR0 4YY.

Contents

Contributors

Aldo Aviña, University of North Texas Health Science Center, 3500 Camp Bowie Blvd, Fort Worth, TX 76107, USA. E-mail: aldo.avina@unt.edu

Nathaniel Bell, University of South Carolina, College of Nursing, 1601 Green Street, Columbia, SC 29208, USA. E-mail: natejbell@gmail.com

Robert Bergquist, Ingerod, Brastad, Sweden. E-mail: robert.bergquist@yahoo.se

Francis P. Boscoe, Department of Epidemiology and Biostatistics, School of Public Health, University at Albany, Rensselaer, New York, NY 12144-3456, USA. E-mail: fboscoe@albany.edu

Jarvis T. Chen, Department of Social and Behavioral Sciences, School of Public Health, Harvard University, Landmark Center, Room 403-N West Wing, Boston, MA 02215, USA. E-mail: jarvis@hsph.harvard.edu

Jin Chen, AT&T Shannon Laboratory, Florham Park, New Jersey, USA. Correspondence address: 9 Meat Ct, Summit, NJ 07901, USA. E-mail: jinchen1000@gmail.com

Myles Cockburn, Department of Preventive Medicine, University of Southern California, 1441 Eastlake Ave., MC 9175, Los Angeles, CA 90089-9175, USA. E-mail: myles@med.usc.edu

Andrew Curtis, GIS Health and Hazards Lab, Department of Geography, Kent State University, 413 McGilvrey Hall, Kent, OH 44242, USA. E-mail: acurti13@kent.edu

Jacqueline W. Curtis, GIS Health and Hazards Lab, Department of Geography, Kent State University, 413 McGilvrey Hall, Kent, OH 44242, USA. E-mail: jmills30@kent.edu

Daniel W. Goldberg, Department of Geography, Texas A&M University, Room 810 Eller O&M Building, TAMU Mail Stop 3147, College Station, TX 77843-3147, USA. E-mail: daniel.goldberg@tamu.edu

Kevin A. Henry, School of Public Health, Rutgers, The State University of New Jersey, 683 Hoes Lane West, Room 327, Piscataway, NJ 08854, USA. E-mail: medicalgeography@yahoo.com

Geoffrey M. Jacquez, Department of Geography, State University of New York at Buffalo, 112 Wilkeson Quad, Buffalo, NY 14261, USA. E-mail: gjacquez@buffalo.edu

Kaila McDonald, Department of Geography, University of Utah, 260 S. Central Campus, Salt Lake City, UT 84112, USA. E-mail: kaila.mcdonald@yahoo.com

Narelle Mullan, Department of Spatial Sciences, Curtin University and Cooperative Research Centre for Spatial Information (CRCSI), GPO Box U1987, Perth, Western Australia 6845, Australia. E-mail: n.mullan@curtin.edu.au

Adam T. Naito, Department of Geography, Texas A&M University, Room 810 Eller O&M Building, TAMU Mail Stop 3147, College Station, TX 77843-3147, USA. E-mail: adam.naito@tamu.edu

Christopher F.L. Saarnak, Department of Veterinary Disease Biology, Faculty of Health and Medical Sciences, University of Copenhagen, Thorvaldsensvej 57, DK-1871 Frederiksberg C, Denmark. E-mail: cls@sund.ku.dk

Anna-Sofie Stensgaard, Center for Macroecology, Evolution and Climate, Natural History Museum of Denmark, University of Copenhagen, 2100 Copenhagen Ø, Denmark. E-mail: asstensgaard@bio.ku.dk

Chetan Tiwari, Department of Geography, University of North Texas, 1155 Union Circle #305279, Denton, TX 76203-5017, USA. E-mail: chetan.tiwari@unt.edu

Jürg Utzinger, Department of Epidemiology and Public Health, Swiss Tropical and Public Health Institute, Socinstr. 57, PO Box 4002, Basel, Switzerland. E-mail: juerg.utzinger@unibas.ch

Xiao-Nong Zhou, National Institute of Parasitic Diseases, Chinese Center for Disease Control and Prevention, 207 Ruijin Er Rd, Shanghai 200025, People's Republic of China. E-mail: ipdzhouxn@sh163.net

Introduction

Francis P. Boscoe

Geographic Health Data: Fundamental Techniques for Analysis is a survey of the latest techniques for the collection, analysis and display of geographic health data. Unlike other books that are tailored towards large, complex and expensive commercial geographic information system (GIS) software, most of the methods described here only presume that the reader has access to an Internet-linked computer, preferably but not necessarily one with a Windows operating system. As computing power has increased and storage costs have plummeted in recent years, it has become increasingly feasible to conduct sophisticated spatial analyses using free and/or open source tools. In fact, several of the authors of this book have been at the forefront of the development of such tools. Commercial GIS software continues to serve a useful role for organizations that have already invested substantially in them, and for certain highly complex or highly specialized applications. For the rest of us, the techniques presented in this book will serve most purposes.

A major reason for focusing on free software, of course, is cost. In the past, the benefits of free software were often negated by its tendency to be unwieldy, poorly documented and/or not compatible with other software. Today, through the benefits of international collaboration via the Internet, this is much less of a concern. Numerous researchers have attested to the vital role that free software is playing in the strengthening of public health capacity, particularly in resource-poor areas. For example, an international team of researchers in the USA, Mexico, England and South Africa used free Google Earth imagery and editing tools to build a dengue fever surveillance system (Lozano-Fuentes *et al.*, 2008). Raoul Kamadjeu (2009) of the US Centers for Disease Control and Prevention used Google Earth as the foundation of a polio eradication campaign in the Democratic Republic of Congo, in a part of the country with no accurate maps. Comparable projects have focused on rural South Africa (Cinnamon and Schuurman, 2010) and Indonesia (Fisher and Myers, 2011).

Another major reason to focus on open source software is its transparency. Geographic data sets tend to be large and complex, and spatial analytical methods can be highly sensitive to choices of parameters and quality of the source data. In order to ascertain the accuracy, reproducibility and sensitivity of some analytical result, it is important for the researcher to have as much control as possible over the process. This condition is not met when using proprietary software, which is closed source and may operate as a 'black box' (Neteler *et al.*, 2012). There do remain some techniques that are only accessible in 'black box' mode, such as some of the advanced location–allocation modelling methods (see Chapter 10), but the gaps are filling rapidly.

Some of the chapters in the book make use of techniques that involve writing computer code and/or entering statements on a command line. Readers weaned on a diet of drop-down menus, toolbars, keyboard shortcuts and other graphical user interfaces (GUIs) may find this intimidating. I hope that the chapters that follow will convince you otherwise. Certainly, for simple tasks that have to be repeated large numbers of times, such as making small adjustments to point locations on a map display, GUI shortcuts are indispensable. But many GIS analysis tasks tend to be of the opposite variety – complex tasks that only need to be executed a small number of times, or even just once. For such tasks, a coding or command-line approach facilitates sharing between researchers, reproducibility of results and minor modifications to input parameters. It also facilitates a deeper level of thinking about spatial data – a recognition and awareness that just about any problem can be broken down into a number of small steps or algorithms, and that these algorithms tend to be similar across problems. For example, in reading this book, take note of how often square grids are used as a means of simplification and efficiency. As a well-known technical writer put it recently, 'knowing how to code will improve your life even if you don't ever program anything useful … I rarely take up coding in my job, but I learned enough to alter the way I approach problems. And that's the most interesting thing about taking up programming: It teaches you to think algorithmically. When faced with a new challenge—whether at work or around the house—I find myself breaking down the problem into smaller, discrete tasks that can be accomplished by simple, repeatable processes' (Manjoo, 2012).

What is in this book?

This book is designed to help public health professionals and students answer some of the most fundamental and recurring questions that arise about the collection, analysis and display of geographic health data. The 11 chapters, which are from ten different primary authors working in the field of GIS and public health, draw from their original, cutting-edge research across the globe. The first chapter, 'Points, Lines and Polygons', begins with the fundamental relationships between these spatial objects – relationships that form the core of GIS and spatial analysis. The algorithms used to determine such relationships as adjacent, near, inside and shortest path are explained. GIS users take these concepts for granted, even without necessarily being able to explain how or why they work, while non-GIS users tend towards 'brute force' versions of these algorithms. The aim of this chapter is to lead both groups towards improved spatial thinking.

The next three chapters are concerned with geographic data collection. Chapter 2, 'Geographic Data Acquisition', focuses on the rapid enhancements in geographic data availability and ease of use, from both a top-down and bottom-up perspective, where top-down refers to government-provided and commercially available data and bottom-up refers to citizen-supplied data, also known as volunteered geographic information (VGI). The authors use a US-based Emergency Operations Center as a running example, with a special focus on the Joplin, Missouri tornado of 2011. Chapter 3, 'Virtual Globes and Geospatial Health: The Public Health Potential of New Tools for the Control and Elimination of Infectious Diseases', reviews the potential applications of virtual globes (specifically, Google Earth) in infectious disease surveillance, with the primary example being the schistosomiasis elimination programme currently being undertaken in China. Chapter 4, 'Geocoding and Health', describes the process by which textual address information is converted into geographic coordinates and used in public health investigations. The authors describe several open access geocoding resources, including one developed by the lead author himself.

Chapter 5, 'Visualization and Cartography', is concerned with how epidemiological data can be assembled into thematic maps and accompanying statistical graphics. This is distinct from the primarily feature-based and locational maps covered up to this point. The authors demonstrate how to construct a thematic map using Quantum GIS, a free and open source software package, using malaria incidence data from Colombia. Moving on from spatial data display, the remainder of the book is concerned with methods of spatial data analysis. Chapter 6, 'Spatial Overlays', covers the most fundamental form of spatial analysis, which is combining layers of points, lines and polygons to identify possible associations. The authors work through a detailed example that assesses pesticide exposure in California's Central Valley, starting with layers of population, crop, pesticide and climatological data.

Geographic health data tends to be noisy, meaning that it exhibits a lot of local spatial variation. The next two chapters describe methods for identifying patterns within such data. Chapter 7, 'Spatial Cluster Analysis', describes techniques for identifying areas where unusually high or low concentrations of some phenomena may be found, using the example of cervical cancer mortality data in the USA. Chapter 8, 'Methods for Creating Smoothed Maps of Disease Burdens', describes methods for combining data from neighbouring locations to reduce variability. The author illustrates the technique by revisiting the malaria incidence data from Chapter 5 using his self-written open source software.

The final three chapters cover more advanced spatial techniques. Chapter 9, 'Geographic Access to Health Services', reviews methods for assessing the extent to which a population is able to satisfy its demand for health care. An important goal of this line of inquiry is to identify underserved areas – those where travel distances pose an important barrier, or where demand for a service outstrips supply. The techniques are illustrated using an example of colorectal cancer screening in the state of Utah. The following chapter, 'Location–allocation Modelling for Health Services Research in Low Resource Settings', goes beyond simply identifying underserved areas to figuring out how actually to serve them. This is done through the creation of new health care resources (location) or the rearrangement of existing ones (allocation). The methods are illustrated with a case study from Romania and commercial GIS software – in contrast to the rest of the book, no free or open source solution presents itself in this instance. The final chapter, 'Multilevel and Hierarchical Models for Disease Mapping', considers a class of mathematical models for describing disease rates that account for multiple scales of causal influence (such as individuals residing in households in neighbourhoods in cities in states, all of which can contribute to health outcomes). Readers will notice a familiarity with the earlier chapter on creating smoothed maps – while the maths is more involved, the same basic concept applies: the health conditions in a location are necessarily influenced by the conditions in surrounding locations. Here, the methods are illustrated using lung cancer mortality data in Boston, Massachusetts.

Finally, please note that while this book does not contain any colour images, some of the maps and graphics are best seen in colour. These images have been placed on a web site (www.albany.edu/~fboscoe/gisbook) that the reader is encouraged to visit.

References

Cinnamon, J. and Schuurman, N. (2010) Injury surveillance in low-resource setting using geospatial and social web technologies. *International Journal of Health Geographics* 9:25. Available at: http://www.ij-healthgeographics.com/content/9/1/25 (accessed 12 March 2013).

Fisher, R.P. and Myers, B.A. (2011) Free and simple GIS as appropriate for health mapping in a low resource setting: a case study in eastern Indonesia. *International Journal of Health Geographics* 10:15. Available at: http://www.ij-healthgeographics.com/content/10/1/15 (accessed 12 March 2013).

Kamadjeu, R. (2009) Tracking the polio virus down the Congo River: a case study on the use of Google Earth™ in public health planning and mapping. *International Journal of Health Geographics* 8:4. Available at: http://www.ij-healthgeographics.com/content/8/1/4 (accessed 12 March 2013).

Lozano-Fuentes, S. *et al.* (2008) Use of Google Earth™ to strengthen public health capacity and facilitate management of vector-borne diseases in resource-poor environments. *Bulletin of the World Health Organization* 86, 718–725.

Manjoo, F. (2012) You need to learn how to program: make a free weekly coding lesson your New Year's resolution. *Slate*, January 4, 2012.

Neteler, M., Bowman, M.H., Landa, M. and Metz, M. (2012) GRASS GIS: a multi-purpose open source GIS. *Environmental Modelling and Software* 31, 124–130.

1 Points, Lines and Polygons

Francis P. Boscoe*
Department of Epidemiology and Biostatistics, University at Albany, New York, USA

1.1 Introduction

Any natural or human-created feature on or near the earth's surface can be represented as a zero-, one- or two-dimensional object. In this book we refer to these objects, respectively, as points, lines and polygons; commonly encountered synonyms include nodes, arcs, and areas, respectively. (While it is also possible to represent features as three-dimensional objects, this is rarely called for in public health, and is beyond the scope of this book.) The type of object that is chosen to represent a particular feature depends on the scale of interest. At the scale of a nation, rivers are typically represented as lines and cities as points, but at a fine scale both can be represented as polygons.

The relationships between points, lines and polygons are the domain of a branch of mathematics and computer science known as computational geometry. Scientists working in this sub-field concern themselves with finding efficient algorithms for computing these relationships. These algorithms form the core of geographic information system (GIS) software packages, and are also integral to the rendering of computer graphics in films and video games and navigation problems in robotics.

University courses in GIS tend to gloss over these algorithms. Instead, students are shown the menus or toolbars needed to compute and display the underlying relationships; the inner workings of the software remain a mystery. As discussed in the introduction, this approach has its limitations.

The purpose of this chapter is to provide a glimpse of the inner workings of GIS software by reviewing some of the basic algorithms governing the relationships of points, lines and polygons. These relationships are universal and can be implemented in just about any programming language or statistical software package that one chooses. When I receive GIS-related questions in my capacity as an employee of a state health department, it is often the case that the questioners possess the knowledge and skills needed to answer the question, but have been blinkered by the belief that they lacked some essential piece of specialized software.

While the specialized journals within the sub-field of computational geometry can be densely mathematical, many of the basic concepts require only rudimentary spatial thinking and common sense, and can be communicated with a minimum of mathematical notation. That is the approach I take here. I also focus on more easily explainable solutions, as

* E-mail: fboscoe@albany.edu

opposed to optimal solutions, to the extent that they differ. For a more rigorous treatment of the material presented here, I recommend the textbook *Computational Geometry: Algorithms and Applications* (de Berg *et al.*, 2000).

1.2 Referencing Locations

Before continuing any further, it is first necessary to discuss how locations on the earth's surface are expressed. This book mainly makes use of latitude and longitude. Latitude describes the distance north or south of the equator, with values ranging from 0 degrees (0°) at the equator to 90° at the poles. By convention, values in the northern hemisphere are positive and those in the southern hemisphere are negative. The distance from the equator to the poles is very close to 10 million m (indeed, the metre was originally defined in the 18th century as one ten-millionth of this distance), so a degree of latitude is about 111 km or 69 miles, about an hour's drive on an empty highway. This is true at all locations on the earth, as latitude lines are parallel.

Longitude describes the distance east or west of the prime meridian, a line connecting the north and south poles that passes through England, France, Spain and several West African countries. Values range from 0° to 180°, with positive values east of the prime meridian and negative values west of it. As longitude lines are not parallel, the distances between them vary – distances are greatest at the equator and shrink to zero at the poles, where all longitude lines converge. A simple way to find the distance between two longitude lines at a given latitude is to multiply 111 km by the cosine of the latitude. For example, at 45° north or south latitude, a degree of longitude is 111 times the cosine of 45° (0.707), or about 79 km (49 miles). Traditionally, latitude and longitude values were recorded in units of degrees, minutes (′) and seconds (″), with 60 minutes per degree and 60 seconds per minute. More recently, it has become standard practice to use decimal degrees (for example, 60.4167° rather than 60°25′). Clearly, this is more convenient in our decimal-based maths system.

The use of latitude and longitude, or any coordinate reference system, requires some assumptions about the shape of the earth. The earth is very close to a perfect sphere, and calculations and measurements based on this assumption will yield only small errors, which are acceptable for many purposes. However, because some measurements, such as property surveys, demand the greatest possible precision, more exact definitions of the earth's shape have been widely developed and used over the last two centuries. Historically, these have been country or region specific. More recently, the widespread adoption of the global positioning system (GPS) has encouraged the use of a single definition of the earth's shape applicable to the entire globe, specifically, the World Geodetic System of 1984 (WGS84). Locations in WGS84 typically differ by tens of metres from the earlier systems. Most commercial GIS software can make the necessary conversions, though as time goes on, data sets using the earlier reference systems are encountered less frequently. In any event, issues of geodetic precision are seldom relevant to public health data sets. This topic is covered in more detail in Chapter 5.

Besides latitude and longitude, the most often seen coordinate system in current use is the Universal Transverse Mercator (UTM). The UTM system divides the inhabited earth into 60 zones of 6° of longitude each. Within each zone, distortion of distance is less than one part per thousand. Locations are given as *x*-and *y*-coordinates called eastings and northings, in units of metres. In the northern hemisphere, the northing describes the distance from the equator; in the southern hemisphere, it describes the distance from the South Pole. The easting describes the distance from the central meridian within the UTM zone. To avoid negative numbers, the central meridian is assigned the easting value 500,000. Hence, the location of the Sydney Opera House can be given as 56S/N 6,252,309/E 334,897, where 56 is the zone number, S stands for the southern hemisphere, N and E stand for northing and easting, 6,252,309 is the distance from the South Pole in metres (and thus about 62.5% of the distance from the South Pole to the equator), and 334,897 indicates that the point is about 165 km west of the central meridian of zone 56 (obtained by subtracting 334,897 from 500,000).

The mathematics of converting latitude and longitude to UTM or vice versa are quite involved, but most GIS software has this functionality built in. For those working outside a GIS, there are a number of calculators online, including one I have written for SAS software, which can be accessed by visiting www.sascommunity.org and searching on the term 'UTM' (sascommunity.org, 2013).

1.3 Point in Polygon

I begin our brief tour of useful geographic algorithms with the *point-in-polygon* relationship. Given a set of point locations, it is often helpful to know which polygons, if any, the points are contained within. This is most commonly encountered in the calculation of disease rates for geographic areas. A disease rate is simply the number of disease cases divided by the population. Disease cases are often recorded as point locations, typically at the residence at the time of diagnosis, while populations are expressed as polygons, such as states or districts or census units. The point-in-polygon relationship is illustrated in Fig. 1.1, which shows an irregular 17-sided polygon and three points of interest, **X**, **Y** and **Z**. Obviously, points **X** and **Z** are inside the polygon, while **Y** is not, but how does GIS software know this?

The answer is obtained by extending a ray from the point of origin in any direction, and counting the number of intersections with the polygon concerned. For this reason, this method is known as the ray-tracing method. If the number of intersections is odd, the point is inside the polygon; if the number is even, the point is outside. This property, often simply called the 'even–odd rule', is a cornerstone of computer graphics. In Fig. 1.1, the rays have been extended to the left in the 17-sided polygon. From points **X** and **Z** there are three intersections, so these points must be inside the polygon. From point **Y** there are four intersections, so it must be outside.

Computer software keeps track of the number of intersections of the ray by comparing the locations of the nodes forming each of the 17 sides of the example polygon with each of the three points of interest. If a pair of nodes both have a higher *x*-coordinate than one of the points of interest, then that line segment of the polygon is to the right of the point of interest and so there is no intersection with the ray. For point **X**, this is true of sides CD, DE, EF, MN and NO. A second test is applied to the *y*-coordinates to eliminate those segments that are entirely above or below the point of interest. For point **X**, this is true of sides AB, BC, HI and QA, among others. What remains are the sides that do intersect: FG, GH and JK. One way to summarize this process is through *pseudocode*, a list of computer-code-like instructions that is not written in any particular computer language, and may even be written in plain

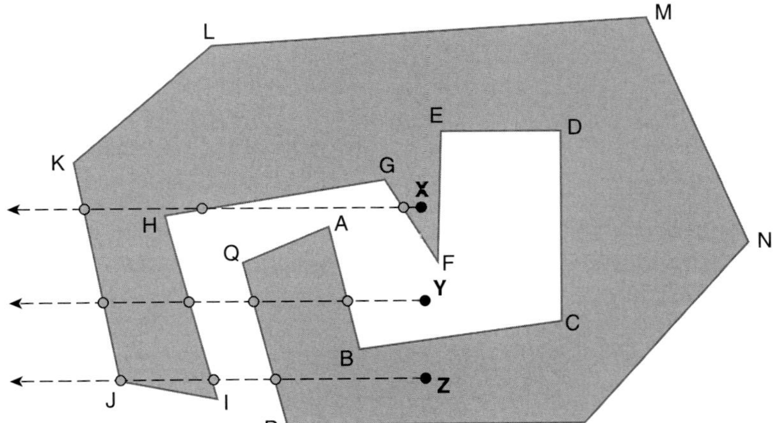

Fig. 1.1. Determining whether a point falls within a polygon.

English. For example, plain-English pseudocode for the point-in-polygon match could be written as:

- For each point of interest, do the following:
- For each line segment within the polygon, do the following:
- Perform *x*-coordinate test:
  - If the *x*-coordinates of both points comprising the line segment are greater than the *x*-coordinate of the point of interest, then there is no intersection
- Otherwise, perform *y*-coordinate test:
  - If the *y*-coordinates of both points comprising the line segment are greater than *or equal to*, or less than, the *y*-coordinate of the point of interest, then there is no intersection
- Otherwise, the segments intersect:
  - Increase intersection count by 1
- If final intersection count is odd, then the point is in the polygon
- Otherwise, the point is outside the polygon

Note the italicized phrase 'or equal to' in the description of the *y*-coordinate test. This was added to address the situation where a ray intersects a node exactly, as in the case of point J in Fig. 1.1. As the *y*-coordinates of points **Z** and J are equal, neither IJ nor JK would count as an intersection using the original logic. Under this revised logic, JK counts as intersecting but IJ does not, thus yielding the correct result. This special situation is known as a *degenerate case*. For most algorithms, it is useful to first find a general solution and then to modify it to incorporate degenerate cases. Another degenerate case not yet covered by this algorithm describes the situation when a point lies on the exact edge of a polygon. Should such a case be counted as inside, outside or neither? One could argue that this instance could be safely ignored as it is highly unlikely to occur – people are residents of particular countries, provinces and so on, and it is not possible to occupy their exact borders. However, in my experience, if something can occur in a spatial data set, it probably will, and so good programming practice dictates that this instance be accounted for by the algorithm as well. Because I would be suspicious about the accuracy of any such points, I would be inclined to place them into a special category for later manual review and correction.

Geographic coordinates tend to be reported with very high precision, often to at least six decimal places, or 11 cm of latitude. While such precision is rarely scientifically appropriate, it does have the advantage of minimizing degenerate cases; here as long as all points are positioned at least 11 cm from all polygon edges, there will be no problems.

The pseudocode above could be readily translated into virtually any computer language in existence. On my personal web page (www.albany.edu/~fboscoe/gisbook), I have developed an example using the R language, using the 14 departments of El Salvador as polygons and their capitals as points. R is a computer language that lends itself well to simple algorithms such as this one: it is clear and simple, it is a popular choice for beginners, it runs on all platforms and it is free and open source. The web page provides the necessary instructions on how to obtain the program and how to view and run the code. The data source used for the polygons was the GADM database of Global Administrative Areas (GADM, 2012), a free spatial database of the world's administrative boundaries for use in GIS and similar software. All subsequent examples in this chapter may also be found here.

1.4 Many Points and Many Polygons

The algorithm just described works fine when there are a small number of points and a small number of polygons. But what happens if the number of points and polygons is large? Imagine a medium-sized country with 50,000 disease cases and 5000 different census units to which they can belong, with each census unit described by an average of 100 points. (Lest this sound unusually detailed, there are examples of spatial units in the 2010 United States Census that are described by tens of thousands of points.) The number of necessary calculations then reaches to the billions. One could still go ahead and do it this way – taking what is known as the *brute force approach* – as long as computing power is sufficient and speed is not critical. There are a variety of shortcuts, however, that can dramatically improve the efficiency of this type of calculation.

One type of shortcut involves creating a layer of regular square cells superimposed over the polygons. Each cell must be either entirely inside a polygon, entirely outside all polygons, or intersect one or more polygons. Following the approach of Žalik and Kolingerova (2001), I will refer to the inside cells as black, the outside cells as white and the intersecting cells as grey. Each point is then matched to the cell it belongs to, rather than to the polygon it belongs to. Points falling in black or white cells can immediately be classified as being inside a specific polygon or outside all polygons. Points in grey cells require a simple additional step. While this method does have more steps than the brute force approach, it requires vastly fewer calculations.

The method is illustrated in Fig. 1.2. There are five polygons, which are labelled with Roman numerals I–V and covered by a 22 × 20 grid. The grid cells are 1 km on a side and locations are given in UTM coordinates. We begin by designating the grey cells, beginning with point A in the first polygon. Given the coordinates of point A of (E 573,590/N 985,920), it can be readily determined that cell (4,4) is grey, as there is a direct mathematical correspondence between coordinates and cell number. Similarly, cell (8,1) is grey, based on the location of point B. We continue winding clockwise around each polygon until the nodes of all polygons have been coded in this manner.

Note that the line segment AB also passes through cells (5,4), (5,3) and several others. A simple test can be employed to identify which cells were passed through in this manner, and these can also be counted as grey. This test consists of first identifying all instances when *x*- or *y*-coordinate values changed by at least 2 units, as happened when moving from (4,4) to (8,1). Next, identify the *x* values of the cells that were skipped (in this case, *x* = 5, 6 and 7). For each of these *x* values, retrieve the *x*-coordinates of both the left and right edges of

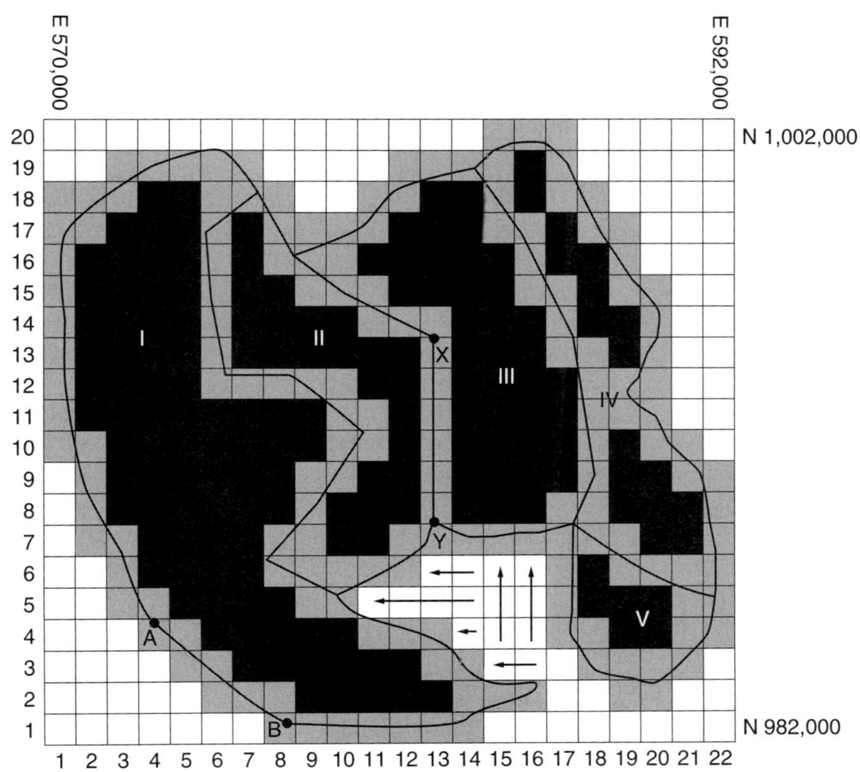

Fig. 1.2. Relating many points and many polygons.

the cell (for cell 5, that would be E 574,000 and E 575,000). Then, using the point-slope formula of a line, find the corresponding *y*-coordinates to these points, and then convert them back to grid values (here (5,4) and (5,3)). In the event that the *y* value is constant (such as the segment connecting (8,1) and (14,1)), this calculation can be skipped and the skipped pairs ((9,1), (10,1), ... (14,1)) filled in directly. In the course of performing these steps, retain a record of which grey cells correspond with which polygons, as this will be used later.

The next step is to assign the white cells. As long as the grid has been defined to extend beyond the polygons in all directions, then an edge cell can only be white or grey. So, begin this step by assigning all non-grey cells along the edges (rows 1 and 20, columns 1 and 22), to white. Next, beginning with row 1, cycle through all remaining unassigned cells, and assign as white all such cells that share a row or column with a white cell and are also adjacent to a white cell. This will assign cells (2,2), (3,2), (4,2) and so on as white. However, it will not assign (15,3) as white, because when this cell is first reached, none of its white neighbours will have yet been defined. This is also true of cell (16,3). Cell (17,3) will be assigned as white because of its adjacency with (17,2). Designate all white cells assigned during this cycle as 'active' white cells. Next, consider all active white cells, and search for adjacent unassigned cells in all four directions. Identify any such cells as newly active white cells. Repeat this process until there are no remaining active white cells. In the lower centre of Fig. 1.2, arrows indicate the three iterations that are required before the white cells are fully identified. All remaining cells can then be assigned as black.

The final task is to determine which black cells belong to which polygons. Here we can make use of the previously stored information about which grey cells correspond to which polygons. Beginning with row 1, proceed sequentially until the first black cell is encountered, here (9,2). From here, proceed westward (left) until the first grey cell is encountered. If this cell is only associated with one polygon, then the black cell must also belong to that polygon. In this example, that is indeed the case, as cell (8,2) is only associated with polygon I, and so it must be inside polygon I.

If the first grey cell encountered is associated with more than one polygon, then one or more additional directions must be attempted to resolve the ambiguity. For example, with cell (11,9), the first grey cell encountered to the west is (10,9), which is associated with both polygons I and II. Heading eastward, cell (12,9) is encountered, and this is associated with polygons II and III. As polygon II is common to both searches, the cell must fall within polygon II. In the degenerate case where a polygon is entirely contained within another polygon, the same result will be obtained in all directions. In this instance, extending the search to the second grey cell, beginning in the westerly direction, will allow the correct result to be deduced.

To summarize:

1. Construct a regular grid encompassing the entire geographic space.
2. Identify polygon nodes, and assign the cells containing them to grey.
3. Assign remaining grey cells by interpolating between the polygon nodes.
4. Assign white cells around the edge of the grid.
5. Assign remaining white cells based on adjacency; remaining cells are black.
6. Assign black cells to specific polygons by testing against neighbouring grey cells.

We now have a situation where points falling into black or white cells can be resolved with minimal computation. Points falling into grey cells require the full point-in-polygon test described in the previous section (Section 1.3), but only on a small number of candidates. For example, cell (8,1) only needs to be tested to see if it is inside polygon I, because otherwise it must be outside all polygons. Cell (9,8) also only needs to be tested against polygon I, because if it is not inside polygon I, then it can only be inside polygon II. Cell (17,7) represents the worst-case scenario of any of the cells here, as it needs to be tested against polygons III, IV and V. However, it can be seen that the large majority of grey cells require only one test.

Going back to our original example of 50,000 disease cases and 5000 census units, the grid-based method calls for a six-step preprocessing procedure followed by about 25,000 point-in-polygon tests, assuming that half the cases fall in grey cells that require one test each.

The brute force approach, in contrast, requires about 2500 tests for every case, or 125 million tests! Put into real-world geographic terms, to find the country containing some arbitrary point in Europe, the brute force approach requires us to first test whether it is in Ireland, then Portugal, then Spain and so on, which will be a very long process if the point happens to be in Greece. With the grid-based method, the number of candidate countries is immediately reduced to one, two or, at most, three.

I once had a researcher approach me with a version of this exact problem: she had a database of locations of plant species collected by volunteers using GPS, and wanted to assign these to the towns they were found in. Town boundaries are not important from an ecological perspective, but for people advocating wildlife conservation it is useful to be able to deliver a message such as 'wild lupin was found in 23 fewer towns in 2010 than in 1990'. The researcher assumed she needed to buy GIS software and/or take a training course. In this particular instance, I was able to explain how she could do this in the database software environment she was already familiar with by using the language and logic of computational geometry.

1.5 Identifying Neighbours (Polygons)

Another frequently encountered problem in the geographic analysis of health data is how to identify neighbours, or the set of geographic objects that are close to a given geographic object. 'Close to' can mean intersecting, sharing a boundary with or being within a specified distance of. Neighbours can also be defined as the closest *n* objects, regardless of distance. The definition of neighbours is an essential ingredient in a wide range of geographic analysis techniques, from clustering (Chapter 7) to smoothing (Chapter 8) to location–allocation modelling (Chapter 10). Here I focus on an algorithm for identifying whether polygons are adjacent, which is the most common way that polygon neighbours are defined.

If polygons are adjacent, it means that they share a common boundary, which can be defined as having at least one point in common or at least one line segment in common. By the first definition, polygon V in Fig. 1.2 is adjacent to polygons III and IV; by the second definition, it is only adjacent to IV. Using an analogy from the movement of chess pieces, the first type of neighbours are known as queen neighbours, while the second type are known as rook neighbours. More precisely, these are first-order rook and queen neighbours. Sometimes it is also useful to identify second-order neighbours, or those polygons that are adjacent to a common polygon. An example is polygons I and III, which are both adjacent to polygon II but not to each other.

The identification of rook neighbours requires the identification of line segments that are common to multiple polygons. In Fig. 1.2, points X and Y, for example, are nodes in both polygons II and III, meaning that line segment XY is an edge in both polygons. A brute force approach suggests itself here: simply compare the line segments from every polygon with those from every other polygon and identify all matches. Like most brute force approaches, this is highly inefficient. Suppose the goal is to identify which European countries border one another and the comparison is between Ireland and Greece. With their rugged coastlines and many islands, both countries may contain thousands of line segments. The comparison of just these two countries alone will take significant computing time, when they are obviously on opposite sides of the continent and ideally would not need to be compared at all.

A more efficient solution makes use of what is known as the bounding box rectangle. This consists of the rectangle with edges at the northernmost, easternmost, southernmost and westernmost points of the polygon (Fig. 1.3). These can be rapidly derived from each polygon by obtaining and storing the minimum and maximum *x* and *y* values from the list of points defining the polygon. To test whether two bounding box rectangles intersect is simple. First, sort the polygons by their *x* values. The one with the lowest *x* value is the farthest west; for each example in Fig. 1.3 this is polygon I. Next, compare the maximum *x* value (easternmost point) from this polygon with the minimum *x* value (westernmost point) from each of the other polygons. If the easternmost point is less than the westernmost point, then the two polygons cannot be adjacent, as in the lower right example. Applying this rule to Ireland, it

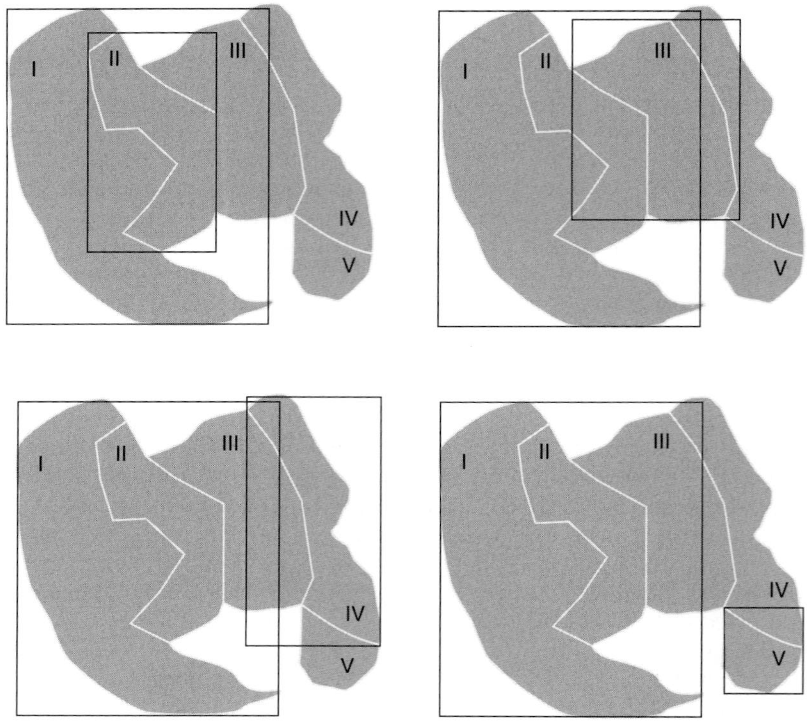

Fig. 1.3. Determining whether polygons intersect.

can quickly be shown that its only possible neighbours are Portugal, Spain, France and the UK. A similar test performed in the *y*-direction eliminates all but the United Kingdom.

This result does not mean that these two polygons are necessarily adjacent; for example, the top right and lower left images in Fig. 1.3 show polygons with overlapping bounding boxes that are not adjacent. When bounding box rectangles intersect, the individual segments still must be sorted and compared, but the number of times this has to be done is relatively few compared with the brute force approach. The efficiency can be improved further still by limiting the comparisons to just the portions of the bounding boxes that intersect. In the top right image, just a small portion of polygon I needs to be considered, while in the lower left image, polygon I can be eliminated entirely and so no testing is actually required.

The bounding box method requires what is known as 'clean topology', meaning that there are no incidental gaps or overlaps between polygons. These can accrue when polygon shapes are drawn inexpertly, such as when geographic boundaries are only drawn to a river's edge, leaving a gap in between. Areas on opposite sides of the river would, therefore, not be considered adjacent. There are specialized algorithms that can address these situations (Klajnšek and Žalik, 2005).

I have witnessed this scenario in my career. A statistical model for evaluating hospital care required the calculation of all adjacent postal code areas in New York State. The brute force solution was implemented using SAS statistical software, which took a long time to run and, inadvertently, did not count areas across the Hudson River from one another as neighbours, and so led to inaccurate results.

1.6 Identifying Neighbours (Points)

The identification of neighbours in a point data set is also important and useful. With points, the concept of adjacency does not apply; instead, neighbours are determined by proximity. Proximity can be variously defined as the single nearest neighbour, the *n* nearest neighbours or all neighbours within a specified distance, each of which uses distinct algorithms. Here I describe a method for finding the single nearest neighbour to a point.

As usual, a brute force solution comes quickly to mind: make a matrix of all point pairs, calculate the distance from every point to every other point, sort by distance and retain the smallest value for each point. As with the other brute force solutions so far, this is very inefficient, as the number of comparisons is the square of the number of points in the file – 50,000 points means 2.5 billion comparisons, more than enough to cripple the typical personal computer. Now, it is true that once we compare A with B, we do not need to compare B with A, so half of the comparisons can be instantly eliminated, but this still leaves us in the billions. If our goal is to compile a list of nearest neighbours of all European towns and cities of more than 5000 people, we would prefer to not have to waste effort comparing places in Ireland with places in Greece.

A more efficient solution is known as the spiral search (Bentley *et al.*, 1980). A square grid is imposed over the geographic space and all points are assigned to their respective cells. Then the point for which we are trying to find the nearest neighbour is tested to see whether there are any points in its own cell. If so, the distances to all of these points are calculated and sorted, and the smallest of these is retained. We next define a square centred over the point of interest with a side length equal to twice this smallest distance. We determine which cells are intersected by this square, calculate the distances to any points found in these cells and see if any are smaller than the previously retained smallest value. (A circle might seem to be a more obvious choice here, but determining the intersecting cells in a circle is more complicated.) The spiral search approach is illustrated in Fig. 1.4, which shows the principal towns and cities of El Salvador. To identify the nearest city to point A in cell (3,2), we first look for points within this cell, and find both Santa Tecla and San Salvador, with the latter closer at a distance of 13 km. We then construct a square centred on point A that is 26 km across, thus including San Salvador. This square intersects three additional cells that together contain three cities, none of which are within 13 km. For point B, as no cities share its cell, the search is expanded to its eight first-order queen neighbours. This yields four candidate cities, the closest of which is Usulután, 27 km to the south. A 54 km square centred on point B intersects no additional cells, so no further calculations are required.

If no points are found in the eight first-order queen neighbours, then the search is expanded

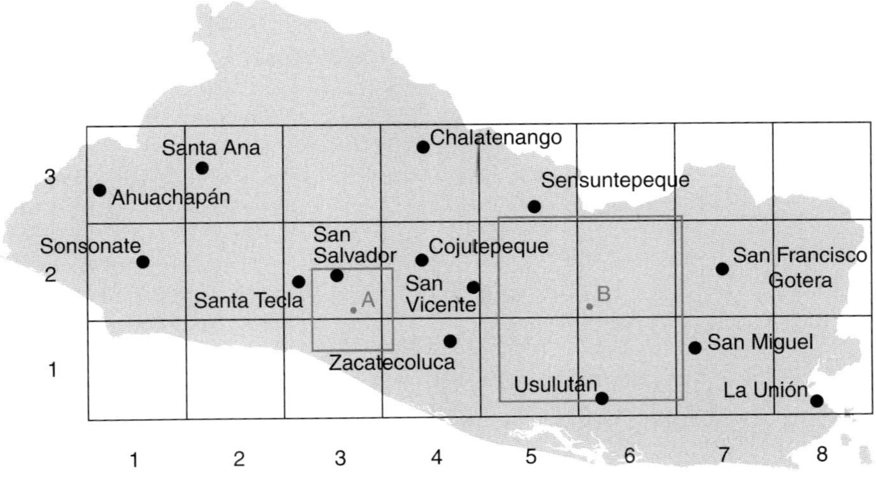

Fig. 1.4. Finding the nearest neighbour to a point, using cities in El Salvador.

to the 16 second-order neighbouring cells, 24 third-order neighbours and so on. The method works best when the resolution of the grid is such that a few points can be expected in a typical cell. Imagine at one extreme a grid consisting of just one cell – all points would need to be tested. At the other extreme, a very fine grid would require searching many orders of neighbours until a candidate point was found. The 'spiral' in the name of this method refers to the path that can be followed to visit and test grid cells at increasing distances from the point of interest. However, the process does not literally require the following of a spiral.

I encountered this problem while a technical adviser to a software development project, one goal of which was to identify the nearest *n* hospitals for any address, in order to facilitate research on health care choice and accessibility. An early meeting was spent debating whether it was feasible to identify the nearest *n* hospitals or whether it should instead be the nearest *single* hospital, and which of these was actually specified in the contract. I think it should be clear that expanding the method just described from one neighbour to *n* neighbours is trivial, and I suspected this was true at the time, but still being somewhat of a closed source 'black box' GIS user at the time, I was unable to convincingly articulate this. The project team settled on the nearest single hospital, though in the end the programmer included the nearest *n* hospitals upon realizing that this expansion was indeed trivial.

1.7 Converting Between Points and Polygons

Of the various spatial analysis methods presented throughout this book, some require point layers and others require polygon layers, and so there is often a need to convert between the two. Converting from polygons to points is the simpler case, as all that is needed is to select a single representative point for each polygon. Often the centroid of the polygon is chosen as this is a representative point. In physics, a centroid of a two-dimensional object is the centre of mass, or the point on which it would balance. For the complex and irregular polygons that are typical of geographic analysis, calculation of the exact centroid can be prohibitive, so the centre of the bounding box rectangle is often used as a shortcut (Fig. 1.5a). This can readily be calculated as the average of the extreme *x* and *y* values in the polygon.

For some polygons, the bounding box centroid does not actually lie within the polygon. (Fig. 1.5b). This is a problem because if we assume that the centroid is representative of the polygon, then it should actually belong to that polygon. GIS software typically builds in a correction that moves the centroid to a location in the polygon. For example, a ray could be extended from the centroid in each of the four cardinal directions until an intersection is found; the closest of these intersections could be used as the centroid. Some researchers advocate the use of population-weighted centroids as more representative than geometric centroids, though

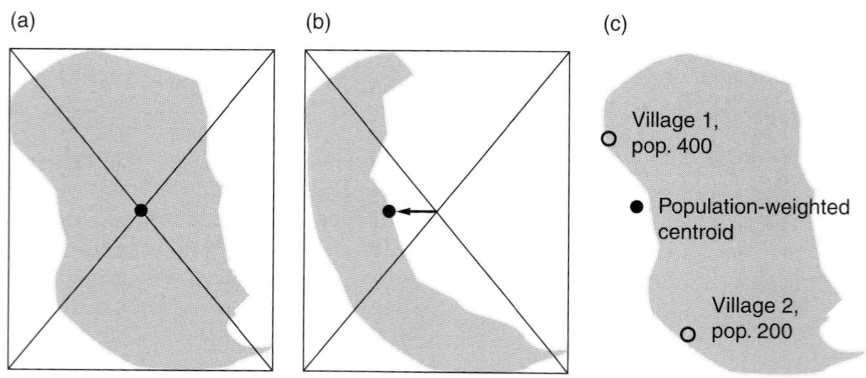

Fig. 1.5. Characteristics of centroids (pop., population).

in practice this adds negligible value to an analysis and still does not guarantee that the point will fall within the polygon (Fig. 1.5c).

It is important to remember that when converting from polygons to points, the points are representative of the polygon as a whole, not of the area immediately surrounding the point. For example, the geographic centroid of Switzerland lies high in the Alps south of Lucerne. Obviously one would not conclude from this that the entire county is unpopulated and at a high elevation. Yet I have witnessed this very error at finer geographic scales, where a postal area or even an entire city is assigned the characteristics of its central point, which may arbitrarily fall within a business district, an economically disadvantaged neighbourhood or even a park.

Converting points to polygons is a bit more complex. The usual procedure is known by several names, reflecting their independent discovery by multiple scientists. In the GIS community, the end products are most often called Thiessen polygons, after the American meteorologist Alfred Thiessen, or Voronoi polygons, after the Ukrainian mathematician Georgy Voronoy. For clarity, I will use the term Voronoi polygons from here on.

Voronoi polygons happen to represent the solution to a famous problem known as Knuth's Post Office problem: given a set of post office locations, how do we determine which is the closest post office to every house? (To translate this into a health or safety context, think in terms of hospital or trauma centre or fire station locations.) The brute force solution that comes to mind would be to measure the distance from every house to every post office, sort the results and choose the smallest distance. As usual, this is unwieldy.

Let us go back to El Salvador and see how we might try something more efficient. If we begin with Ahuachapán in the west, clearly all the points to the north and west of here will be part of its polygon, because there are no other closer cities. To the south, we eventually reach the midway point to Sonsonate, and to the east, the midway point to Santa Ana. We draw boundaries along these midway lines until we have a complete polygon surrounding Ahuachapán. Continuing in this manner for the remaining cities would not be too difficult, but of course we want the computer to be doing this work for us. While multiple algorithms to solve this problem exist, the optimal one is known as Fortune's algorithm (Fortune, 1987). Unlike the algorithms described up to this point, this one is a bit more involved; the explanation here is somewhat streamlined.

Fortune's algorithm maintains what are called a 'sweep line' and a 'beach line', both of which move west to east (left to right) as the algorithm progresses. The sweep line is a straight vertical or north–south line. The beach line is a complex curve behind the sweep line (that is, to the west of it) consisting of pieces of parabolas. The parabolas represent the curves that are equidistant from the cities and the sweep line. As the sweep line progresses from west to east, new parabolas emerge every time a new city is encountered, while old parabolas converge and disappear. The points at which parabolas intersect form the lines in the Voronoi polygons, while the points at which parabolas converge and disappear form the vertices. It is perhaps easier to visualize this process than to describe it; an elegant Java application that does this may be found at http://www.diku.dk/hjemmesider/studerende/duff/Fortune/, within an article by Odgaard and Nielsen (2000). A more thorough treatment, including pseudocode, is given Section 7.2 of de Berg *et al.* (2000). Figure 1.6 shows an in-progress, nearly completed Voronoi diagram for El Salvador.

Among other things, Voronoi polygons provide a general solution to the nearest neighbour problem covered earlier. From Fig. 1.6, it is clear that the polygons describe the nearest city for every point in the entire country. Taking this approach to finding neighbours means that you would need to know which points belonged to which Voronoi polygons – which is an application of the point-in-polygon algorithms that we began with. Generally speaking, there is usually more than one efficient algorithmic path to solving a spatial problem. This brings us to our final section, on finding the shortest path between two points.

1.8 Shortest Path

Here, the shortest path refers to the shortest route between two points in a network, such as a road or trail network, where one is obligated

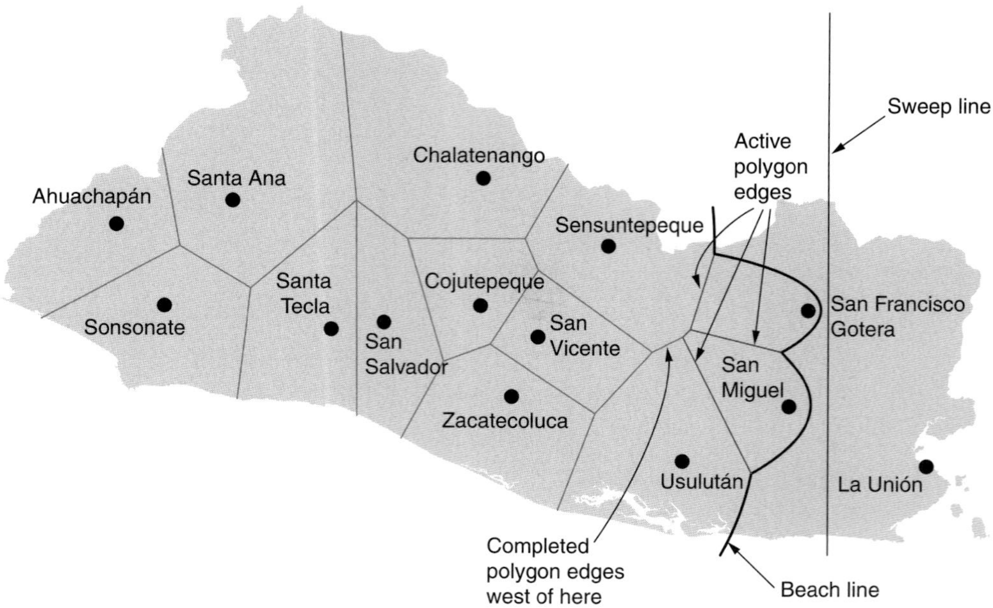

Fig. 1.6. Fortune's algorithm for building Voronoi polygons. See text for further explanation.

to remain on the network. (This is not the same as the shortest possible path, which is a somewhat simpler case known as the great circle distance and is covered in Chapter 9.) The most well-known solution to this problem is known as the Dijkstra Algorithm, after Dutch computer scientist Edsger Dijkstra, who discovered it in the 1950s. He originally viewed it as interesting but trivial, certainly not something that would be widely used for decades to come. 'What's the shortest way from Rotterdam to Groningen?' he recounted. 'One morning I was shopping in Amsterdam with my young fiancee, and tired, we sat down on the café terrace to drink a cup of coffee and I was just thinking about whether I could do this, and I then designed the algorithm for the shortest path ... it was a 20-minute invention' (Misa, 2010). Given the algorithm's simplicity and the lack of an obvious application for it, Dijkstra did not publish the result for some time. Eventually, he saw an application to answering the question of how to minimize the amount of copper wire in an early computing device. Now the algorithm is widely used in countless fields, and the very short paper describing it (Dijsktra, 1959) was cited over 500 times in 2011 alone.

Here I apply the algorithm to find the shortest path across El Salvador from west to east using the 14 department capitals (Fig. 1.7). The map has been simplified to include only straightforward routes linking the cities. The numbers represent travel times in minutes, as obtained from Google Earth. In the first step, the westernmost city Ahuachapán is assigned a distance value of zero and all other cities are assigned a value of infinity. Every city is assigned a status of 'unvisited'. We next consider all of Ahuachapán's unvisited neighbours and calculate a tentative distance to them. For Santa Ana, this is 42 min and for Sonsonate, it is 41 min. If these values are less than the current values, then those values are replaced; otherwise the existing value is retained. As the current values are infinity, they are replaced with 42 and 41, respectively. We are now finished with Ahuachapán. Its status is changed to 'visited' and it will not be involved in any further calculations (other than by including its distance from either Santa Ana or Sonsonate in those calculations).

We then move eastward to the next unvisited node, which is Sonsonate, and calculate tentative distances from (Ahuachapán to)

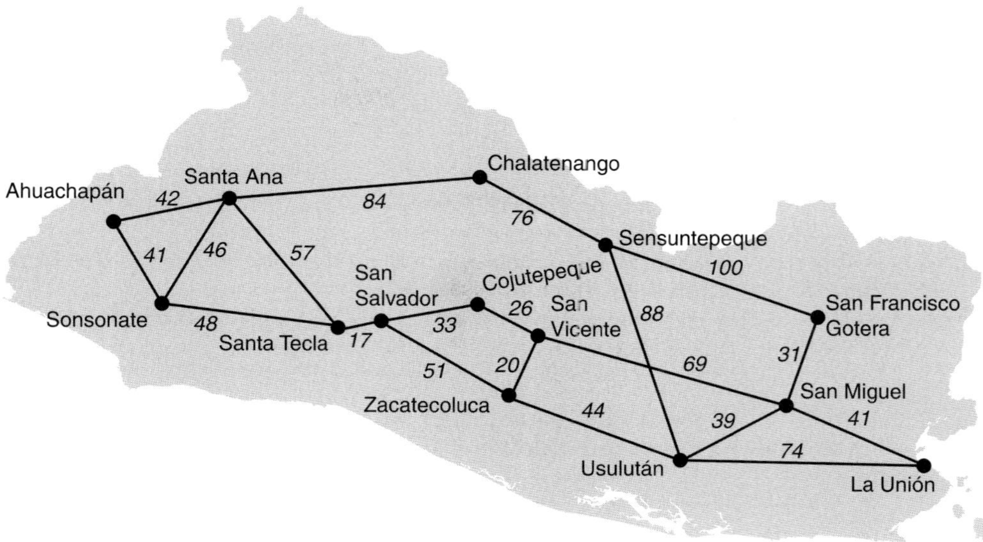

Fig. 1.7. Finding the shortest path across El Salvador from west to east using the 14 department capitals. The numbers in italics are travel times in minutes obtained from Google Earth.

Sonsonate to its unvisited neighbours. For Santa Ana, this is 87 min (41 plus 46) and for Santa Tecla it is 89 min (41 plus 48). Santa Ana's existing value of 42 is retained while Santa Tecla's infinite value is replaced with 89. Sonsonate has now been visited.

Next up is Santa Ana, with two unvisited neighbours: Chalatenango, with a value of 126 min (42 plus 84), and Santa Tecla, with a value of 99 minutes (42 plus 57). Santa Tecla's existing value of 89 is less than 99, so this is retained. Santa Ana has now been visited.

Repeating this process for the remaining cities yields a final minimum travel time of 274 min, which is the route from Ahuachapán to Sonsonate to Santa Tecla to San Salvador to Cojutepeque to San Vincente to San Miguel to La Unión. The alternative route through San Salvador, Zacatecoluca and Usulután is just 1 min slower, at 275 min. Note that the algorithm not only found the shortest path across El Salvador, but it also found the shortest path from Ahuachapán to every point in between.

1.9 Conclusion

The aim of this introductory chapter has been to emphasize the fundamental building blocks of geographic analysis – points, lines and polygons – and show how they are fundamentally related through a collection of algorithms collectively known as 'computational geometry'. You most likely will never have the need to code any of these fundamental geographic algorithms from scratch, as it is nearly always beneficial to take advantage of software tools and code that already exist. Still, there are advantages to understanding the algorithmic details. They give you an idea of the relatedness of many spatial analytic problems and the kinds of solutions that are called for, so that you can at least put the proper terms into an Internet search query to see how others have solved the problem.

Some time ago, I had a non-GIS-using student who needed to calculate measures such as poverty rates and educational attainment from United States Census data. Because her units were different from the census units, what she had was a polygon overlay problem – the intersection of two dissimilar polygon layers (this is covered in Chapter 6). I was able to give her some simple SAS code to get started. When I heard from her a few days later, some of measures seemed to be correct but others were obviously nonsensical. It quickly became clear that, not understanding the code I had given her, she had taken a brute force approach to the code itself, trying out numerous combinations of syntax and punctuation, stopping only when there were no longer any errors in the log. Hopefully this chapter, and those that follow, will convince you that there really is no substitute for having a solid understanding of the tools that are at your disposal.

References

Bentley, J.L., Weide, B.W. and Yao, A.C. (1980) Optimal expected-time algorithms for closest point problems. *ACM Transactions in Mathematical Software* 6, 563–580.

de Berg, M., van Kreveld, M., Overmars, M. and Schwarzkopf, O. (2000) *Computational Geometry: Algorithms and Applications*, 2nd edn. Springer, Berlin, Heidelberg, Germany.

Dijkstra, E.W. (1959) A note on two problems in connexion with graphs. *Numerische Mathematik* 1, 269–271.

Fortune, S. (1987) A sweepline algorithm for Voronoi diagrams. *Algorithmica* 2, 153–174.

GADM (2012) GADM database of Global Administrative Areas, version 2.0 (January 2012). Available at: www.gadm.org (accessed 11 March 2013).

Klajnšek, G. and Žalik, B. (2005) Merging polygons with uncertain boundaries. *Computers and Geosciences* 31, 353–359.

Misa T.J. (2010) An interview with Edsger W. Dijkstra. *Communications of the ACM* 53, 41–47.

Odgaard, A. and Nielsen, B.K (2000) A visual implementation of Fortune's Voronoi algorithm. Available at: http://www.diku.dk/hjemmesider/studerende/duff/Fortune/ (accessed 11 March 2013).

sasCommunity.org (2013) Latitude/longitude to UTM conversion (and vice-versa). Available at: http://www.sascommunity.org/wiki/Latitude/longitude_to_UTM_conversion_%28and_vice-versa%29 (accessed 11 March 2013).

Žalik, B. and Kalingerova, I. (2001) A cell-based point-in-polygon algorithm suitable for large sets of points. *Computers and Geosciences* 27, 1135–1145.

2 Geographic Data Acquisition

Andrew Curtis* and Jacqueline W. Curtis
Department of Geography, Kent State University, Ohio, USA

2.1 Introduction

Since the mid-2000s, access to spatial data and spatial technology has become ubiquitous. In the USA, geoportals and spatial data clearing houses, which are access points to geospatial information, are available from multiple sources, ranging from federal agencies to academic departments. From a disaster perspective, a geoportal would more frequently be used to access pre-event data layers, while a clearing house is sometimes created for a specific event. The availability of spatial data in the USA also permeates the governmental hierarchy at all levels, from cities, to counties, to states. One such example of municipal spatial data availability is the Los Angeles County GIS Data Portal (see http://egis3.lacounty.gov/dataportal/index.php). In addition, most major universities have some type of online data access point, either for local information, as exemplified by Louisiana State University's 'Atlas: The Statewide GIS' (see atlas.lsu.edu), or as a global spatial resource, as with the Harvard Geospatial Library (see hgl.harvard.edu).

In the past, finding such varied data sources was a time-intensive process. Now though, with the power of Internet search engines, a series of keyword searches often lead to readily available shapefiles or georeferenced imagery. It is almost impossible to keep abreast of all available data locations because these spatial data sources are so varied and dynamic. Even the latest version of the most popular GIS (geographic information system) software, Esri's ArcGIS 10.1 (see www.esri.com), has an online search function that links the user into a daily expanding geospatial data community.

It is not just pre-packaged GIS vector data (meaning points, lines and polygons) that are so readily available. It is also easier to acquire the components for users to create their own spatial data layers. For example, high-resolution imagery is accessible through an array of geoportals, such as the National Climatic Data Center (NCDC) of the US National Oceanic and Atmospheric Administration (NOAA), or with a little manipulation, from freely available software such as Google Earth. Aerial photography makes the creation of new data in a GIS a relatively easy prospect through the technique of digitizing; examples are the creation of map layers of wells, damaged infrastructure or areas of green space, all of which might have relevance to a disaster or public health investigator. Using a GIS, such characteristics of the built environment can be identified on the imagery and then 'drawn' into the GIS with their real-world location.

* E-mail: acurti13@kent.edu

However, it is not only spatial data availability that has improved, but also the technologies and formats of viewing and manipulating these data. Google Earth and its Keyhole Markup Language (KML) files are arguably the most important of these at the time of writing. New geospatial technologies like these facilitate the dissemination of information and ideas because they enable the public at large to develop an appreciation for spatial information. For professionals who deal with disasters and health, this medium enables them to share spatial data among themselves to enhance situation awareness and to facilitate decision support (Mills *et al.*, 2008), as well as to disseminate information to the public (Mills and Curtis, 2008; Mills, 2009). For example, Fig. 2.1 shows imagery for Joplin, Missouri as accessed through Google Maps on 22 August 2012. This photography clearly shows the scars of homes that had been damaged or destroyed by the tornado of 2011 and have since been removed, as well as a few homes where the remnants of the basement are still visible, and those of the 'pioneer' returnees who have moved back and rebuilt. This imagery is a compelling visual description of conditions in this post-disaster environment.

While the aerial perspective displayed in Google Earth or Google Maps is a useful tool on its own, when overlaid with spatial data in KML, it has the ability to become a platform for giving context in real time or near real time. An excellent example of how a federal agency uses online spatial displays to disseminate information, and in so doing connect the public with real world events in real time, is the KML output of seismic activity from the Earthquake Hazard Program of the United States Geological Survey (USGS) (http://earthquake.usgs.gov/earthquakes/map/).

As a result of imagery such as that shown in Fig. 2.1, or the display of data output used by USGS, both the public and GIS users are now more aware of and connected to spatial

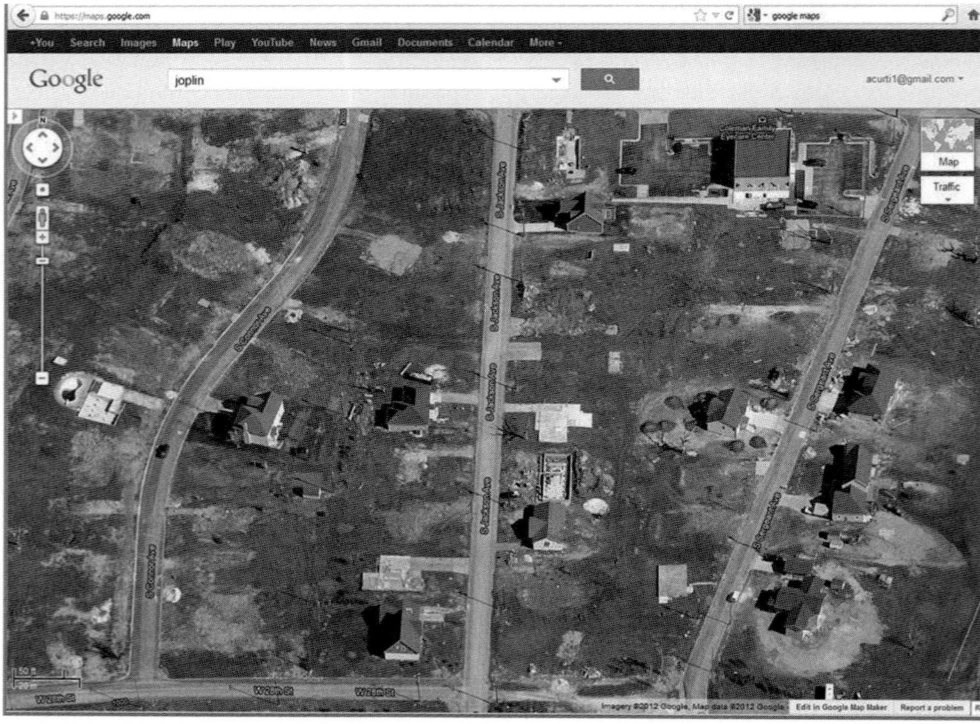

Fig. 2.1. Post-tornado imagery for Joplin, Missouri, USA, 22 August 2012. Source: Imagery © 2012 Google, Map data © 2012 Google.

data. These maps also allow for the creation of new GIS data, especially if multiple time periods are available. For example, the location and amount of recovery could be mapped from such readily available sources.

Advances in GPS (global positioning system) technology also encourage the public to participate in this spatial revolution, from in-car navigation to different smartphone functions ranging from navigation to geotagging photos. In academia, researchers are now exploring the collection of primary data through different mobile mapping platforms, especially individual GPS units that can be linked to people, sometimes in conjunction with other biometric sensors to 'map' stress or physical activity, or to map animals to understand spatial behaviour and its relationships with different habitats. In general, these technologies facilitate research into fine-scale spatial processes, and allow for data to be created for previously information-poor environments, such as developing countries and places recently affected by natural disasters. For example, the spatial video approach described later in this chapter was applied in 2012 to assess water risks in the cholera-affected areas of Haiti, an environment which is both challenging from a fieldwork perspective and deficient in typical spatial data.

This chapter will touch on some of these new data sources as seen through the lens of disaster response and, to a lesser degree, recovery. The reader will be led through the typical operations of an Emergency Operations Center (EOC) working at the height of a disaster, before describing the ways in which spatial damage data is collected and coded. One novel data collection approach, a spatial video unit, which has been used to capture disaster assessment and recovery, and also health data, will be described later in the chapter as well. A detailed worked exercise for the Joplin, Missouri tornado of 2011 will show how this imagery can be used to gain spatial insight and facilitate map-making.

However, before delving into more detail, we should also acknowledge the upswell in 'bottom-up' or grassroots spatial data generation that often occurs in conjunction with an externality such as a disaster or other social upheaval. Although there are several examples, the reader is pointed to the efforts of Ushahidi (see www.ushahidi.com/), a non-profit technology company that specializes in developing free and open source software for information collection, visualization and interactive mapping and Crisis Mappers (see http://crisismappers.net/), a technology network for powering effective early warning for rapid response to complex humanitarian emergencies, and to the work of Liu and Palen (2010).

2.2 Responding to a Disaster with Spatial Data: The Role of the EOC

In the USA, disaster response is managed through an Emergency Operations Center (EOC). The EOC coordinates all aspects of the response which, if it is a large tornado, may cover only an area of several square miles, or, in the case of Hurricane Katrina, most of the southern part of Louisiana and Mississippi, including all of New Orleans and its metropolitan area. A typical EOC contains multiple desks for federal, state, city and non-profit organizations such as the American Red Cross (ARC). The purpose of bringing everyone together under one roof is to streamline the organizational process, coordinate efforts, share resources and data, and effectively strategize each step of the response.

Now imagine just the spatial aspects of the response, which basically means the geospatial support of all of the above. In an episode of the British television show *Spooks* (called *MI5* in the USA) the (paraphrased) order given is 'bring out the big map' during an emergency in their EOC. There are plenty of big maps during a disaster response: maps showing the dynamic conditions on the ground (maybe the flooded area), the locations of critical infrastructure, city sections which had been covered that day by search teams or possible potential subsequent hazards. The 'big map' may be tactile, such as a plotted output that becomes the centre of morning briefings either to the media or to EOC personnel. It can also be digital and projected on to one of the many media screens found in most EOCs. But small maps and onscreen cartography are also important, especially for performing tasks such as putting together field team navigation packets, or using

Google Earth to find key coordinates. To create these maps, geospatial technologies and skill sets are vital, as is the access to readily available spatial data.

2.3 Spatial Data in the EOC

So what data are needed? Even though an 'all hazards approach' stipulates that theoretically the same approach should work irrespective of hazard, in practice there is a regional geography to potential risk (Bokman, 2003). Think about the disasters that have occurred in your region during the last 10 years, and then add in the unlikely scenarios.

Different hazards generate different spatially supported actions and therefore require different spatial data. Wildfires are relatively slow moving when compared with a tornado, so a response is more likely to focus on evacuation and shelter. But as we saw with the fires in the state of Colorado in 2012, these wildfires can be more geographically extensive, which means that response logistics will be stretched far thinner. Tornadoes are quick moving, with warnings often only giving residents minutes to make life or death decisions. As a result, for the worst of these events, activities facilitated through the EOC would primarily involve searching for the injured, recovering bodies and sheltering those who had lost their homes. Hurricanes are also slow moving, but as we saw with Katrina in 2005, not everyone evacuates. So we are left with the similar aspects of both wildfires and tornadoes – evacuating and sheltering large populations both before and after impact, while also caring for the injured and searching for bodies in the immediate aftermath. Finally, there are the events that are not tied to a specific geography, situations that could emerge anywhere, such as an epidemic (for example, a more virulent strain of avian influenza), a zoonotic outbreak (an economically devastating event such as foot-and-mouth disease) or a human-infrastructure catastrophe, including a terrorist attack.

For each of the above disasters there are hazard-specific spatial data that are required, some of which are readily available, while others require a modelling frame needing dynamic updates. Flood models for coastal areas (for example the Sea, Lake and Overland Surges from Hurricanes – SLOSH), or locally generated tsunami inundation maps will show which areas are likely to be worst affected and this, in turn, should help to prioritize evacuation or warnings. These models are sometimes available locally as standalone outputs; in the USA, they are incorporated in the all-encompassing Federal Emergency Management Agency (FEMA) geospatial methodology for estimating potential losses from disasters, Hazus (details available at http://www.fema.gov/plan/prevent/hazus/).

The EOC cannot just rely on existing data or model outputs, as many situations are dynamic, often changing daily or even by the hour. For example, wildfire growth models already contain the underlying topography but these require daily updates of fire location and of wind direction and speed.

Other spatial data are not so hazard specific but are still invaluable, such as population data, critical infrastructure (important buildings such as a hospital or power station), state lands on which shelters can be located and routes to provide effective navigation support. The key to these ubiquitous data layers is ease of access and pre-creation wherever possible. Anyone who has navigated through the web site of the United States Census Bureau (see www.census.gov/) knows that the appropriate time to put together social vulnerability data (which basically means cohorts that are disproportionately at risk during a disaster) for an affected area is not when the disaster is occurring.

So how are these data sets used in an EOC? The primary role of the GIS desk is to provide mapping support for all aspects of the response, from helping search and rescue teams navigate through the disaster area to creating graphics of the current situation for press conferences. One dynamic data set that is always generated during an emergency is 911 calls (the emergency telephone number for the North American Numbering Plan, or NANP). Just as in non-disaster situations, these have to be answered, mapped and prioritized to field teams. But in this case, each call is part of a larger unfolding picture that may be stretching all resources. Part of the EOC GIS support is to navigate search and rescue teams to these call locations. To achieve this, a GIS desk worker needs to be able to turn different data strands into actionable information, such as mapping out where 911 calls fall within flood zones that are updated hourly, or which teams have covered different disaster sectors, or if certain roads were blocked. During Hurricane Katrina, many search and rescue teams from outside the area had no knowledge of New Orleans, and simple street maps were less than effective as most roads (and street signs) were underwater. User-friendly handheld and vehicle GPS units obviously make this easier, though an effective geospatial team should also be ready to think outside the box. The message here is that while these new mobile technologies may appear to make things easier, for the worst events there is still the likelihood that creativity and flexibility will be needed at the GIS desk.

In order for the EOC geospatial response to be effective, four interlinked areas have to be considered: (i) spatial data; (ii) GIS personnel; (iii) technology; and (iv) logistics. Spatial data are the building blocks of the maps that will be created in the EOC. They include base layers that are static and can be prepared before a disaster event, such as political boundaries. Dynamic, event-generated data, such as flood extent and depth, will then be overlayed with the base layers. GIS personnel are those who will make the maps in the EOC. Not only must these people have technical GIS skills, but also the temperament and personality to work under pressure in extreme conditions. Technology refers to the hardware and software needed to acquire, store and communicate the final map products. Finally, logistical considerations include having an organizational structure to people's roles, workflow and data protocols.

2.3.1 Spatial data availability and requirements

We have already mentioned how different hazards require different responses which, in turn, require different data. It is imperative that any EOC has as much data at hand as possible. For some locations, such as California, the constant number of wildfires means that the Los Angeles County Fire Department (LACFD) GIS team has a robust experience set, so both base data layers (such as census and neighbourhood information), as well as scientific output (fire growth models) are readily available.

Unfortunately, for other EOCs, especially in locations where disasters are uncommon, problems in data availability are likely to only emerge during the response itself. These problems might include the interuption of data flow (maybe from a server), the physical loss of data (the flooding of a building) or not having the relevant pre-packaged data layers available – which means that additional and unnecessary data processing is needed in a stressful environment. As an example from Hurricane Katrina, searches were needed of state land data to help with locating potential shelter sites. Luckily, the geospatial response was handled primarily by Louisiana State University (LSU) teams which already had easy access to many data sources through university and interpersonal connections. It is important to brainstorm in advance all possible scenarios in terms of what data might be needed and where it might be found. In general, the EOC should not be reliant on any one data source but have multiple backup sites at the ready.

Some data, as has been mentioned, will be dynamic; 911 call data is the obvious example and emergency systems are usually well adept at handling this source of information. Other dynamic data may include reports from the field, especially in the form of daily debriefs by field teams, remotely sensed data that is processed daily and even social media feeds. Although it is fascinating to read tweet trends from within a disaster zone, as of yet these contain little spatial information that can be used in a real time or near real time way by an EOC. Research is ongoing to determine how this information might be used, such as how to extract spatial meaning from the messages or how to intepret on-the-ground social information in a systematic way (Goodchild and Glennon, 2010). The potential benefits are obvious; this is real time information (some of which is) originating from inside the disaster area; but we are not there yet.

Another form of daily data that is usually 'donated' during a disaster is high resolution aerial photography, as well as airborne oblique photography, with the latter providing the most comprehensive 'picture' of an on-the-ground feature from all angles. These data are a rich source of information, but problems can still arise from their use, such as lack of the skill and time to process or rectify the images (luckily, many are now donated already rectified) and of the ability to effectively use the information beyond showing an impressive backdrop to the ongoing situation.

2.3.2 GIS desk personnel

The second aspect of a geospatial response that is integral to the effective use of data in a GIS environment is the personnel. Every EOC will be slightly different. The team working the GIS desk during Hurricane Katrina provides a reasonable non-professional example (meaning spatial experts and technicians assigned to the EOC rather than those employed in-house, as in the case of LACFD). A supervisor can help to take 'jobs' and prioritize tasks to two or three other workers. These individuals manipulate, create and distribute spatial information, usually in the form of a map, by either accessing existing sources (finding maps for certain areas), plotting dynamic data (911 calls), recombining data layers (overlaying flood zones on to road networks) or, sometimes, even creating new data, such as the heads-up (interactive on-screen) digitizing of gunfire reports from criminal elements in New Orleans based on daily debrief reports from search and rescue teams returning from the damaged areas. Most of these tasks only require rudimentary GIS skills; what is more important is the character of the individual doing them – someone who can work for long hours, under stressful conditions, while still performing tasks effectively, which means quickly and accurately.

Three personnel problems can emerge. First, no one knows how anyone will perform under stressful conditions, and although simulated exercises are useful, they cannot capture what it is like to be in an EOC in full flow. Secondly, additional stressors on the workers may affect performance, especially if the disaster is local, as friends and family may be in the disaster area. Finally, with the worst events, such as with Katrina, the logistics of how many workers are needed come into play. The Katrina response lasted over 2 weeks. In an ideal situation, there should be three shifts of four people per day (12 people in total) with substitutes ready to offer breaks every few days. I doubt if any EOC has that size of geospatial team, which is a good reason why partnerships that bridge government agencies, the private sector and universities are necessary for such catastrophic events (Curtis *et al.*, 2006c). These relationships may be formalized pre-event through memoranda of understanding (MoUs) or may develop through more informal networks, such as being alumni of the same university. For Katrina, after the first few days, the vast majority of GIS desk workers were LSU GIS savvy students and alumni.

2.3.3 Geospatial technology

The third data-related aspect of the EOC is technology. The obvious geospatial software is a GIS and ideally everyone at the desk should be familiar with how this works in terms of the most basic operations. However, it is also important to not reinvent the wheel. There is no need to print off street maps if commercial products are available, though adding additional context such as flood layers may make this a valuable task. There is also no need to use a GIS if the spatial operation is simple, such as finding the coordinate of a clinic for a helicopter pilot.

Katrina was the first time Google Earth was used as a widespread tool for a major disaster in the USA. As previously mentioned, Google Earth and other popular spatial technologies, including in-car GPS units and smartphones or tablets, have changed the public's comfort level with geography and spatial data. Society is now more familiar with maps, with the interpretation of features on those maps, with how to extract meaning from an aerial photograph and generally with how to make sense of multiple spatial layers (Butler, 2006; Miller, 2006). This also means that non-GIS users can supplement the EOC team and solve the logistical issue of staffing. For example, during Katrina a typical task would be for a helicopter pilot to sit beside the EOC GIS desk worker and give the name of a clinic. It was easy to type in the address and then give the coordinate back to the pilot, either in decimal degrees or in degrees, minutes and seconds. Not only that, but the pilot could quickly see the area surrounding the clinic and the best place to land. This process was further improved during the response phase by a disaster 'triage' approach that evolved to extract flood data from aerial imagery and turned it into a Google Earth KML layer. This is now a standard manipulation which makes data dissemination even easier, especially to satellite EOCs (there are likely to be several EOCs for federal and local agencies as well as for non-profit organizations working the same disaster) and field teams.

It is also worth noting how important high resolution aerial photography is for creating new data layers, whether in the Google Earth environment or through a normal GIS. Buildings, damage and standing water are just three examples of features that can be extracted from such imagery. We will return to this in more detail in the section on damage assessment (Section 2.4).

2.3.4 Logistical issues

There are several logistical issues in the use of spatial data that have to be considered in an EOC, beyond adequate staffing; for example, how to effectively record all the tasks asked of the GIS desk so that new data and maps can be stored effectively and found and used by subsequent teams. This requires a data flow system and a filing convention: who has taken the job, at what stage is it, has it been completed and where are the manipulated data and final maps stored? An additional consideration is where this work should be done. As previously mentioned, the EOC is a high-stress environment and many normally competent people cannot produce their best work under these conditions. One solution is to move some of the data production tasks to another room, or even another building, and to communicate only the final products in the form of PDFs to be plotted in the EOC. Part of the pre-disaster planning should include this distributed approach and also what technology is needed to allow for the transfer of large data packets.

It would also be remiss not to briefly mention disaster cartography. There is an ongoing debate about how much 'correct cartographic convention' should be followed in a disaster. On the one hand, unless complete convention is followed (scale, title, date, north arrow, etc.) the possibility exists that the map produced may confuse and mislead. On the other hand, the alternative argument is that in a triage situation you do what you have to do to get the message across. For example, students tasked to make several large maps for ARC teams during Katrina were slowed by their inability to decide which features were necessary and what were the most effective colour schemes. This can be somewhat alleviated by having prepared templates ready in a GIS. These templates might also include all the acknowledgements and logos of those who had contributed to the final map, which also helps in negating future arguments about contribution.

Last, it is important to discuss the issue of spatial confidentiality. Much has been written about the vulnerability of spatially analysing and mapping health data (Curtis *et al.*, 2006a,b). Although there are several different components to this problem, possibly the two most important aspects in a post-disaster environment are the release of what would normally be considered confidential data, and then the actual revealing of those data displayed in a map form.

It is accepted that there probably will be a lessening of normal data protocols in an emergency response. The addresses of people with certain health conditions either reported before the event or realized through doctors' records or 911 calls will be shared with the GIS desk in order to support the response. It is to be hoped that these data will remain within the confines of the EOC, though the constant movement in and out of people and data storage devices means that this is a difficult aspect to police.

Related issues are data that are not exactly confidential but may still be sensitive, which brings us to the second aspect of disaster related confidentiality: revealing sensitive data in a mapped form. There is an ethical responsibility for any cartographer to think about the implications of a map that is created. For example, vital records (mortality locations) are not confidential in the strictest definition, but is it right to map deceased addresses for public consumption? This raises an interesting ethical dilemma: if these data are available through web sites or printed maps (in newspapers), is it right for spatial scientists to use them? The problem lies in the skill of the GIS scientist in making these data more accessible, or adding more contexts to them. Previous work has shown that a map of points (death locations) displayed on even the coarsest of backgrounds can be re-engineered back to actual or proximate addresses (Curtis *et al.*, 2006b). If this process is possible, then any map made, whether digital or paper, could at a future time be used as a data source. Again, during a response this is not the first thought of those trying to save lives. It is therefore necessary to develop a set of universally accepted guidelines for such situations. It is worth spending a little time thinking what other confidential spatial layers might be of concern for the EOC GIS desk during a disaster response.

Now that we have provided a thumbnail sketch of geospatial data sources and use in an EOC, we will turn our attention to one particular task that is essential to effective disaster response in the EOC, or in the earliest days of the recovery phase. That task is damage assessment, in particular, how to assess building scale damage from a disaster.

2.4 Damage Assessment

A disaster related spatial data layer that cannot be pre-prepared is the amount and location of building damage. Having accurate spatial damage data is important for many tasks, from helping prioritize the paths for search and rescue teams, to organizing debris clear-up. These damage layers are used by multiple sectors; researchers need these data to understand what happened, both in terms of the effectiveness of the evacuation or the science behind the actual event, and as base layers to assess recovery. Municipalities need damage assessment as the first part of assessing the impact on their community. Insurance companies need these data to process claims, and both FEMA and the ARC use building level damage to help with the distribution of aid.

There are three usual ways to acquire geospatial damage data after a disaster: (i) remote sensing; (ii) ground surveys; and (iii) mobile mapping. Each has advantages as well as drawbacks. One central question is: how quickly and effectively can each assessment type be performed?

2.4.1 Remotely sensed data

The quickest form of spatial damage acquisition is through using remotely sensed data, of which there are three main types: high resolution overhead aerial photography; oblique aerial photography; and multispectral satellite imagery.

High resolution overhead aerial photography is often available soon after the disaster and can show broad swathes of damage. The resolution of these images is usually such that considerable detail can be seen for each home. Two drawbacks emerge: the physical labour needed to turn these photographs into a GIS damage score for each property; and the related issue of the ability of the coders to *get it right* by correctly assessing the amount of damage per property, especially when the damage is not catastrophic.

Oblique aerial photography offers even more detail, with the ability to view a damaged property from all sides almost in a three-dimensional perspective. Although there are still issues of coding success with this, the real drawback involves access to the imagery and the software to use it. In the USA (and for some overseas disasters), this may be donated by the company Pictometry during the event, but as with most donated products, a cost will become involved at some point along the response to recovery continuum.

Multispectral satellite imagery can also be used to identify broad areas of impact, such as the extent of flooding or a path of a tornado. While there is the potential benefit of automated or semi-automated classification of these, for example using variations in reflectance from pre- and post-tornado paths to identify where damage occurred (Jedlovec *et al.*, 2006; Gerke and Kerle, 2011), current spatial resolution is not fine enough to allow for building level damage assessment.

2.4.2 Ground surveys

Ground surveys of some form happen after any disaster in the USA. For example, the ARC usually completes street sheets, which are paper forms on clipboards that volunteers use to assess building damage from within a car (a windshield survey). These records are used in ARC centres to support the decision to release monetary support for affected families. Other teams performing similar surveys might be tasked by the municipality, by insurance companies and, if we use the example of a tornado, from federal agencies such as the National Weather Service (NWS) to estimate the strength of the tornado by using a damage assessment scale or the National Institute of Standards and Technology (NIST) to assess structural deficiencies.

The benefit of this data collection approach is having an expert assessment in front of the damaged structure, which usually means seeing more of the damage actually in context. But even here, there can be variation in how two people may view the same degree of damage. Problems also arise in terms of the logistics of sending enough people into the field to collect data, including the on-the-ground challenges of moving through affected streets, some of which may still be treacherous and filled with understandably unhappy people. A further problem with this method is the reliance on accurate reporting from the field team with little hope of validation, though this is being improved with the use of handheld GPS which are both easy to use and allow for geotagged photography. From a research perspective, another issue is the financial cost of mobilizing ground surveys to cover large geographic areas, which are needed if it is hoped for any spatial analysis of the area. This is particularly challenging given the need for such surveys to be conducted in the days, or at most weeks, following the event.

2.4.3 Mobile mapping

The third type of damage data collection involves mobile mapping, such as the spatial video, which is defined as location encoded video imagery (Mills *et al.*, 2010; Curtis and Mills, 2011). Different approaches exist, for example encoding a GPS signal as a series of audio beeps on to camcorder recording media. Each camcorder is mounted on a window of the data collection vehicle, which is usually just a car or SUV. The track from a typical camera can be seen in Fig. 2.4. After software specific processing, these video tracks can be displayed either in a GIS style window, or actually incorporated into the GIS as an extension. This technology has recently improved as a result of the popularity of extreme sports. Tiny high definition cameras now carry an internal GPS, which when recorded on to a 32GB micro SD (secure digital) memory card means that up to 4 h of high quality video can be collected at a time and then spatially displayed on freely available software. This allows for the camera system to be easily shipped to an affected area, where little expertise is needed, and where as long as an Internet connection is available, the results can be seen immediately.

In June 2012, we took one such system to Haiti to help work on the cholera epidemic there. Even given the logistical issues of working in such a challenging environment, it was still possible to view the collected video linked to a map at the end of every day. Figure 2.2 shows video from a downward facing camera designed to capture water 'risks' within the town of Petit Goave, Haiti. In this image, a child is standing in one of the roadside drains. The figure also shows the location on a map. This Internet based software, which is called Contour Storyteller (http://contour.com/software/storyteller), is freely available, thus allowing for the easy dissemination of the video.

In summary, there are three main advantages to this particular geospatial data collection approach: it is easy and relatively cheap; large areas can be covered quickly (even up to speeds of 35 mph with little image degradation); and more of a spatial context can be captured than by simply treating each structure as a single data entry, as is the case with normal field surveys. This new way of collecting spatial data also has further applications: (i) the collection of temporal data; (ii) the creation of primary spatial data; and (iii) its potential as a geonarrative tool.

First, because this method is cheap, temporal data can be collected so that the way an

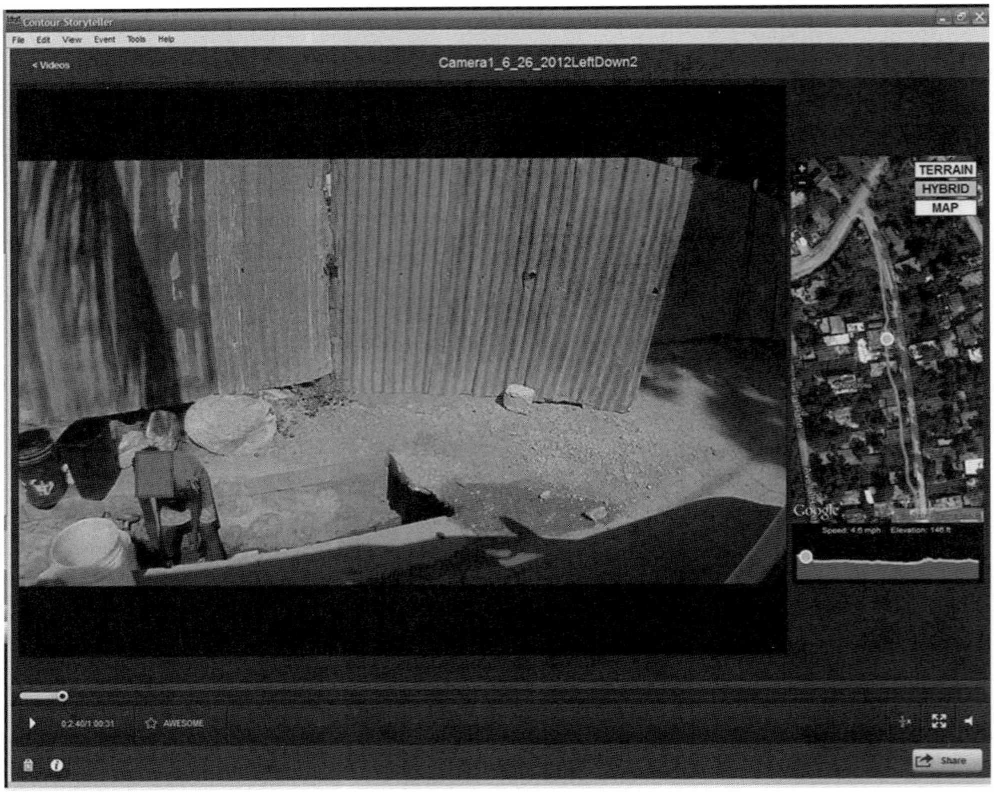

Fig. 2.2. Video-still image from a downward facing camera designed to capture water 'risks' within the town of Petit Goave, Haiti, during the cholera epidemic.

environment recovers after the disaster can be monitored. For example, 'The Changing Landscape of the Lower Ninth Ward', a tour of the evolving landscape of this ward of New Orleans following Hurricane Katrina, which was presented by the *New York Times* (and is available at: http://www.nytimes.com/interactive/2010/08/27/us/lower9th-5year-anniversary.html), is a useful illustration of why the capture of temporal change is important. This multimedia presentation makes available spatial video data collected by the authors of this chapter that display two roads in the Lower 9th Ward for four separate time periods. The user can progress forward along each road to see what changes have occurred in the 5 years following Katrina. In this way, the lack of recovery and patterns of rebuilding can be identified and then turned into actual GIS layers for spatial analysis. From a public health perspective, other health data can be layered on top of such urban change maps. For example, two areas of possible investigation are the access to playgrounds for children of returning families, and the link between domestic violence and the stress associated with the isolation of recovery. As of 2012, the Lower 9th Ward in New Orleans largely remains unoccupied, with whole city blocks covered in dense vegetation. There are, however, pockets of return. These returnees face multiple challenges, including the general lack of service provision, poor infrastructure, the loss of their neighbourhoods and community in general, and even crimes such as the dumping of tyres, cars and sometimes bodies, all because of the general lack of community oversight. It is not surprising in such a stressful living environment that hotspots of domestic violence sometimes coincide with these pockets of return.

Secondly, spatial video can be used to create primary spatial data, with the added benefit of providing a visual archive to delve back into when location specific events occur, such as a crime or an infant death. The possibilities of this approach are in many ways only limited by the creativity of the researcher and by his/her coding scheme. In New Orleans, we use this approach to look at the condition of and access to public parks and play spaces; in other declining cities, it is the growth (literally) of urban gardens; and in Los Angeles it is to map gang graffiti and support a new progressive diabetes clinic.

Thirdly, one further advantage of this technology is its potential as a geonarrative tool. By recording the comments of a ride along expert, such as a patient talking about his/her neighbourhood and the day-to-day living challenges, or a gang member interpreting graffiti, or a community resident describing known safe water locations, invaluable information can be encoded with a spatial location and then mapped in a GIS. So not only are we collecting primary data, but the data also provide a conduit to spatial insights that have previously been hard, if not impossible, to acquire.

To fully appreciate the possibilities and uses of these types of spatial data, the following exercise has been designed to replicate both the conditions of post-disaster response, and also the type of task that is performed.

2.5 Coding Data: An Exercise in How We Use Spatial Video Data

The following exercise has been designed to replicate the typical conditions following a disaster. It involves a team of disaster assessment coders working together from a common data source, collaborating and then producing a final document.

2.5.1 Overview

The purpose of this exercise is to work as a team to assess the level of damage following a disaster, in this case, the Joplin tornado. The task will be conducted digitally and not in person.

Objective 1. To learn how to work efficiently as a team under unusual circumstances.

Objective 2. To perform an accurate damage assessment of a disaster landscape.

Objective 3. To map the degree of damage in Joplin, Missouri.

Objective 4. To make comparisons between damage maps and describe features of interest.

The *final product* will be a PDF report of your work, including tables, maps and a written summary. This report will also include a group self-diagnosis of your ability to work together and of whether everyone played the same active role.

Your instructor will send you an e-mail which includes the identity of four people in your group. E-mail contact addresses will be provided. A nominal 'leader' is also identified. It is the task of this leader to make an initial contact to all other members of the group and to arrange a group communication (using whatever medium/software you prefer but not in person). If the leader has not made contact by [date], another member of the group should take over the responsibility.

Your instructor will also contact you about electronic 'meeting' times when you can ask questions.

Steps 1 and 2 should be completed over the course of 2 weeks. As you are not physically meeting, the danger is to not spend enough time on the tasks; time management is an important part of disaster response. Do not think of Step 1 as being the first week's task as Step 2 is longer. You will have to communicate with your group members to make sure the tasks proceed at an appropriate pace.

2.5.2 Step 1

Step 1 is to perform a damage assessment of the building damage in the PDF file 'Images (which is available at http://www.albany.edu/~fboscoe/gisbook/images.pdf). You will need to discuss with each other the logistics of how this step will be completed.

The purpose of this first step is to 'train' your group to think in the same way in terms of your damage score. This exercise will give you the chance to see where differences lie in your individual perceptions of damage.

The file Images contains 42 pictures of buildings damaged in the Joplin tornado. Using the Modified Enhanced Fujita (MEF) scale to assess the amount of damage that has been caused to a building by the tornado, each member of the group will score every building. In addition, you will rank each score from 1 to 5. This ranking indicates the level of confidence that you place in your score, on the following scale:

1 = extremely not confident
2 = somewhat not confident
3 = neutral
4 = somewhat confident
5 = extremely confident

The MEF damage scale assesses the amount of damage to a building as follows:

1 = No visible damage.
2 = Minor visible damage (usually loss of roof tiles, guttering, etc.).
3 = More substantial roof loss and/or boarded windows and doors.
4 = Large sections of roof material have been lost and less rigid sections of the house such as car ports have collapsed.
5 = The building has shifted on its foundations and/or sizeable holes have been knocked through walls or the roof.
6 = The roof has been removed.
7 = Exterior walls have collapsed.
8 = Exterior walls have collapsed leaving just a few inner walls standing.
9 = The entire structure has been reduced to rubble.
10 = Even the debris has been blown away leaving just dirt or a concrete slab.

Scores 1–3, though causing damage, should not result in loss of life, especially if the resident was not proximate to outer walls that might have been penetrated by projectiles.
Scores of 4 and 5, though not necessarily causing injury, carry more of an injury risk (albeit slight under normal precautions) as part of the outer shell of the building may have been penetrated.
Scores 6 and 7 both result in considerable damage to the home, which could easily result in injury or loss of life. This is especially true for the upper reaches of a score of 7 if multiple walls have collapsed. A building crushed by a tree would also score a 7.
Scores 8–10 are likely to result in injury or death unless there is an inner reinforced storm room or basement.

Two examples each of MEF scores 5, 6, 7 and 8 are shown in Fig. 2.3, which are images taken by the first author just after the Tuscaloosa tornado of 2011. For MEF 5, the buildings show multiple scarring to the roof and walls but the shell remains intact. For MEF 6, the first example shows a well constructed middle class home with large sections of the roof missing. In the second example, the smaller home has most of the roof missing although the walls remain intact. For the MEF 7 examples, both buildings have lost their roofs and sections of the exterior walls. For the MEF 8 examples, the majority of the outer shells of the buildings have gone, leaving just the fragile remains of the inner walls. MEF 9 and 10 are not displayed as these would just show debris or a scoured concrete slab.

One member of the group should collect all the scores and summarize these in an Excel table (for each image, both score and confidence rank for each group member). For the six buildings that generate the most disagreement in the group, either in terms of score or confidence, arrange to 'meet' using whatever medium you prefer and discuss these variations. Then you will write a group summary.

Deliverables from Step 1

1. Excel sheet showing the individual ranking and confidence score for each group member for every image.
2. A half page summary identifying and describing those buildings with the greatest difference.
3. A brief report describing the percentage effort contributed by each group member to the component parts of Step 1.

2.5.3 Step 2

Step 2 is to make two damage maps for Joplin based on three video routes. This actual task

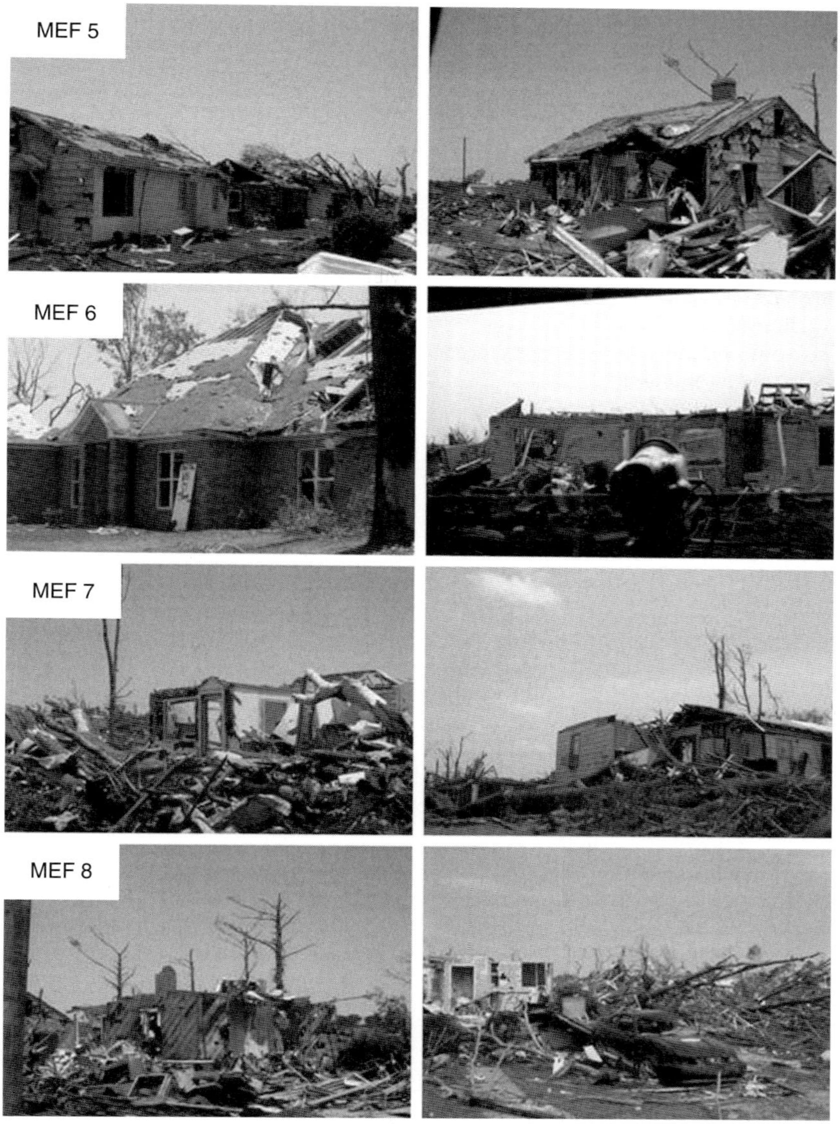

Fig. 2.3. Two examples of MEF (Modified Enhanced Fujita scale) scores 5, 6, 7 and 8 to rate building damage caused by a tornado. Images taken by the first author just after the Tuscaloosa, Alabama tornado of 2011.

involves the group in making these two damage maps using the same MEF score system as used in **Step 1**. The maps are to show patterns of damage and you will use them to answer questions. Area 1 has just one video run (Route 1), while Area 2 comprises two video runs (Routes 2A and 2B); if you don't have enough time, or if you only have three group members, then just map Route 2B. You will again need to meet (through whatever medium you prefer, but not in person) and decide who is working on what. It is up to you how you partition the workload.

What you need

You are provided six video segments in YouTube (three routes, left and right sides). These routes can be found by searching for:

route1left (or http://www.youtube.com/watch?v=R1iwcjXksDg)
route1right (or http://www.youtube.com/watch?v=p51lGRJYYkA)
route2Aleft (or http://www.youtube.com/watch?v=ffWTtqOFOMY)
route2Aright (or http://www.youtube.com/watch?v=QxOhiDWNIYo)
route2Bleft (or http://www.youtube.com/watch?v=iCS2YXJZQzQ)
route2Bright (or http://www.youtube.com/watch?v=X4ifi224uV4)

These video routes correspond to the Google Earth Kmz file 'damage_routes_for_class.kmz' (which is available at http://www.albany.edu/~fboscoe/gisbook/damage_routes_for_class.kmz). By opening this in Google Earth, you can see the path of the video, as well as aerial photography of the damage (see Fig. 2.4). Both Route 1 and Route 2a start from the south; Route 2b starts from the north.

Your task is to make a damage assessment map for each of the areas (1 and 2) by matching the video in YouTube to the path in Google Earth, and also using the background damage imagery in Google Earth. You should also consult Google Street View to help you determine what the buildings looked like before the tornado (work out your locations using Google Earth). You will also be provided with two building outline emf files: Route 1 Building outlines and Route 2 Building outlines (which are available at http://www.albany.edu/~fboscoe/gisbook/route_1_building_outlines.emf and http://www.albany.edu/~fboscoe/gisbook/route_2_building_outlines.emf). These can be opened in MS Paint and coloured according to your damage scheme.

Think about proper map design!

Decide as a group how you will make these maps – split the component tasks among yourselves. Once completed, you will also have to write a one page summary that includes answers to the following questions:

Q 1. Compare the damage between the two areas.
Q 2. Are there any patterns you notice about the damage? (think spatial patterns and damage associated with certain building types).
Q 3. What other interesting features on the landscape have you seen in the video?
Q 4. What have you seen in the video that relates to recovery?
Q 5. Find a local media story that has association with the damage information on your maps.

Deliverables from Step 2

These are:

1. Your finished maps for both areas.
2. Your answers to the questions.
3. A brief report describing the percentage effort contributed by each group member to the component parts of Step 2.

2.5.4 Final deliverables from Steps 1 and 2

All of the deliverables for Steps 1 and 2 combined into a single PDF report and emailed to your instructor. Edit the final report together as a group – it represents you all.

2.6 Conclusion

This chapter highlights issues of spatial data acquisition and use in responding to a disaster. From static base layers prepared in advance of an event to dynamic field data gathered in the hours and days following that event, geospatial technologies and GIS can play an important role in the effective management of a disaster. This chapter would be incomplete though without stressing that the success of such technologies is dependent upon the human network in which they operate. Ultimately, people are the key to managing disaster response. They must have awareness of the importance of the spatial data and the technologies needed to leverage data into actionable information.

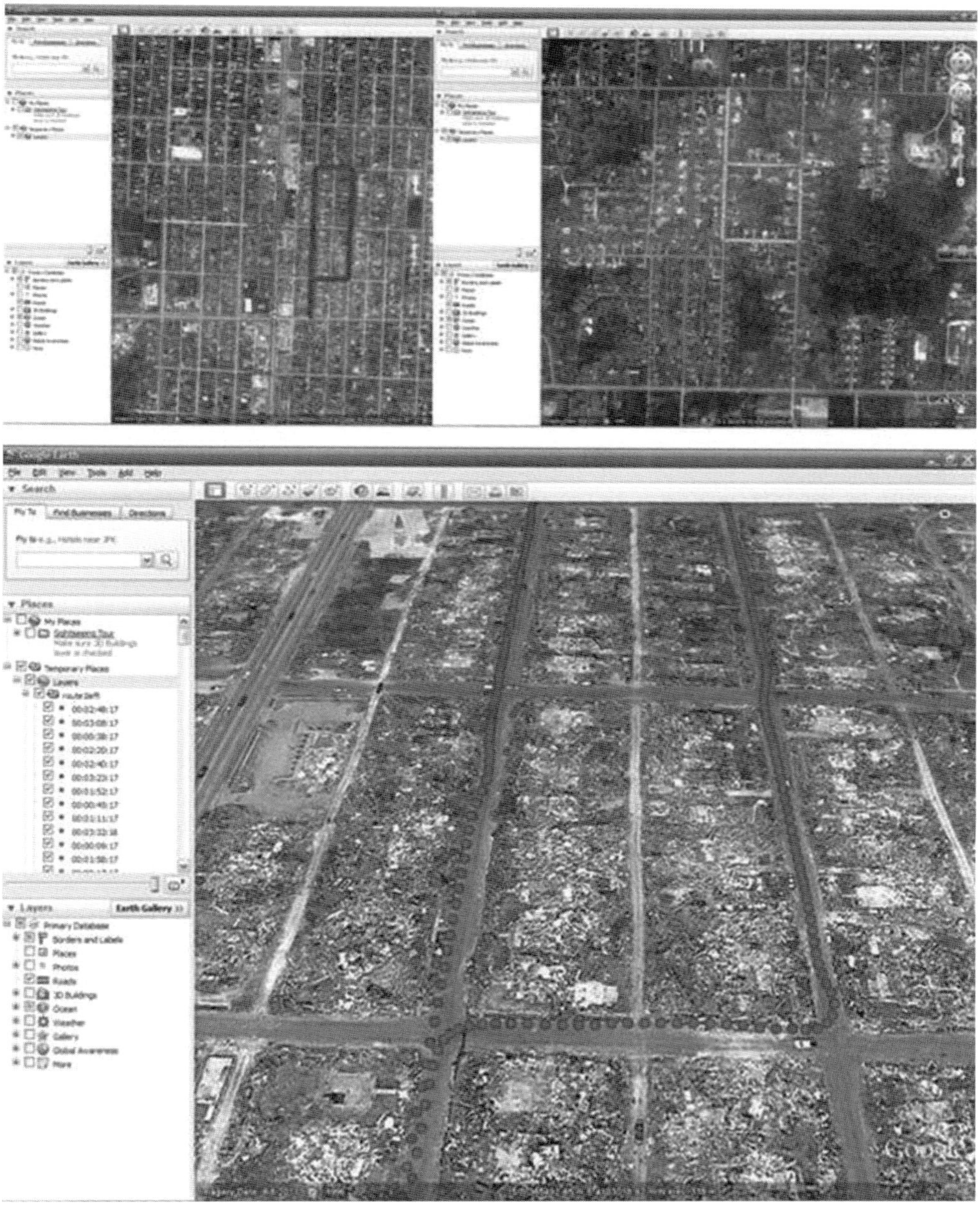

Fig. 2.4. Example of GPS tracks for video. Source: © 2012 Google

This requires political will and financial investment. It also requires people to be educated in the technical, creative and critical thinking skills to properly utilize these technologies and data. With each disaster response, the reliance on spatial data and geospatial technologies grows and new developments are made in data formats and platforms for use. However, the basic components covered in this chapter do not change, nor does their dependence on individuals in the human network for effective use in helping people at a time of great need.

References

Bokman, H. (2003) All-hazards planning: what does it mean? *Natural Hazards Observer* 27(4), March 2003, 10–11. Available at: http://www.colorado.edu/hazards/o/archives/2003/mar03/mar03.pdf (accessed 12 September 2012).

Butler, D. (2006) The web-wide world. *Nature* 439, 776–778.

Curtis, A. and Mills, J.W. (2011) Spatial video data collection in a post-disaster landscape: the Tuscaloosa tornado of April 27th 2011. *Applied Geography* 32, 393–400.

Curtis, A., Mills, J.W. and Leitner, M. (2006a) Keeping an eye on privacy issues with geospatial data. *Nature* 441, 150.

Curtis, A., Mills, J.W. and Leitner, M. (2006b) Spatial confidentiality and GIS: re-engineering mortality locations from published maps about Hurricane Katrina. *International Journal of Health Geographics* 5:44. Available at: http://www.ij-healthgeographics.com/content/5/1/44 (accessed 14 March 2013).

Curtis, A., Mills, J.W., Blackburn, J.K., Pine, J.C. and Kennedy, B. (2006c) Louisiana State University geographic information system support of Hurricane Katrina recovery operations. *International Journal of Mass Emergencies and Disasters* 24, 203–221.

Gerke, M. and Kerle, N. (2011) Automatic structural seismic damage assessment with airborne oblique Pictometry imagery. *Photogrammetric Engineering and Remote Sensing* 77, 885–898.

Goodchild, M.F. and Glennon, J.A. (2010) Crowdsourcing geographic information for disaster response: a research frontier. *International Journal of Digital Earth* 3, 231–241.

Jedlovec, G.J., Nair, U. and Haines, S.L. (2006) Detection of storm damage tracks with EOS data. *Weather and Forecasting* 21, 249–267.

Liu, S.B. and Palen, L. (2010) The new cartographers: crisis map mashups and the emergence of neogeographic practice. *Cartography and Geographic Information Science* 37, 69–90.

Miller, C.C. (2006) A beast in the field: the Google Maps mashup as GIS/2. *Cartographica* 41, 187–199.

Mills, J.W. (2009) Spatial decision support in a post-disaster environment: a community-focused approach. *Cartographica* 44, 17–31.

Mills, J.W. and Curtis, A. (2008) Geospatial approaches for disease risk communication in marginalized communities. *Progress in Community Health Partnerships: Research, Education, and Action* 2(1), 61–72. Available at: http://muse.jhu.edu/ (accessed 12 March 2013).

Mills, J.W., Curtis, A., Pine, J.C., Kennedy, B., Jones, F., Ramani, R. and Bausch, D. (2008) The clearinghouse concept: a model for geospatial data centralization and dissemination in a disaster. *Disasters* 32, 467–479.

Mills, J.W., Curtis, A.J., Kennedy, B., Kennedy, S.W. and Edwards, J. (2010) Geospatial video for field data collection. *Applied Geography* 30, 533–547.

3 Virtual Globes and Geospatial Health

Christopher F.L. Saarnak,[1]* Anna-Sofie Stensgaard,[1,2] Robert Bergquist,[3] Xiao-Nong Zhou[4] and Jürg Utzinger[5]

[1]Department of Veterinary Disease Biology, University of Copenhagen, Frederiksberg, Denmark; [2]Center for Macroecology, Evolution and Climate, Natural History Museum of Denmark, University of Copenhagen, Denmark; [3]Ingerod, Brastad, Sweden; [4]National Institute of Parasitic Diseases, Chinese Center for Disease Control and Prevention, Shanghai, People's Republic of China; [5]Swiss Tropical and Public Health Institute, Basel, Switzerland

3.1 Introduction

This chapter reviews recent advances in the application of the Google Earth virtual globe (and its web pendant, Google Maps) and aims to show how it can be a useful tool as well as a strong vehicle for the dissemination of primarily health oriented research. As a result it turn, will provide public health stakeholders and decision makers with improved tools for targeting health campaigns. The specific objectives are:

1. To give examples on the current (2012) usage of virtual globes in health research and dissemination.
2. To illustrate the applicability of the technology within the context of schistosomiasis research, including the elimination programme that is currently underway in the People's Republic of China (2012).
3. To examine the full potential of virtual globe technology for surveillance, control and eventual elimination of vector-borne and other infectious diseases that depend on intermediate hosts.

These issues are discussed and a set of conclusions drawn from the examples is presented.

3.2 How It All Started

A virtual globe is essentially a three-dimensional (3-D) representation of the earth, usually based on satellite imagery, upon which various types of information with a spatial character can be superimposed. It provides the users with the ability to append their own data, to share the added data layer with other interested users and to freely move around in the virtual environment by zooming in and out, and changing the position and viewing angle. In 1998, Al Gore, then Vice President of the USA, made a speech at the California Science Center in Los Angeles, where he presented a vision of a Digital Earth, in which satellite imagery, databases and georeferenced information were

* E-mail: cls@sund.ku.dk

all stored and made accessible through the Internet. Offline versions of a virtual globe had been available since the previous year through Microsoft's Encarta product. Still, Gore was very much ahead of his time, and he could imagine a near future where this information was publicly accessible for each and every one. Further, given the limits in bandwidth and home computer CPU speeds, it would be a service of libraries and museums to show the Digital Earth to the public:

> Imagine, for example, a young child going to a Digital Earth exhibit at a local museum. After donning a head-mounted display, she sees Earth as it appears from space. Using a data glove, she zooms in, using higher and higher levels of resolution, to see continents, then regions, countries, cities, and finally individual houses, trees, and other natural and man-made objects. Having found an area of the planet she is interested in exploring, she takes the equivalent of a "magic carpet ride" through a 3-D visualization of the terrain. Of course, terrain is only one of the many kinds of data with which she can interact. Using the systems' voice recognition capabilities, she is able to request information on land cover, distribution of plant and animal species, real-time weather, roads, political boundaries, and population. She can also visualize the environmental information that she and other students all over the world have collected as part of the GLOBE project. This information can be seamlessly fused with the digital map or terrain data. She can get more information on many of the objects she sees by using her data glove to click on a hyperlink. To prepare for her family's vacation to Yellowstone National Park, for example, she plans the perfect hike to the geysers, bison, and bighorn sheep that she has just read about. In fact, she can follow the trail visually from start to finish before she ever leaves the museum in her hometown.
>
> (Gore, 1998)

This vision is a perfect example of what virtual globes are capable of today, except that now they are pretty much accessible on most home computers with an up-to-date bandwidth connection. In fact, it was only 6 years on from Gore's speech, in 2004, before the first online virtual globe was launched by NASA (the US National Aeronautics and Space Administration). This was NASA's World Wind (see http://worldwind.arc.nasa.gov/), which was developed at the NASA Ames Research Center in Iowa. World Wind was followed in 2005 by Microsoft's MSN Virtual Earth (see Microsoft, 2005) and Google Earth. Microsoft's Virtual Earth was later rebranded as Bing Maps (available at http://www.microsoft.com/maps/). The smartphone industry is also at the forefront, Nokia having released its virtual Earth 'app', and one could speculate that it is probably only a question of time before Apple launches its version, as in 2010 it acquired the Poly9 group, an independent Canadian virtual Earth provider, followed in 2011 by acquisition of the Swedish company C3 Technologies, which creates 3-D maps with virtually no input from humans (Gurman, 2011). For a more in-depth review on the summary of current usage of virtual globes in the earth sciences, we refer the reader to Stensgaard *et al.* (2009) and Yu and Gong (2012).

It is outside the scope of this chapter to describe all the currently available virtual globe technologies or to discuss their strengths and limitations in a comprehensive and comparative manner. Instead, due to its current dominance among the virtual globe technologies, we have put the emphasis on Google Earth and its possibilities. Launched without great publicity in 2005, the prominence of Google Earth is now manifested by having been downloaded more than 1 billion times (McClendon, 2011). Perhaps Google Earth's biggest impact is the opening of the exploration of spatially explicit data to a large audience of mainly non-specialists. The application was originally called Earth Viewer and was developed by Keyhole Inc., a company acquired by Google in 2004; it was launched as a virtual globe the following year. Essentially, Google Earth maps the world by superimposing satellite raster imagery, aerial photography, vector maps and other layers, in a single and integrated tool, thus allowing users to interactively 'fly' in 3-D space, zooming in from the global to regional and local levels.

Although Google Earth is primarily aimed at the general public, and is for use mainly as a search tool, it has also attracted a large community that uses the application for a wider array of applications and purposes. Google Earth is a stand-alone application, and the user is required to install the software on personal computers before it can be used. Google Maps, the web-based pendant to Google Earth, is a complete web page with no need to install any additional software to browse the maps displayed by the provider. Like Google Earth, Google Maps can include satellite imagery, but the view is limited to two dimensions (2-D) and it does not have Google Earth's 3-D 'tilt' feature. Google Maps does not, therefore, essentially constitute a virtual globe; nevertheless, it is included in this review as it is often used in parallel with Google Earth on research project web pages to maximize outreach by targeting a wider audience. The primary method for visualizing data in Google Earth is through the creation of Keyhole Markup Language (KML) files, which are an Extensible Markup Language (XML) notation for expressing geographic visualization and annotation. Version 2.2 of KML was released in 2008 and by then it contained most of the features that are relevant to scientific data, such as large data support and the ability to time stamp features and to create animations. KML has been declared the standard for virtual globe visualization by the Open Geospatial Consortium (OGC), and is supported by a number of virtual globe applications and geographic information system (GIS) packages.

There are numerous ways to produce KML files for Google Earth, with detailed documentation and tutorials freely available online (at http://www.google.co.uk/intl/en_uk/earth/learn/). New tools and add-ons to existing software packages are increasingly being developed to make this task as quick and easy as possible. Below, we highlight some of the most prominent new tools and add-ons:

- Users of ESRI's ArcGIS products (version 9.2 and onwards) can now export their vector and raster layers or complete map projects directly into KML file format.
- Quantum GIS, a popular free GIS software program (available at http://www.qgis.org) converts shape files to KML files and vice versa.
- Users of the Matrix Laboratory (MATLAB) platform can export results of geostatistical analysis to Google Earth by using the Google Earth toolbox.
- Online, user friendly tools, such as GPSvisualizer (see http://www.gpsvisualizer.com), convert georeferenced data files to KML format and displays it on a Yahoo or Google map. In this latter application, the source file can be either in spreadsheet format or directly imported from a handheld global positioning system (GPS) receiver.

3.3 Mapping and Visualizing Epidemiology

Epidemiology is the discipline that deals with disease patterns at the population level. In spite of focusing on exposure and outbreaks, proximal or distal, and on single or cumulative risk factors using screening and surveillance as monitoring tools, epidemiology traditionally did not have strong visual support. However, modern spatial epidemiology deals with the description and variation of the geographic distribution of a disease as a function of behavioural, demographic, environmental, genetic and socio-economic determinants and risk factors. This generally encompasses disease mapping and prediction, geographic correlation studies and cluster analysis. To understand the increasingly important role of visualization in epidemiology, we start by contemplating mapping in general, because mapping joined the visual arts long before epidemiology found it convenient to use this medium. Maps are inextricably linked to the representation of spatial relationships and the history of cartography is the history of making spatial knowledge visible.

The visualization of epidemiological data is particularly required in the current era of global change – unprecedented movement of people and trade, and globalization – in order to show on maps the present and future scenarios of epidemics. Such information is needed for the establishment of early warning systems (EWS). Areas into which certain diseases can be expected to expand have been noted for schistosomiasis in the northern part of the People's Republic of China (Yang *et al.*, 2006; Zhou *et al.*, 2008) and for malaria, leishmaniasis and dirofilariasis in northern Europe (Genchi *et al.*, 2005, 2009). Other important drivers for the (re)-emergence and spread of vector-borne parasitic diseases include vector habitat changes (Bhunia *et al.*, 2011), pollution, resistance to pesticides and drugs and the general fallout from globalization (Harrus and Baneth, 2005). The changing distribution of previously strictly localized endemic human and livestock infections include the diseases of babesiosis, bluetongue, chikungunya, dengue, Lyme borreliosis (or Lyme disease), tick-borne encephalitis, trypanosomiasis and West Nile virus disease, and there are many more (Takken and Knols, 2007).

Aerial photography revolutionized cartography in the mid-1900s but the real breakthrough for remote sensing did not come until around 1975 when satellites equipped with photographic sensors came into wider use. Cartographers and meteorologists were the first to put these tools into civil use, while it took epidemiologists longer to appreciate the full potential of these new opportunities. Indeed, original research papers in this area did not start to appear regularly until around the late 1980s, but remote sensing, GIS and GPS are now well-known tools of the trade and few scientists working in the field can do without them. Earth-observing satellites were originally put in place for military purposes, but the information relayed back to the earth today also provides insights on climatic, ecological and anthropogenic factors related to the transmission levels and patterns of many communicable diseases (Brooker *et al.*, 2000; Rinaldi *et al.*, 2006). However, although remote sensing can clearly be of great use for epidemiological research, including disease control and elimination efforts, a bibliographic analysis reveals some risks. For example, the selection of images is often done by price and availability, resulting in poorly addressed and oversimplified data, which is sometimes not fully relevant to the research under consideration (Herbreteau *et al.*, 2006, 2007).

The study of risk factors for an infection and disease-related morbidity and mortality is an important aspect of epidemiology. The identification of causal pathways between risk factors and disease, in turn, allows the design and implementation of preventive and control measures that aim to reduce disease burdens. Infectious diseases are often considered to be 'environmental' diseases because a considerable fraction of their burden can be attributed to environmental factors (Listorti and Doumani, 2001; Prüss-Üstün and Corvalán, 2007). Hence, distribution patterns of infectious diseases are strongly associated with the spatially heterogeneous environment in which they are embedded (Woolhouse *et al.*, 1997; Brooker and Clements, 2009). Visualization of this heterogeneity, at different spatial scales, is paramount in revealing new insights into the patterns of disease. Indeed, it is only the simultaneous visualization of health data with environmental data obtained from a diversity of sources that can further our understanding of environmental health linkages and provide data for articulating new hypotheses on the distribution of diseases.

GIS are designed for this purpose and contain an increasing number of sophisticated capabilities for data display and analysis. The use of GIS in spatial epidemiology in human and animal health, and in the geospatial health sciences in general, has firmly established the technique as a useful tool for collating, exploring, visualizing and analysing health data in a spatially explicit manner (Rinaldi *et al.*, 2006; Brooker, 2007; Simoonga *et al.*, 2009; Yang *et al.*, 2012). The integration of remotely sensed environmental data into a GIS platform can deepen our understanding of the spatio-temporal dynamics of a wide range of disease systems, especially those with environmental correlates. However, high-resolution, geo-rectified imagery in a digitized format is difficult to visualize and explore without the expertise and availability of sophisticated (and often expensive) GIS software. This remains a hurdle to benefiting from the full advantages that GIS can provide for the elucidation of spatial epidemiology and geospatial health, especially in a resource-constrained developing country context.

None the less, recent advances in the development of virtual globe technology, such as Google Earth, have provided an opportunity for a cheap and accessible method for communicating epidemiological data more effectively to different stakeholders, including non-specialists. Virtual globe technologies are essentially web-based GIS tools, which bring some of the functionality of the sophisticated applied GIS to the non-specialist. Therefore, they are suitable for the display and dissemination of research results where location and spatial variation are critical components. While virtual globe applications have limited analytical functions and are not designed to replace professional GIS software, they may be a useful complement to traditional GIS technologies and geostatistical analyses tools. In our opinion, the virtual globe technology holds a large, hitherto still under-explored potential for applications in the health sciences, especially in low- and middle-income countries.

Since around 2005, virtual globe applications in general, and Google Earth in particular, have increasingly been recognized by the scientific community as far more than just a handy map or a fun toy (Butler, 2006). They are becoming a meeting place for scientists and non-scientists alike, offering a way to connect and share data, and to exchange scientific ideas with one other. Their application pertains to a wide variety of scientific disciplines, including environmental management, biodiversity and conservation biology, urban planning, disaster management, agriculture, land use, community mapping and education, among others. For a full list see Stensgaard *et al.* (2009) and Yu and Gong (2012).

Applications of Google Earth in public health and medicine are becoming frequent. One of the earliest references made to the potential of virtual globe technology for disease mapping was highlighted by Malone (2005) in the context of vector-borne parasites. Another example worth mentioning is the scientific journal *Nature*'s use of Google Earth to track the spread of the H5N1 avian influenza virus around the globe (Butler, 2006). A further example convincingly showing the operational usage of Google Earth in public health was its use to track a polio virus outbreak down the Congo River (Kamadjeu, 2009).

3.4 Health Projects

Health projects, whether driven by a specific research question or public health initiatives, have increasingly applied virtual globes as a powerful tool for monitoring and presenting health-related data. In other words, in addition to its increasingly common use in epidemiological prospective studies, virtual globe technology and Google Earth have also been used retrospectively by creating and publishing Google Earth KML files of key findings to supplement scientific publications and to broaden the dissemination of results. We do not list all the current health projects that use this technology, as the number of different projects is not stable, but brief details of four of these are given below (for a recent list, see Stensgaard *et al.*, 2009 and Duhl *et al.*, 2011).

- *Disease outbreak and real time surveillance.* Butler (2006) won the Association of Online Publishers (AOP) Use of the New Digital Platform Award 2006 for tracking the spread of the H5N1 avian influenza virus around the globe. This Google Earth presentation compiles data on outbreaks of avian flu in birds from 2003 onwards and on confirmed human cases of infection, as well as other relevant spatial data layers, in order to map cases and outbreaks by location and time, with links to relevant web resources from the Food and Agriculture Organization (FAO) of the United Nations, the World Health Organization (WHO) and other organizations (Butler, 2006). This example demonstrates the potential of so-called 'mashups', a term originally used to describe the mixing together of musical tracks, but now referring to web sites that weave data from different sources into a new service (Boulos *et al.*, 2006). Further examples can be found at the Google Earth Outreach initiative web site (http://earth.google.com/outreach/index.html), which contains a continuously updated online overview of health-related showcases.
- *Global warming and disease.* This project was a collaboration between Google and a group of epidemiologists looking at the impact of climate change on vector-borne diseases. Based on the findings from several separate studies (Hales *et al.*, 2002; Tanser *et al.*, 2003; Ezzati *et al.*, 2004; Ebi *et al.*, 2005), the different research groups created a KML animation named 'GlobalWarmingDisease.kml' (Adams, 2008); this shows the projections for the

changes in the global transmission of dengue and malaria in Africa (see Fig. 3.1).

- A third project, *HealthMap*, has been carried forward by a team of researchers, epidemiologists and software developers based at Children's Hospital Boston. This database project was initiated in 2006, and has become a global leader in utilizing online informal sources for disease outbreak monitoring and real time surveillance of emerging public health threats (HealthMap, 2012). Since its inception, the project has now grown and branched out into several sub-projects from flu surveillance to the HN1 influenza A (swine flu) outbreak, as well as cholera cases reported on Haiti and African swine fever (AFS) outbreaks. Details of these are available on the HealthMap web site (healthmap.org/projects/).
- Imperial College London, on its Spatialepidemiology.net web site (http://www.spatialepidemiology.net/), has created interesting mashups combining genetic and epidemiological data on pathogenic microorganisms. This site not only provides a Google Earth map-based interface for the display and analysis of epidemiological data, but also allows users to create their own maps easily through the Google Maps application programming interface (API).

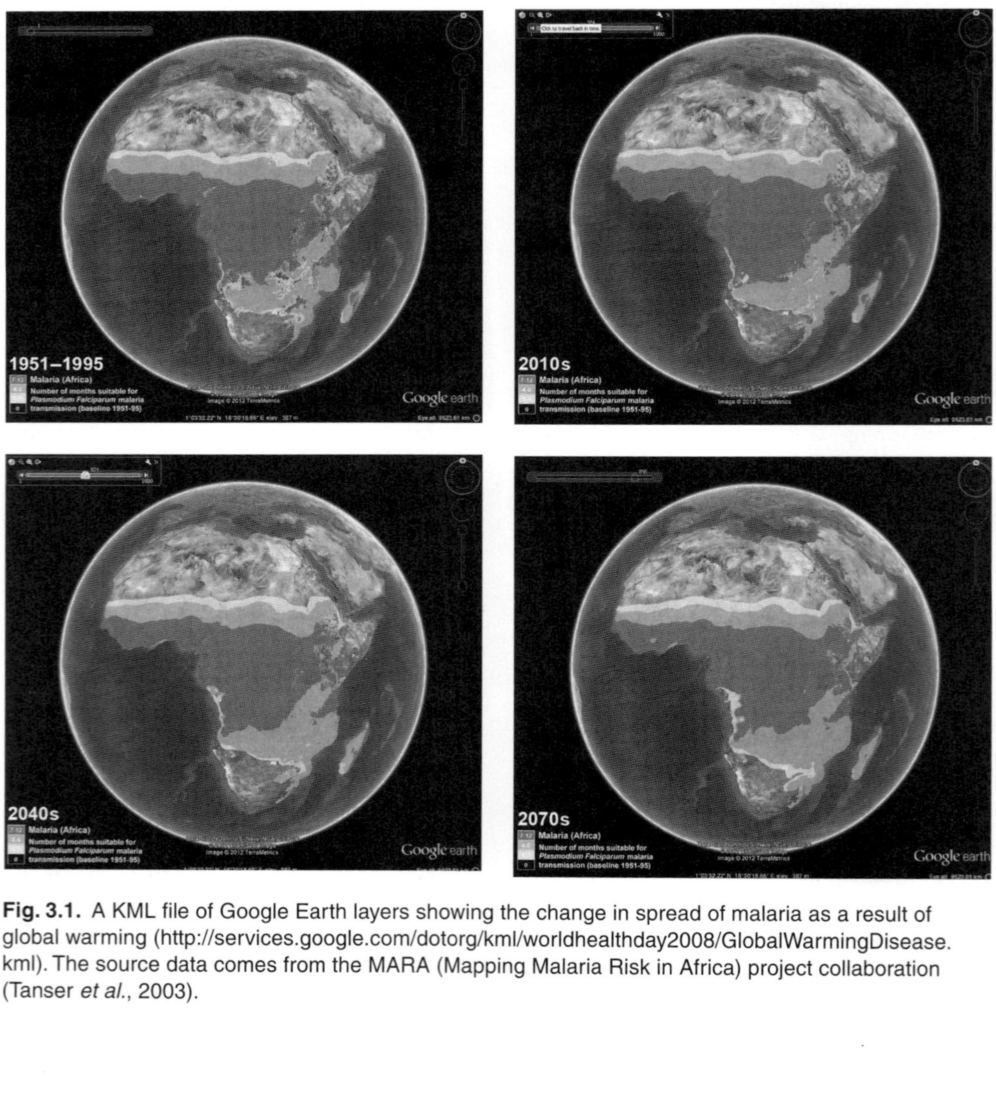

Fig. 3.1. A KML file of Google Earth layers showing the change in spread of malaria as a result of global warming (http://services.google.com/dotorg/kml/worldhealthday2008/GlobalWarmingDisease.kml). The source data comes from the MARA (Mapping Malaria Risk in Africa) project collaboration (Tanser *et al.*, 2003).

The three subsections below discuss three applications of Google Earth to schistosomiasis projects.

3.4.1 Usage of Google Earth in the CONTRAST research project

Google Earth and Google Maps were applied within the framework of a 4-year European Union (EU) funded project under the acronym of CONTRAST (a multidisciplinary alliance to optimize schistosomiasis control and transmission surveillance in sub-Saharan Africa), for which details are available at http://www.eu-contrast.eu/. This EU funded project ran from late 2006 to late 2010 and aimed at building a multidisciplinary research platform to better understand which interventions should be used to control the snail-borne parasitic disease schistosomiasis and how to tailor interventions at the local level. The morbidity of schistosomiasis is predominantly controlled by preventive chemotherapy campaigns (using the anti-schistosomal – anthelminthic – drug praziquantel) (WHO, 2006; Hotez *et al.*, 2007). However, in order to achieve sustained success in reducing transmission and ultimately reaching the goal of elimination, a thorough consideration of the environmental components is essential, because the disease is completely dependent on its freshwater-dwelling intermediate host snail (Stothard *et al.*, 2009; Utzinger *et al.*, 2011a).

A key feature of the CONTRAST project was the highly interdisciplinary team efforts, consisting of a strong research node network across Africa, which brought together key skills and expertise to generate new knowledge on molecular, biological, environmental and socioeconomic risk factors relating to schistosomiasis in different parts of the continent. These nodes worked on establishing innovative molecular tools to characterize both intermediate host snails (Standley *et al.*, 2011) and schistosome parasites (Kane *et al.*, 2011), and the potential genetic consequences of large-scale administration of anthelmintic drugs (Norton *et al.*, 2010). This work has defined the importance of host–parasite dynamics across different eco-epidemiological settings and resulted in the development of new spatial models for disease risk mapping and prediction (Schur *et al.*, 2011b; Stensgaard *et al.*, 2011). An additional aim of CONTRAST was to encourage and assess novel, local control interventions using a social science approach, while ensuring widespread dispersal of and access to information. Virtual globe technology lends itself particularly well to the activities within research projects such as CONTRAST that are concerned with the spatial epidemiology for risk mapping and prediction at non-sampled locations (Hürlimann *et al.*, 2011; Schur *et al.*, 2011a,b). Google's virtual globe technologies were used for a variety of purposes, ranging from partner communication, data visualization and validation to web-based dissemination of project research and key results.

The conceptual diagram in Fig. 3.2 illustrates where and how Google Earth and Google Maps were used in the project, project work flows and stages. The overall communication and assembly of project-related data took place via the CONTRAST web page (stage 1), where Google Earth and Google Maps were used to communicate in a spatially explicit manner. New data collected by the project partners during epidemiological and malacological surveys were entered online using a standardized format managed by the FireFlower data management system (http://www.fireflower.ca). Historical data on schistosome parasites and intermediate host snails for all of sub-Saharan Africa are continuously being collated and digitized using a systematic approach to review extant literature and managed in a relational database with direct KML export capabilities (stage 2 – see Hürlimann *et al.* (2011) for details). Here, the Google Earth display of data can be used for data location, georeferencing, validation and gap identification. The development of predictive models of disease distribution takes place via advanced spatial and geostatistical analysis (stage 3). As Google Earth has no analytical capabilities, this process essentially occurs through statistical software packages (e.g. STATA, from the Stata Corporation, College Station, Texas, version 9.2; WinBUGS, from Imperial College and the Medical Research Council, London, UK, version 1.4.2;

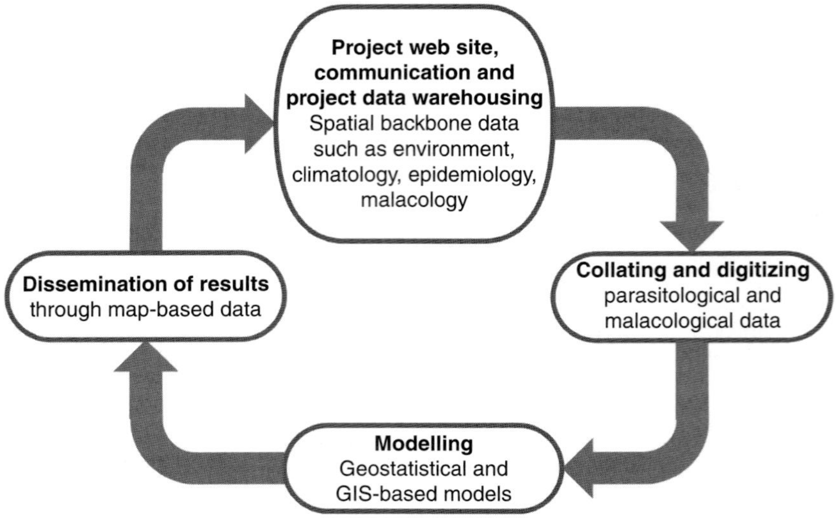

Fig. 3.2. Conceptual diagram showing the work-flow and stages in the EU-funded CONTRAST project (an alliance for optimizing schistosomiasis control and transmission surveillance in sub-Saharan Africa), relating specifically to spatial epidemiology for schistosomiasis risk mapping and prediction at non-sampled locations. Google Earth's virtual globe technologies are applied in all but the modelling stage.

and R, see http://www.R-project.org), as well as more conventional GIS packages. Finally, in addition to the common dissemination of results through scientific literature, models and other research results are illustrated via Google Earth (stage 4). The extensive public interest in such visualizations makes the scientific information widely accessible to general users. To underscore this issue, the Hürlimann *et al.* paper, published in December 2011, was accessed over 5400 times by mid-June 2013. Also of note, personal data and results can be combined with other spatial data and thereby stimulate scientific debate and the articulation of new research questions and hypotheses.

Data visualization is also useful for decision support, particularly in the spatial targeting of disease control measures, but also for the identification of knowledge gaps and the stimulation of further data collection. Figure 3.3 shows a screen shot of one of the Senegalese field sites – Temeye, on the lake Lac de Guiers – where schistosomiasis transmission is widespread.

3.4.2 Developing a digital, interactive atlas of the distribution of schistosomiasis and intermediate host snails

Another example of the use of Google Earth in a schistosomiasis project pertains to its role in efforts to develop a digital, interactive atlas of the distribution of schistosomiasis and its intermediate host snails (Hürlimann *et al.*, 2011). This is thus a logical continuation of the initial efforts made by the University of Bordeaux (France) and WHO in the 1980s, which resulted in the publication of the first global, printed atlas of schistosomiasis (Doumenge *et al.*, 1987). However, because this atlas appeared just before the 'age of the Internet', it cannot be updated continuously as new data become available.

Since the inception of the CONTRAST project in October 2006, considerable efforts have gone into digitizing and georeferencing historical records of schistosomiasis prevalence data and intermediate host snail species. These data are being assembled in

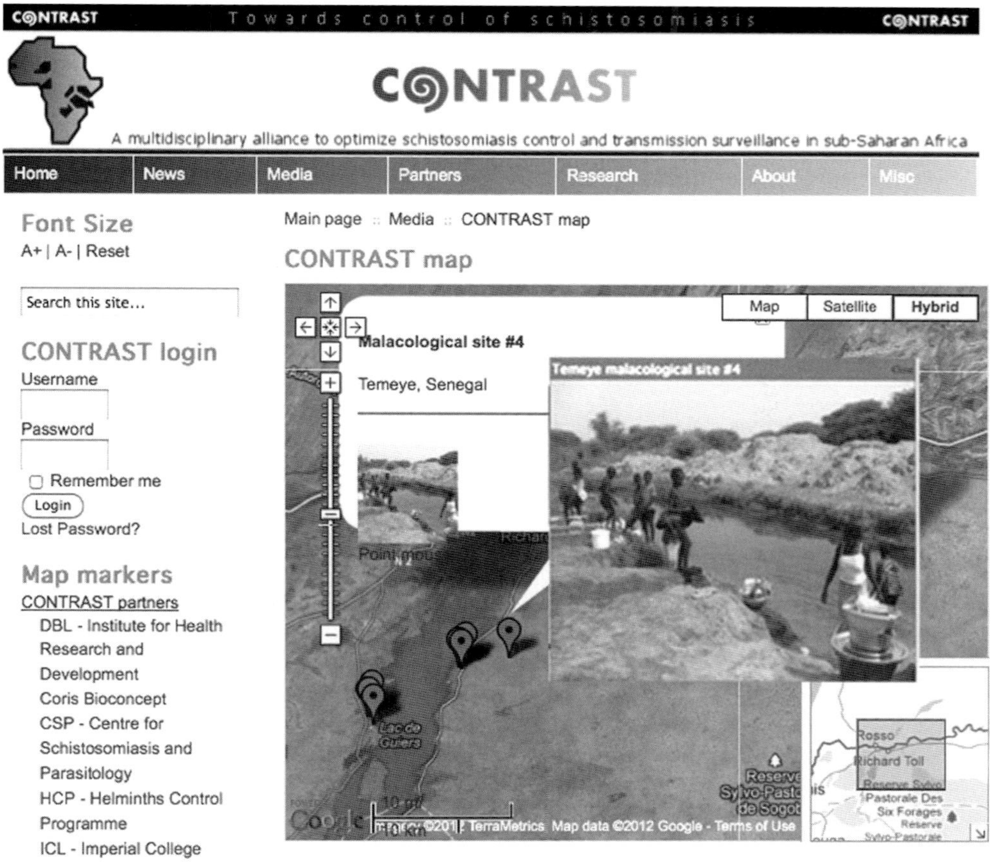

Fig. 3.3. A screenshot displaying the use of Google Maps as applied for presenting a field site (Temeye, Senegal) in the CONTRAST project.

the open source MySQL relational database management system, and are continuously updated. As of 1 June 2012, the database consists of more than 12,000 georeferenced locations with associated parasite prevalence data, along with information on the distribution of the intermediate host snail species associated with the transmission of schistosomiasis. Geocoding, the process of converting text descriptions of locations to computer-readable geographic locations (e.g. latitudes and longitudes, see Chapter 4), is carried out using gazetteers such as the BioGeoMancer (http://www.biogeomancer.org/ https://sites.google.com/site/biogeomancerworkbench/) (Guralnick *et al.*, 2006).

The CONTRAST database, with an initial focus on schistosomiasis in Africa, has been extended geographically and in terms of its disease portfolio to include other neglected tropical diseases (NTDs). Indeed, towards the end of 2011, the database has been made publicly available under the name of the GNTD Database 'gntd.org' (Fig. 3.4). Future plans are to utilize Google's virtual globe technology as part of the database interface. An advantage of this approach is that any person working with the database can directly export any chosen data selection directly from the database to a KML file for instant viewing in Google Earth. The files can be emailed to colleagues (who may have no knowledge of, or access to, GIS), and then simply be 'dragged and dropped' by the recipient on to their own desktop Google Earth display, where the layer is immediately draped over the Google Earth landscape. This simple and instant mapping in Google Earth

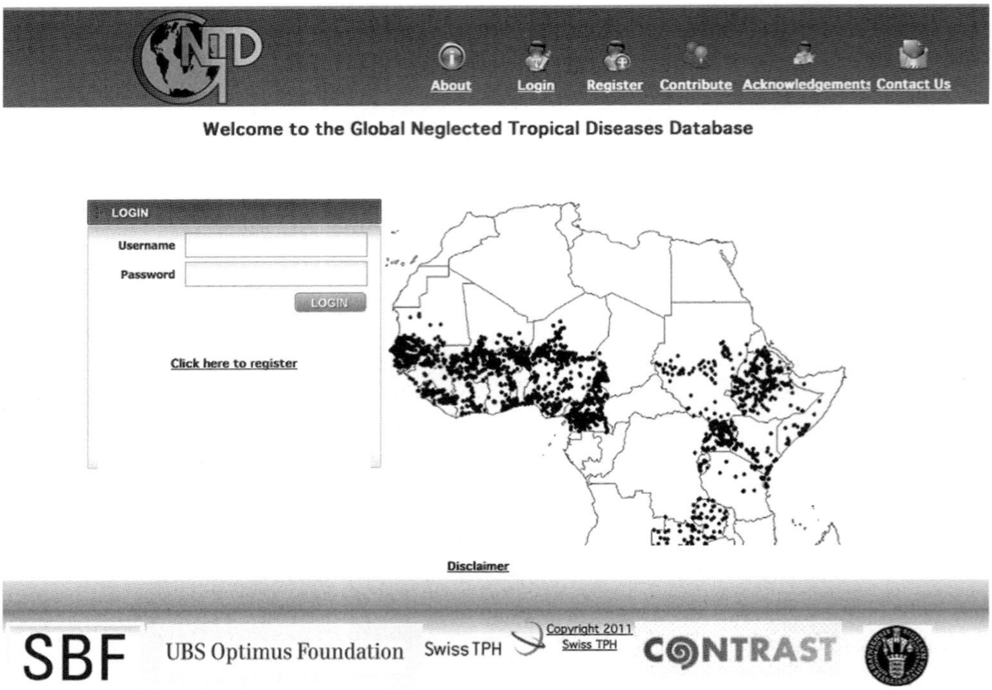

Fig. 3.4. A screenshot of the front page of the Global Neglected Tropical Diseases (GNTD) Database (available at http://www.gntd.org).

serves several purposes. It has made it possible to quickly identify spatial data gaps and it has been helpful in identifying areas where further epidemiological and malacological surveys are warranted. It has also proven instrumental in validating the global position of the thousands of localities (small rural settlements, towns, etc.) that have been retrospectively georeferenced; partners in various geographic regions can quickly identify geocoding errors, and hence assist with improving the precision of the geographic coordinates.

3.4.3 Going from science to operational public health management: a Web GIS platform to monitor and forecast schistosomiasis in the People's Republic of China

The Internet has undeniably played an integral part in giving scientists and decision makers access to near real time data. The presentation of data based on interactive, computer-generated map applications represents a straightforward way of visualizing large numbers of data sets in a geographic context. In the People's Republic of China, combining spatial data from Google Earth with a GIS package has developed a basic Web GIS framework for the rapid assessment of the risk for schistosomiasis (see Fig. 3.5). This framework provides dynamic information on an important endemic disease in near real time and has the added function of an EWS as it can quickly locate high-risk areas. The system retrieves all-important data needed as well as providing detailed and up-to-date information on the performance of the control programme for the disease. In this way, the epidemiological status of schistosomiasis can be shared in near real time, not only with the individual researchers around the country who are at work extending the evidence base but, most importantly, with decision makers and disease control managers.

The Chinese Web GIS platform includes remotely sensed data and GIS analysis as well

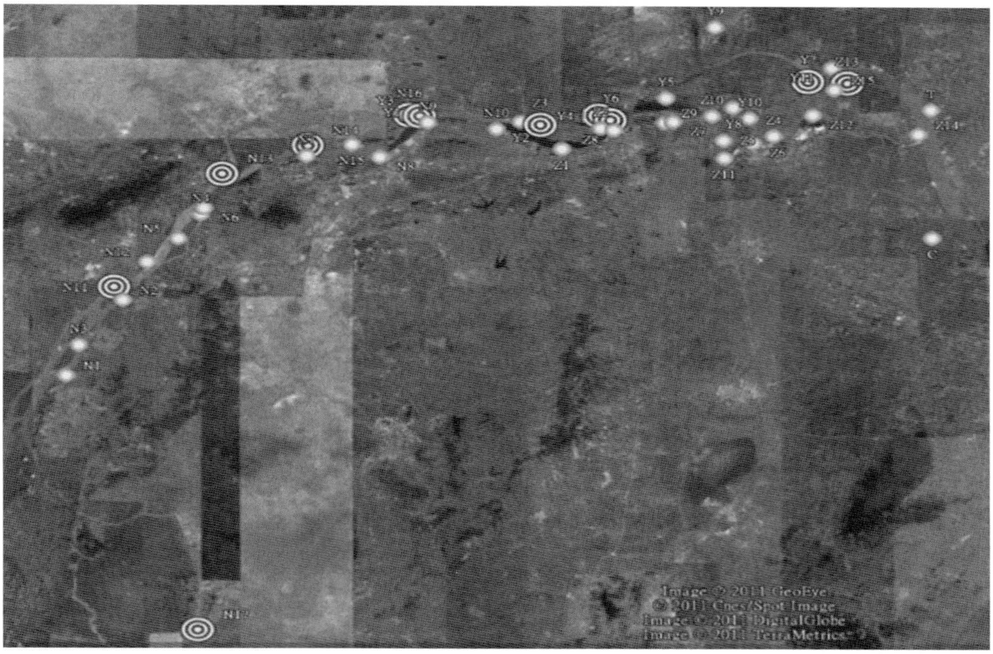

Fig. 3.5. Chinese Web GIS showing the 45 surveillance sites for schistosomiasis monitoring in Jiangsu Province. The sites are located approximately 10 km from each other along both banks of the lower reaches of the Yangtze River. The surveillance period was May–September for 3 years (2009–2011), and the surveys were done each month at high tides. Target (bull's eye) symbols indicate positive sites.

as visualization of the distribution of schistosomiasis and intermediate host snail habitats. The latter information is not only provided by searches using Google Earth but is also collected through field surveys. Furthermore, it includes advanced risk forecasts based on data stored in the server processed by spatio-temporal modelling, e.g. the WinBUGS (Bayesian inference Using Gibbs Sampling) programme (available at http://www.mrc-bsu.cam.ac.uk/bugs/).

The available layers of the Web GIS platform include information on:

- the current endemic status of schistosomiasis
- prevalence in humans and livestock (most importantly water buffalo)
- snail distribution, snail density and percentage of infected snails
- control measures implemented
- high-risk regions

Users can request maps by e-mail or download them in KML format for importation into their own GIS software packages. They can also obtain information about historic endemic situations and field information in the form of pictures or videos; the system permits results in the form of annotated maps to be generated and printed as well.

The Web GIS uses common industry standards, including widely accepted data descriptions and communication protocols to facilitate interoperability and portability, thereby permitting communication and data transfer between units running on different platforms and using different technologies, e.g. the different versions of Internet Explorer and Firefox, as well as the Linux-based operating systems and MacOS. The components that make up the platform were chosen so they could be bundled together without having to write specific computer programs. The database was designed with consideration to the environmental parameters influencing the prevalence of schistosomiasis in humans, reservoir animals and the intermediate host snail, as well as the risk for outbreaks due to the continuous population flux between rural and urban areas – the importance of which for the transmission of various diseases has been pointed out by many authors (Engels *et al.*, 2002; Taylor, 2008; Wang *et al.*, 2008).

The design of the platform is capable of providing analyses based on remotely sensed data and GIS applications. Active control programmes are constantly generating updated information and the platform should be capable of following and incorporating these developments in near real time, the necessity of which has been pointed out many times (Taylor, 2008; Wang *et al.*, 2008, 2009; Zhou *et al.*, 2008). Ongoing field operations require constant guidance and the platform must be ready to respond to queries on the effectiveness of a particular intervention approach in certain settings, or the feasibility of interventions in relation to the resources available, i.e. when and where to intervene and how to identify and locate high-risk areas. The experience of using the platform is encouraging and it has the potential to improve present support systems and strengthen schistosomiasis control activities, in particular for surveillance EWS and current efforts towards the elimination of schistosomiasis. What makes this development particularly interesting is that the approach chosen can be used for the validation and surveillance of any disease, and even outside the area of communicable infections.

The combination of GIS, remote sensing and Google Earth technologies offers new opportunities for the rapid assessment of endemic areas, provision of reliable estimates of populations at risk, prediction of disease distributions in remote areas that lack baseline data and guidance of intervention strategies so that scarce resources are allocated in the most cost-effective manner possible (Yang *et al.*, 2005; Chen *et al.*, 2007; Zhou *et al.*, 2009). The Web GIS approach makes it possible to analyse complex geospatial data and communicate them in a user-friendly graphical format, thus solving the problem of presenting and explaining the epidemiological situation for decision makers and the general public in a case-by-case manner (Theseira, 2002; Croner, 2003; Kamadjeu and Tolentino, 2006; Maclachlan *et al.*, 2007; Syed-Mohamad, 2009).

As the technology for Web GIS development becomes more and more readily available, including access to software systems for data management, geographic data visualization through the Internet (e.g. MapServer), geographic data analysis (e.g. ArcGIS), spatial statistics and Internet server management (e.g. Apache, http://httpd.apache.org/ABOUT_APACHE.html), then general purpose applications will become more common. The XML-based standard Geography Markup Language (GML) is becoming the world standard language for encoding geographic features and geoprocessing service requests (Boulos, 2004). By comparison, many agencies, particularly in the USA, have an extensive Web GIS presence presenting a multitude of digital geospatial data from various areas, e.g. improving hospital bed availability in community health and bioterrorism surveillance services (Boulos, 2004), and the information on West Nile Virus at the United States Geological Survey (USGS) web site (http://diseasemaps.usgs.gov/wnv_us_human.html).

The challenge for real time surveillance platforms is to adapt technologically advanced and costly concepts for disease management to resource-poor environments by developing low-cost tools and solutions (Hrster and Wilbois, 2007; Choo, 2009). Alhough satellite imagery has been available for over half a century, its broader use was limited until the Landsat programme was initiated in 1972 (http://landsat.gsfc.nasa.gov/). Due to cost and quality issues, though, the satellite technology has remained in the industrial world and spread only slowly to the developing countries. However, the past few years have seen this 'monopoly' give way to a more global use, at least for the satellite imagery produced.

3.5 A New Generation of 'vHealth' Papers

The old adage 'A picture is worth a thousand words' was discussed at a symposium held during the 60th Annual Meeting of the American Society of Tropical Medicine and Hygiene in Philadelphia in December 2011 in connection with new ways of visualizing health data using geospatial tools, including remote sensing, GIS and Google Earth (Utzinger *et al.*, 2011b). Ideas discussed and further consolidated during this symposium were subsequently translated into the concept of 'vHealth' papers ('v' standing for visualization). In an editorial published in the May 2012 issue of the journal *Geospatial Health*, the launch of vHealth papers is featured (Bergquist and Tanner, 2012). The editorial goes hand in hand with three examples, giving a flavour of the potential of geospatial tools, including virtual globes, for visualizing complex public health issues (see Fig. 3.6) (Krieger *et al.*, 2012; Maire *et al.*, 2012; Winkler *et al.*, 2012). The key feature of these vHealth papers is that they contain a link to a video, which can be readily downloaded free of charge or directly viewed on any personal computer connected to the Internet. Importantly, two of these vHealth papers use Google Earth applications. These are briefly summarized here (Krieger *et al.*, 2012; Maire *et al.*, 2012).

Krieger *et al.* (2012) pursued numerous integrated impact assessments of projects with particular emphasis on the health impacts on local communities of large-scale industrial projects in the developing world. These impact assessments usually result in reports of several hundreds of pages, with numerous technical appendices that are difficult to access by non-specialists. In an effort to bring the key findings across to senior management in a more digestible format, the key essence of such impact assessments is captured in short video clips that contain spatially explicit data. For example, the predicted environmental and health risks and accompanying mitigation strategies for a uranium mine in Tajikistan are highlighted. Using Google Earth, the viewer of a 17 min video clip is zoomed from the globe right into the heart of the uranium mine near the town of Adrasman in northern Tajikistan. Aided by 3-D 'fly-through' visuals and sophisticated video sequence generation overlaid on project-specific satellite imagery and GIS products, and assisted by object-based imagery analysis, segmentation and land feature classification, the viewer embarks on a virtual tour of the mining site, quite similar to that predicted by Al Gore in the 1990s. While the current video is designated for senior management of the international finance cooperation and development banks, it can be readily adapted to other stakeholders, including non-literate communities that will be affected by the project.

Maire *et al.* (2012) provided an overview of the development of the Health Resources Allocation Model (HRAM) dating back to the late 1980s, in which they explain how this eLearning tool has been widely and successfully used by health cadres and scientists. Indeed, the HRAM is a powerful tool for introducing the basic concepts of rational district-based health planning and systems thinking under resources constraints. The model was initially developed as a simple DOS program with data from the Kilombero district in Tanzania. It allows the evaluation of resource allocation strategies in relation to key outcome measures (e.g. coverage with insecticide-treated nets, vaccination among under 5 year old children, equity of services achieved and number of deaths and disability-adjusted life years (DALYs) averted by to specific health interventions. Most importantly, the model takes into account geographic and demographic characteristics and the health seeking behaviour of populations. Google Earth is utilized as the platform for spatial data display. Furthermore, HRAM can be extended to other social–ecological and health systems settings in developing countries.

3.6 Discussion and Conclusion

The ease, efficiency and speed of data communication and analyses are paramount to, and characteristic of, any mature science. The key strengths of virtual globe applications are their relatively simple, intuitive nature and ability to incorporate new data in a straightforward manner. GIS software is already an important tool for understanding spatial and temporal factors in a wide range of disciplines, increasingly so in the geospatial health sciences, which investigate links between diseases and the multidimensional environments in which they occur. However, commercial GIS tools have traditionally been an expensive and complex solution, especially in the developing world. They are often not mutually compatible,

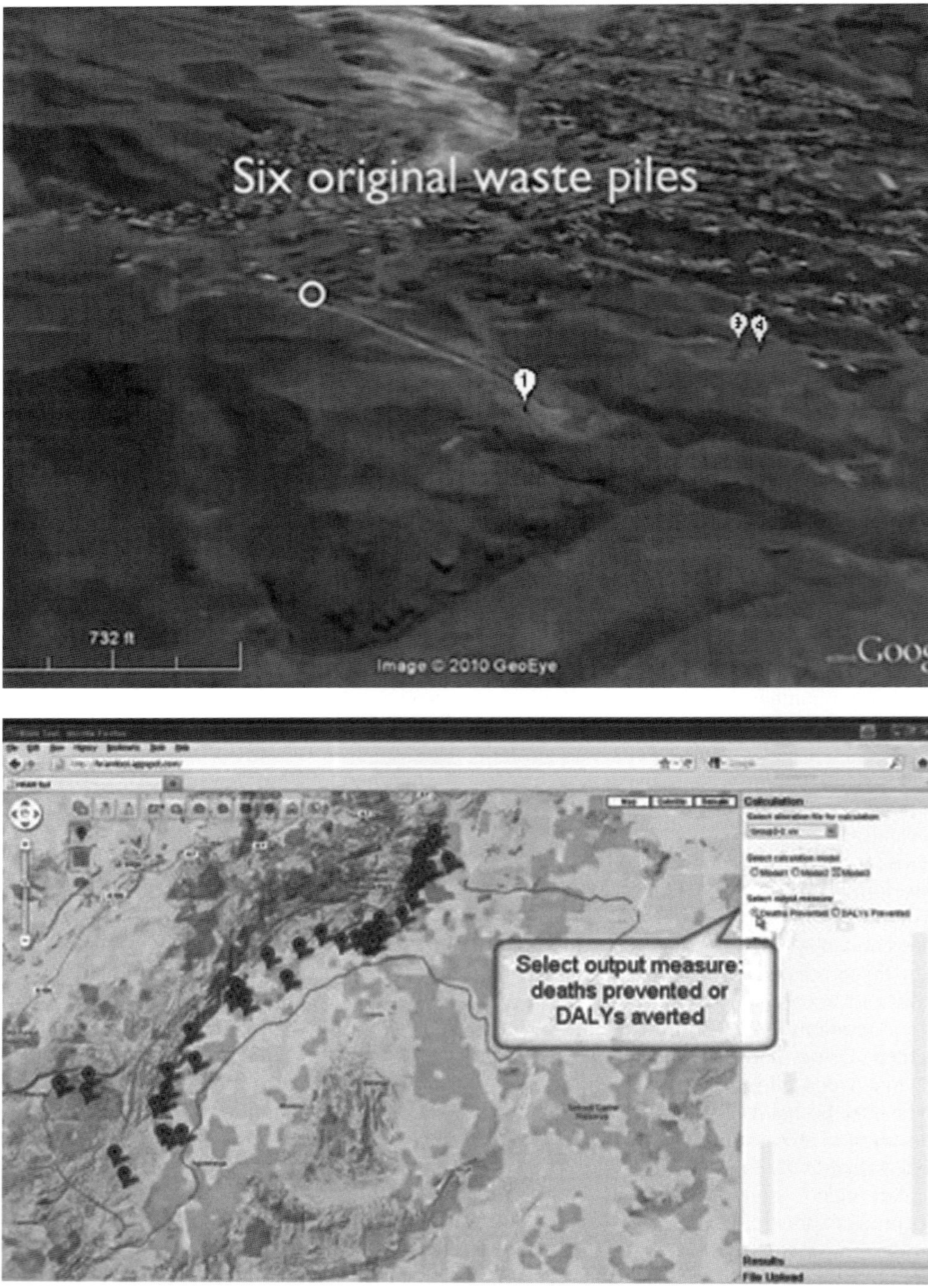
Six original waste piles
732 ft
Image © 2010 GeoEye
Select output measure:
deaths prevented or
DALYs averted

Fig. 3.6. Stills from the 'vHealth' papers in the journal *Geospatial Health* by Krieger *et al.* (2012) and Maire *et al.* (2012). At the top is a 3-D fly-in showing the location of waste piles – a novel way of enhancing environmental impact assessment through visualization. At the bottom is an example of how Google Maps layers are used in the Health Resources Allocation Model (HRAM), an eLearning tool (DALY, disability-adjusted life years).

making it difficult to combine data from different sources in a smooth manner.

Google Earth and other virtual globe applications offer researchers a simpler alternative to GIS software and we envisage that this will lead to increased data sharing (beyond static images), while enabling the implementation of a new and exciting science. Thus, Google Earth has the potential to make mapping accessible to a new set of public health users, including the developing world. The availability and quality of satellite imagery, combined with features such as KML or image overlay, provide a flexible yet powerful platform that set it apart from traditional mapping tools. It should be emphasized, though, that virtual globe applications are engineered to do only a small portion of what a full GIS technology does, and should be viewed as a complement to, rather than a full replacement of, more sophisticated GIS technologies. The following points are offered for discussion of some of the merits and limitations of Google Earth as compared with other virtual globe technologies and GIS.

First and foremost, Google Earth allows easy simultaneous visualization of point data together with many of types of auxiliary environmental data, which makes it well suited for the 'exploratory' phases of scientific work. Users can upload their own georeferenced data (in point, polygon and raster format) and share it with selected users or, alternatively, with the whole impressive network that is the Google Earth community. Although Google Earth does not offer traditional GIS functionality, it can also be used to add content, such as points or lines, to the existing maps, and to measure areas and distances, derive coordinates and ultimately load GPS data.

Secondly, for web-based data sharing, the data is readily located on Internet servers. This means that users do not have to download or install any data locally – although the need to access the Internet (e.g. to capture satellite images of areas of interest) is a limitation that will impede the use of Google Earth for this purpose in some parts of the world.

Thirdly, the base maps in Google Earth (remote sensing images, roads, administrative units, topography, etc.) are extensive and, above all, are frequently updated and constantly improving in quality. Though still far from suitable for all kinds of epidemiological studies, this brings new promise for the improved use of remote sensing applied to epidemiology, which hitherto has been criticized for not fulfilling its promises (Herbreteau *et al.*, 2007). A limitation is that non-urban areas in the developing parts of the world still suffer from poor coverage of high-resolution satellite imagery. This is a limitation that is a particular problem for local studies of many diseases, including schistosomiasis and other NTDs, as well as malaria. Another limitation with acquiring high-resolution imagery through Google Earth is that the exact acquisition date of the image cannot be chosen, which makes it less than perfect for analysis purposes (Monkkonen, 2008; Kamadjeu, 2009). Although Google Earth, with its version 5, has opened the possibility for accessing (and presenting) historical imagery (Hanke, 2009), there is no way to select the date of image acquisition. Especially in regions with strong climatic seasonality, such as the Sahel region of Africa, this poses a problem. If landscape features are to be monitored over time, it is important to retrieve data from the same time of the year.

An important strength of Google Earth is that it uses a single coordinate system, i.e. the world geodetic system (WGS-84) and that the geodata are visualized using a 3-D model rather than a projected 2-D system. This means that the user avoids having to deal with the complexity of understanding and merging maps and layers from different projection systems. The fact that more and more people and organizations are now producing KML versions of their spatial data (as opposed to other spatial data formats that require different types of GIS software) has made it easy for scientists, and the general public alike, to quickly prepare mashups and explore data obtained by different research groups. The use of Google Earth and Google Maps in the CONTRAST project, which is also generally applicable to other research projects with geospatial health components, can be summarized in a few overall categories such as:

- visualization
- communication
- data exploration (e.g. the identification of spatial and temporal disease clustering)

- validation
- dissemination of research results for a wider audience
- support for decision making

A remaining problem, though, is how to attain the proper geocoding of disease-related data, not least for the vectors and the intermediate hosts carrying the infectious agents; this still hinders the full potential of virtual globe applications for these purposes. Failure to include spatial information may eliminate potentially highly productive routes to analysis, including those not yet foreseen. But these data are frequently inadequate or absent, and this remains one of the main obstacles for the direct mapping of, for instance, vector-borne diseases and the exploration of their relationships with the heterogeneous environment in which they exist. Other important issues, not dealt with in this chapter, pertain to the ethics of displaying traceable health information in public space and concerns with confidentiality of the data (Curtis *et al.*, 2006; Mak, 2012). According to some, the type of visualization exemplified by the virtual globe crosses several ethical thresholds in communicating scientific and environmental information, and participatory uses of virtual globes by experts and laypeople carry both benefits and risks (Sheppard and Cizek, 2009). Thus, while the appeal of these techniques is evident, with unprecedented opportunities for public access to data and collaborative engagement over the web there are, none the less, several important ethical aspects that need to be considered before applying these techniques in areas of public interest, such as planning and policy making. At present, Google Earth appears to be primarily used as a geobrowser for exploring spatially referenced data. However, its functionality can be integrated with various analytical tools for spatial analysis (e.g. GIS and open-source statistical packages such as R; Bivand, 2006), while facilitating the sharing of spatially referenced data between international research groups and agencies (Wood *et al.*, 2007).

We hope that this chapter will stimulate further exploration of virtual globe applications for spatial epidemiologists, and that this could also introduce the broader research community to the potential of recording and producing accessible spatial data in appropriate formats. We continue to use Google Earth and Google Maps as an integral part of the next phase of the CONTRAST project and we invite readers to check the project's web site, as well as the web sites of the many other research projects mentioned in this chapter, to witness how virtual globe applications can be used for the display and sharing of data and research relevant to the management and control of vector-borne and other environmental diseases.

References

Adams, C. (2008) Global warming heats up infectious diseases. The Official google.org blog, Monday 4/07/2008 08:32:00 AM. Available at: http://blog.google.org/2008/04/global-warming-heats-up-infectious.html (accessed 13 March 2013).

Bergquist, R. and Tanner, M. (2012) Visual approaches for strengthening research, science communication and public health impact, *Geospatial Health* 6, 155–156.

Bhunia, G.S., Kesari, S., Chatterjee, N., Pal, D.K., Kumar, V., Ranjan, A. and Das, P. (2011) Incidence of visceral leishmaniasis in the Vaishali district of Bihar, India: spatial patterns and role of inland water bodies. *Geospatial Health* 5, 205–215.

Bivand, R. (2006) Implementing spatial data analysis software tools in R. *Geographical Analysis* 38, 23–40.

Boulos, M. (2004) Towards evidence-based, GIS-driven national spatial health information infrastructure and surveillance services in the United Kingdom. *International Journal of Health Geographics* 3:1.

Boulos, M.N.K., Scotch, M., Cheung, K.-H. and Burden, D. (2006) Web GIS in practice VI: a demo playlist of geo-mashups for public health neogeographers. *International Journal of Health Geographics* 7:38.

Brooker, S. (2007) Spatial epidemiology of human schistosomiasis in Africa: risk models, transmission dynamics and control. *Transactions of the Royal Society of Tropical Medicine and Hygiene* 101, 1–8.

Brooker, S. and Clements, A.C. (2009) Spatial heterogeneity of parasite co-infection: determinants and geostatistical prediction at regional scales. *International Journal for Parasitology* 39, 591–597.

Brooker, S., Rowlands, M., Haller, L., Savioli, L. and Bundy, D.A.P. (2000) Towards an atlas of human helminth infection in sub-Saharan Africa: the use of geographical information systems (GIS). *Parasitology Today* 16, 303–307.

Butler, D. (2006) Mashups mix data into global service. *Nature* 439, 6–7.

Chen, Z., *et al.* (2007) Strategy formulation for schistosomiasis japonica control in different environmental settings supported by spatial analysis: a case study from China. *Geospatial Health* 1, 223–231.

Choo, C.W. (2009) Information use and early warning effectiveness: perspectives and prospects. *Journal of the American Society for Information Science and Technology* 50, 1071–1082.

Croner, C.M. (2003) Public health, GIS and the Internet. *Annual Review of Public Health* 24, 57–82.

Curtis, A.J., Mills, J.W. and Leitner, M. (2006) Spatial confidentiality and GIS: re-engineering mortality locations from published maps about Hurricane Katrina. *International Journal of Health Geographics* 5:44.

Doumenge, J.P., Mott, K.E., Cheung, C., Villenave, D. and Chapuis, O. (1987) *Atlas of the Global Distribution of Schistosomiasis.* Presses Universitaires de Bordeaux, Bordeaux, France.

Duhl, T.R., Guenther, A. and Helmig, D. (2011) Estimating urban vegetation cover fraction using Google Earth® images. *Journal of Land Use Science* 6, 1–19.

Ebi, K.L., Hartman, J., Chan, N., McConnell, J., Schlesinger, M. and Weyant, J. (2005) Climate suitability for stable malaria transmission in Zimbabwe under different climate change scenarios. *Climatic Change* 73, 375–393.

Engels, D., Chitsulo, L., Montresor, A. and Savioli, L. (2002) The global epidemiological situation of schistosomiasis and new approaches to control and research. *Acta Tropica* 82, 139–146.

Ezzati, M., Lopez, A.D., Rogers, A. and Murray, C.J.L. (2004) *Comparative Quantification of Health Risks: Global and Regional Burden of Diseases Attributable to Selected Major Risk Factors.* World Health Organization, Geneva, Switzerland.

Genchi, C., Rinaldi, L., Cascone, C., Mortarino, M. and Cringoli, G. (2005) Is heartworm disease really spreading in Europe? *Veterinary Parasitology* 133, 137–148.

Genchi, C., Rinaldi, L., Mortarino, M., Genchi, M. and Cringoli, G. (2009) Climate and *Dirofilaria* infection in Europe. *Veterinary Parasitology* 163, 286–292.

Gore, A. (1998) The digital earth: understanding our planet in the 21st Century. Speech made at Open GIS Consortium at the California Science Center, Los Angeles, California, on January 31, 1998.

Guralnick, R.P., Wieczorek, J., Beaman, R. and Hijmans, R.J. (2006) BioGeomancer: automated georeferencing to map the world's biodiversity data. *PloS Biology* 4(11): e381. Available at: http://dx.doi.org/10.1371%2Fjournal.pbio.0040381 (accessed 13 March 2013).

Gurman, M. (2011) Apple acquired mind-blowing 3D mapping company C3 Technologies, looking to take iOS Maps to the next level. Feature, October 29, 2011/10:26 am, 9to5mac Apple Intelligence. Available at: http://9to5mac.com/2011/10/29/apple-acquired-mind-blowing-3d-mapping-company-c3-technologies-looking-to-take-ios-maps-to-the-next-level/ (accessed 13 March 2013).

Hales, S., de Wet, N., Maindonald, J. and Woodward, A. (2002) Potential effect of population and climate changes on global distribution of dengue fever: an empirical model. *Lancet* 360, 830–834.

Hanke, J. (2009) Dive into the new Google Earth. Google Official Blog. Posted: Monday, February 02, 2009. Available at: http://googleblog.blogspot.dk/2009/02/dive-into-new-google-earth.html (accessed 13 March 2013).

Harrus, S. and Baneth, G. (2005) Drivers for the emergence and re-emergence of vector-borne protozoal and bacterial diseases. *International Journal for Parasitology* 35, 1309–1318.

HealthMap (2012) About HealthMap. Available at: healthmap.org/about/ (accessed 13 March 2013).

Herbreteau, V., Demoraes, F., Hugot, J.-P., Kittayapong, P., Salem, G., Souris, M. and Gonzalez, J.-P. (2006) Perspectives on applied spatial analysis to animal health: a case of rodents in Thailand. In: *Impact of Emerging Zoonotic Diseases on Animal Health: 8th Biennial Conference of the Society for Tropical Veterinary Medicine. Annals of the New York Academy of Sciences* 1081, 17–29.

Herbreteau, V., Salem, G., Souris, M., Hugot, J.-P. and Gonzalez, J.-P. (2007) Thirty years of use and improvement of remote sensing, applied to epidemiology: from early promises to lasting frustration. *Health and Place* 13, 400–403.

Hotez, P., Molyneux, D.H., Fenwick, A., Kumaresan, J., Ehrlich Sachs, S., Sachs, J.D. and Savioli, L. (2007) Control of neglected tropical diseases. *New England Journal of Medicine* 357, 1018–1027.

Hrster, W. and Wilbois, T. (2007) Early warning and risk management: an interdisciplinary approach. *Information Technologies in Environmental Engineering* 7, 343–356.

Hürlimann, E., *et al.* (2011) Toward an open-access global database for mapping, control and surveillance of neglected tropical diseases. *PLoS Neglected Tropical Diseases* 5(12): e1404.

Kamadjeu, R. (2009) Tracking the polio virus down the Congo River: a case study on the use of Google Earth™ in public health planning and mapping. *International Journal of Health Geographics* 8:4.

Kamadjeu, R. and Tolentino, H. (2006) Web-based public health geographic information systems for resources-constrained environment using scalable vector graphics technology: a proof of concept applied to the expanded program on immunization data. *International Journal of Health Geographics* 5:24.

Kane, R.A., Stothard, J.R., Rollinson, D., Leclipteux, T., Evraerts, J., Standley, C.J., Allan, F., Betson, M., Kaba, R., Mertens, P. and Laurent, T. (2011) Detection and quantification of schistosome DNA in freshwater snails using either fluorescent probes in real-time PCR or oligochromatographic dipstick assays targeting the ribosomal intergenic spacer. *Acta Tropica* (in press). Proof available at: http://dx.doi.org/10.1016/j.actatropica.2011.10.019, (accessed 13 March 2013).

Krieger, G.R., Bouchard, M.A., Marques de Sa, I., Paris, I., Balge, Z., Williams, D., Singer, B.H., Winkler, M.S. and Utzinger, J. (2012) Enhancing impact: visualization of an integrated impact assessment strategy. *Geospatial Health* 6, 303–306.

Listorti, J.A. and Doumani, F.M. (2001) *Environmental Health: Bridging the Gaps*. World Bank Discussion Paper No. 422, World Bank, Washington, DC.

Maclachlan, J.C., Jerrett, M., Abernathy, T., Sears, M. and Bunch, M.J. (2007) Mapping health on the Internet: a new tool for environmental justice and public health research. *Health and Place* 13, 72–86.

Maire, N., Hegnauer, M., Nguyen, D., Godelmann, L., Peterhans, B., Hoffmann, A., de Savigny, D. and Tanner, M. (2012) The Health Resources Allocation Model (HRAM) for the 21st century. *Geospatial Health* 6, 295–298.

Mak, S. (2012) Geocoding-protected health information using online services may compromise patient privacy – Comments on "Evaluation of the positional difference between two common geocoding methods" by Duncan *et al. Geospatial Health* 6, 157–159.

Malone, J.B. (2005) Biology-based mapping of vector-borne parasites by geographic information systems and remote sensing. *Parasitologia* 47, 27–50.

McClendon, B. (2011) Google Earth downloaded more than one billion times. Google Lat Long Blog, Wednesday, October 5, 2011 at 6:45 AM. Available at: http://google-latlong.blogspot.co.uk/2011/10/google-earth-downloaded-more-than-one.html (accessed 13 March 2013).

Microsoft (2005) MSN virtual earth gives people an immersive way to search, discover and explore their world online. [Press Release], July 24, 2005. Available at: http://www.microsoft.com/en-us/news/press/2005/jul05/07-24VirtualEarthBetaPR.aspx (accessed 13 March 2013).

Monkkonen, P. (2008) Using online satellite imagery as a research tool. *Journal of Planning Education and Research* 28, 225–236.

Norton, A.J., Gower, C.M., Lamberton, P.H.L., Webster, B.L., Lwambo, N.J.S., Blair, L., Fenwick, A. and Webster, J.P. (2010) Genetic consequences of mass human chemotherapy for *Schistosoma mansoni*: population structure pre- and post-praziquantel treatment in Tanzania. *American Journal of Tropical Medicine and Hygiene* 83, 951–957.

Prüss-Üstün, A. and Corvalán, C. (2007) How much disease burden can be prevented by environmental interventions? *Epidemiology* 18, 167–178.

Rinaldi, L., Musella, V., Biggeri, A. and Cringoli, G. (2006) New insights into the application of geographical information systems and remote sensing in veterinary parasitology. *Geospatial Health* 1, 33–47.

Schur, N., Hürlimann, E., Garba, A., Traoré, M.S., Ndir, O., Ratard, R.C., Tchuem-Tchuenté, L.-A., Kristensen, T.K., Utzinger, J. and Vounatsou, P. (2011a) Geostatistical model-based estimates of schistosomiasis prevalence among individuals aged ≤20 years in West Africa, *PLoS Neglected Tropical Diseases* 5(6): e1194.

Schur, N., Hürlimann, E., Stensgaard, A.-S., Chimfwembe, K., Mushinge, G., Simoonga, C., Kabatereine, N.B., Kristensen, T.K., Utzinger, J. and Vounatsou, P. (2011b) Spatially explicit *Schistosoma* infection risk in eastern Africa using Bayesian geostatistical modelling. *Acta Tropica* (in press) Proof available at: http://dx.doi.org/10.1016/j.actatropica.2011.10.006 (accessed 13 March 2013).

Sheppard, S.R. and Cizek, P. (2009) The ethics of Google Earth: crossing thresholds from spatial data to landscape visualisation. *Journal of Environmental Management* 90, 2102–2117.

Simoonga, C., Utzinger, J., Brooker, S., Vounatsou, P., Appleton, C.C., Stensgaard, A.-S., Olsen, A. and Kristensen, T.K. (2009) Remote sensing, geographical information system and spatial analysis for schistosomiasis epidemiology and ecology in Africa. *Parasitology* 136, 1683–1693.

Standley, C.J., Wade, C.M. and Stothard, J.R. (2011) A fresh insight into transmission of schistosomiasis: a misleading tale of *Biomphalaria* in Lake Victoria. *PLoS ONE* 6(10): e26563.

Stensgaard, A.S., Saarnak, C.F.L., Utzinger, J., Vounatsou, P., Simoonga, C., Mushinge, G., Rahbek, C., Møhlenberg, F. and Kristensen, T.K. (2009) Virtual globes and geospatial health: the potential of new tools in the management and control of vector-borne diseases. *Geospatial Health* 3, 127–141.

Stensgaard, A.-S., Utzinger, J., Vounatsou, P., Hürlimann, E., Schur, N., Saarnak, C.F.L., Simoonga, C., Mubita, P., Kabatereine, N.B., Tchuem-Tchuenté, L.-A., Rahbek, C. and Kristensen, T.K. (2011) Large-scale determinants of intestinal schistosomiasis and intermediate host snail distribution across Africa: does climate matter? *Acta Tropica* (in press). Proof available at: http://dx.doi.org/10.1016/j.actatropica.2011.11.010 (accessed 13 March 2013).

Stothard, J.R., Chitsulo, L., Kristensen, T.K. and Utzinger, J. (2009) Control of schistosomiasis in sub-Saharan Africa: progress made, new opportunities and remaining challenges. *Parasitology* 136, 1665–1675.

Syed-Mohamad, S.M. (2009) Development and implementation of a web-based system to study children with malnutrition. *Computer Methods and Programs in Biomedicine* 93, 83–92.

Takken, W. and Knols, B.G.J. (2007) Epilogue: emerging pests and vector-borne diseases are a reality. In: Takken, W. and Knols, B.G.J. (eds) *Emerging Pests and Vector-Borne Diseases in Europe*. Wageningen Academic Publishers, Wageningen, The Netherlands, pp. 465–474.

Tanser, F.C., Sharp, B. and le Sueur, D. (2003) Potential effect of climate change on malaria transmission in Africa. *Lancet* 362, 1792–1798.

Taylor, M. (2008) Global trends in schistosomiasis control. *Bulletin of the World Health Organization* 86, 738.

Theseira, M. (2002) Using Internet GIS technology for sharing health and health related data for the West Midlands region. *Health and Place* 8, 37–46.

Utzinger, J., N'Goran, E.K., Caffrey, C.R. and Keiser, J. (2011a) From innovation to application: social–ecological context, diagnostics, drugs and integrated control of schistosomiasis. *Acta Tropica* 120 (Supplement 1), S121–S137.

Utzinger, J., Rinaldi, L., Malone, J.B., Krauth, S.J., Kristensen, T.K., Cringoli, G. and Bergquist, N.R. (2011b) Geospatial Health: the first 5 years. *Geospatial Health* 6, 137–154.

Wang, L.D., Utzinger, J. and Zhou, X.-N. (2008) Schistosomiasis control: experiences and lessons from China. *The Lancet* 372, 1793–1795.

Wang, L.D., *et al.* (2009) A strategy to control transmission of *Schistosoma japonicum* in China. *New England Journal of Medicine* 360, 121–128.

WHO (2006) *Preventive Chemotherapy in Human Helminthiasis: Coordinated Use of Anthelminthic Drugs in Control Interventions: A Manual for Health Professionals and Programme Managers*. World Health Organization, Geneva, Switzerland.

Winkler, M.S., Krieger, G.R., Divall, M.J., Singer, B.H. and Utzinger, J. (2012) Health impact assessment of industrial development projects: a spatio-temporal visualization. *Geospatial Health* 6, 299–301.

Wood, J., Dykes, J., Slingsby, A. and Clarke, K. (2007) Interactive visual exploration of a large spatio-temporal dataset: reflections on a geovisualization mashup. *IEEE Transactions on Visualization and Computer Graphics* 13, 1176–1183.

Woolhouse, M.E.J. *et al.* (1997) Heterogeneities in the transmission of infectious agents: implications for the design of control programs. *Proceedings of the National Academy of Sciences of the United States of America* 94, 338–342.

Yang, G.J., Vounatsou, P., Zhou, X.N., Utzinger, J. and Tanner, M. (2005) A review of geographic information system and remote sensing with applications to the epidemiology and control of schistosomiasis in China. *Acta Tropica* 96, 117–129.

Yang, G.J., Vounatsou, P., Tanner, M., Zhou, X.N. and Utzinger, J. (2006) Remote sensing for predicting potential habitats of *Oncomelania hupensis* in Hongze, Baima and Gaoyou lakes in Jiangsu province, China. *Geospatial Health* 1, 85–92.

Yang, K., Sun, L.P., Huang, Y.X., Yang, G.J., Wu, F., Hang, D.R., Li, W., Zhang, J.F., Liang, Y.S. and Zhou, X.N. (2012) A real-time platform for monitoring schistosomiasis transmission supported by Google Earth and a web-based geographical information system. *Geospatial Health* 6, 195–203.

Yu, L. and Gong, P. (2012) Google Earth as a virtual globe tool for earth science applications at the global scale: progress and perspectives. *International Journal of Remote Sensing* 33, 3966–3986.

Zhou, X.N., Yang, G.J., Yang, K., Wang, X.H., Hong, Q.B., Sun, L.P., Malone, J.B., Kristensen, T.K., Bergquist, N.R. and Utzinger, J. (2008) Potential impact of climate change on schistosomiasis transmission in China. *American Journal of Tropical Medicine and Hygiene* 78, 188–194.

Zhou, X.N., Lv, S., Yang, G.J., Kristensen, T.K., Bergquist, N.R., Utzinger, J. and Malone, J.B. (2009) Spatial epidemiology in zoonotic parasitic diseases: insights gained at the 1st International Symposium on Geospatial Health in Lijiang, China, 2007. *Parasites and Vectors* 2,10.

4 Geocoding and Health

Daniel W. Goldberg,[1]* Geoffrey M. Jacquez[2] and Narelle Mullan[3]
[1] *Texas A&M University, College Station Texas, USA;* [2] *State University of New York at Buffalo, Buffalo, New York, USA;* [3] *Curtin University and Cooperative Research Centre for Spatial Information (CRCSI), Perth, Western Australia, Australia*

4.1 Introduction

Geocoding is commonly considered to be the process of converting postal address data into geographic coordinates in the form of a latitude/longitude pair (Boscoe, 2008). This process plays a critical role in health science research because geocoded data are widely used in spatially based research investigations (Rushton *et al.*, 2006; Goldberg and Cockburn, 2012). Health science researchers have employed geocoding for such diverse topics as determining accessibility and other measures to identify underserved populations (Grumbach *et al.*, 2003; Gordon-Larsen *et al.*, 2006), quantifying individual-level environmental exposures to understand the links between environmental factors and health outcomes (Rose, 2001; Brody *et al.*, 2002; Rull *et al.*, 2006; Ritz and Rull, 2008; Turabelidze *et al.*, 2008) and understanding infectious disease transmission paths (Myers *et al.*, 2006). In each of these and numerous other examples geocoding places an individual or population within a geographic context, enabling researchers to elucidate the role and impact that spatial relationships between the subject(s) and aspects of his/her environment play in ultimate health outcomes (Meliker *et al.*, 2005; Zandbergen, 2009).

This chapter explores the geocoding process in the context of health science research from both the theoretical and applied viewpoints. First, the many roles that geocoding plays in health science research are illustrated to show the breadth of scenarios where geocoding technologies have an impact. Secondly, technical details of the geocoding process are covered to provide a baseline level of knowledge – from the types of input data that health science researchers may put through a geocoding system, to each of the components of geocoding systems that manipulate these data, and then to the eventual output data and the means by which the quality of these data are represented and reported. Thirdly, the geocoding resources available to the health science community are described, and a vision for the future of geocoding in health science is presented to foster research and technology development. The chapter concludes with a review of the salient findings for health science researchers who wish to employ geocoding in their investigations, applications and policy decisions.

4.2 The Role of Geocoding in Health Science Research

Spatially based health investigations are now often undertaken by researchers around the globe. In these studies, researchers place individuals,

* E-mail: daniel.goldberg@tamu.edu

groups and features such as treatment service locations within a geographic context for analysis (Jacquez, 1998). As described elsewhere in this book, this approach – the employment of geographic thought and spatial reasoning within health investigations – helps investigators to shape research questions, use specific analysis techniques and understand how the geographic relationships between objects influence behaviour and system processes (Rushton, 2003).

Spatial health investigations require spatially referenced data. These spatial data may be representations of the locations of people, transportation networks, government services, food outlets, parks and open spaces, and/or instances of crime, just to name a fraction of the types of data that can be employed. Studies in the spatial health arena are as diverse as the types of data that are used. From investigating associations between environmental contaminants and human health outcomes (Brody *et al.*, 2004; Morgenstern *et al.*, 2007; Nuckols *et al.*, 2007; Jerrett *et al.*, 2008; Cockburn *et al.*, 2011), to quantifying accessibility to treatment options for determining underserved populations or communities (Grumbach *et al.*, 2003; Boscoe *et al.*, 2011; Henry *et al.*, 2011), to evaluating the impact of neighbourhood characteristics on mental health outcomes (Kruger *et al.*, 2007), the ways in which spatial thinking, techniques and data contribute to health science research are many and have led to significant advances in our understanding of human health and its determinants.

Geocoding is one tool available to health science researchers that facilitates spatially based health investigations. Just like the full complement of modern spatial analysis techniques described elsewhere in this book, geocoding plays a specific role in the health science research pipeline (Fig. 4.1). In the simplest terms, it produces the spatial data used by spatial analysis techniques to undertake spatially based health research (Goldberg *et al.*, 2007). As detailed below, the process of geocoding takes textual data, most commonly in the form of postal addresses, and converts them into spatial information that can be used within geographic information systems (GIS) for analysis, visualization and mapping.

The importance of geocoding in spatially based research cannot be understated because it is typically the first operation performed on the data (Goldberg and Cockburn, 2012). Regardless of the data source – disease registries, administrative lists, surveys, patient-entered information, etc. – if the data contain addresses, then geocoding is the fundamental tool used to put that person, group or object into a geographic context. This relates directly to the infamous 'garbage in, garbage out' scenario: if the quality of the output of a geocoding system is poor, all subsequent analyses performed on the data will suffer and the ultimate conclusions may be suspect.

The primary purpose of this chapter is to introduce the reader to the fundamentals of geocoding systems so that he/she can understand

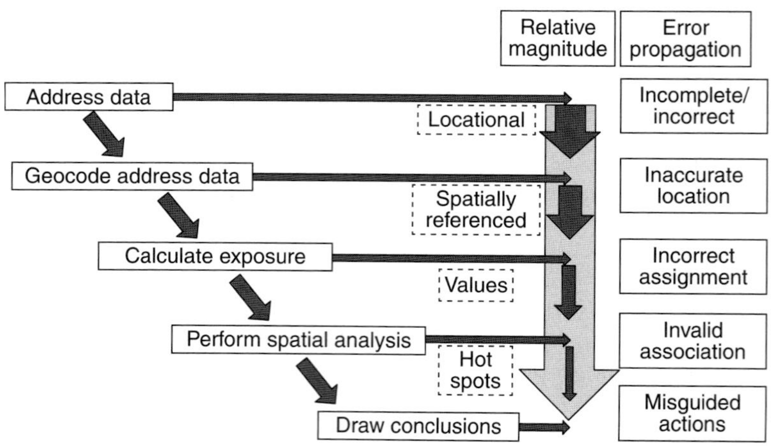

Fig. 4.1. The role of geocoding in spatially based health research; from Goldberg and Cockburn (2012).

how his/her data are produced and enable intelligent decision making when there is a need to geocode data for a particular purpose. This includes empowering the end users of geocoded data with knowledge of the quality of their data and understanding how this quality may have an impact on health science studies, applications and decision making. Although the addresses and examples used throughout this chapter primarily deal with US-based postal address geocoding, the fundamental techniques and issues raised are applicable in most geocoding settings around the globe.

4.3 Geocoding Fundamentals

The process of geocoding is basically an operation that attempts to match one or more geographic objects that have similar attribute values to an input data item (Goldberg *et al.*, 2007). As mentioned previously, the input data processed by geocoding systems are commonly in the form of postal street addresses. The geographic objects that are used as matches to produce one or more geographic outputs (which can be used in spatial analyses, visualization and mapping) include digital geographic objects representing linear street segments, point-based representations such as building centroids, and polygon objects such as parcel boundaries, building outlines and various civil administrative boundaries.

To perform the matching process between an input data item and the database of geographic objects, a geocoding system may try several matching approaches – both to determine which geographic object matches and to provide a score on how well the input matches the geographic reference object(s) selected. When one or more geographic objects are selected as possible matches, the geocoding system then computes where along or within the matching object the output location should be placed. Here, estimation techniques are utilized based on what is known about the input data and the corresponding geographic objects that it was matched to (see schematic in Fig. 4.2). The next sections detail the inner workings common to most geocoding systems: the input data, reference data, address parsing and normalization, matching algorithms, feature interpolation and output data.

4.3.1 Input data

The input data to be geocoded for use in health science research are drawn from many different sources. In the USA, these include administrative

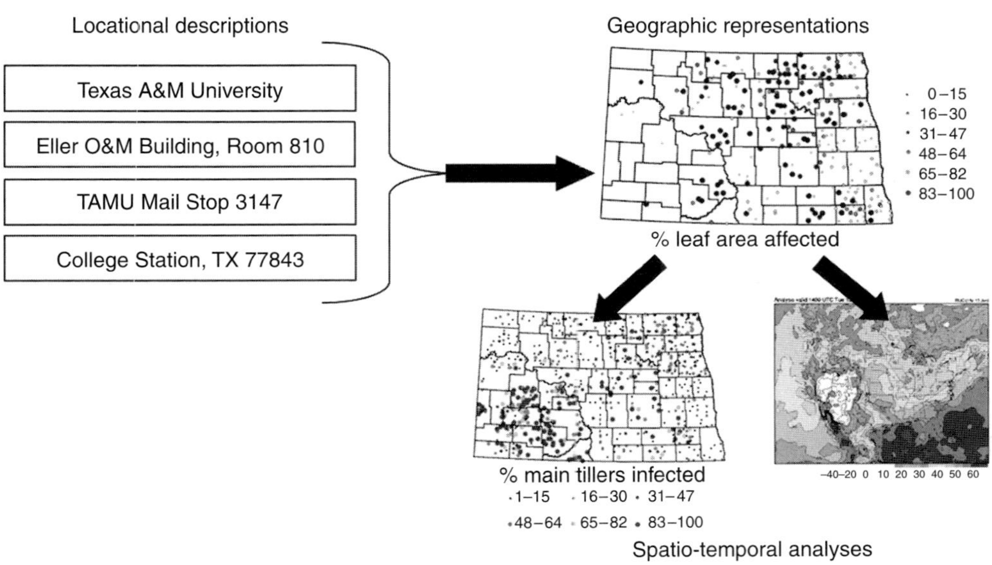

Fig. 4.2. High-level geocoding process schematic.

lists such as a state's Department of Motor Vehicles (DMV) records, Medicare rolls, Social Security databases, housing foreclosure lists, disease registry databases and national death indices (Reynolds *et al.*, 2004). These types of input data sources are common in other countries as well, for example, cancer registry data sets are used for public health surveillance and control activities in many regions of the world. The data may also come from patient-, subject-, or study participant-reported records that have been transcribed into a digital format from handwritten forms or entered by the subject or patient. The potential sources that could be useful in health research are growing as investigators employ novel data sources and collection techniques, and as the applications of geocoded data evolve. Because of the large variety of data sources, formats and types, geocoding systems must process a wide range of input data and geocoding system designers must engineer systems that can handle multiple representations of an individual's location.

Postal address data are the most common form of data that health science researchers process through geocoding systems. In the USA, these data are usually of a form similar to the example address '3616 Trousdale Parkway, Suite B55, Los Angeles, CA 90089-0374'. This address contains several address components, including the street number of the address '3616', the street name and suffix 'Trousdale' and 'Parkway', the suite and suite type 'Suite' and 'B55', the city 'Los Angeles', the state 'CA', and the United States Postal Service (USPS) zip code '90089' along with a four digit zip code extension '0734'. Other potential address attributes are possible as well, including pre- and post-directionals as in '123 North Main Street' and '123 Main Street South', pre- and post-qualifiers as in '123 Old Main Street' and '123 Main Street New', and many other combinations of data elements that vary by region. As noted earlier, although countries around the world use different addressing systems, the material presented in this chapter deals primarily with US-style postal addressing standards, though the majority of the information is applicable to geocoding in other nations.

A second potential type of input data that is less frequently encountered is the rural route address (Vieira *et al.*, 2008). Here, instead of the address indicating a postal delivery drop-off point, it describes a shared mailbox somewhere along a delivery route. A typical address of this type is 'Rural Route 16, Box 12', which indicates the route number and the box within which the postal delivery service would deposit the mail for the addressee. Other variants of this type include highway contract routes and star routes, each of which describes a rural addressing scheme. These types of addresses are notoriously difficult to geocode, mainly because the delivery route used by a postal delivery service does not directly correspond to a geographic reference feature (as described later). In the USA, rural route addressing systems are slowly being replaced by city style address as Emergency 911 (E-911) services are rolled out on a locality by locality basis. The goal of E-911 systems is to ensure that emergency personnel can be directed to a specific location should a call be placed to the emergency services. Facilitating this public service requires that structures be identifiable down to a certain level of spatial accuracy, which is precisely the point of city-style addressing systems.

A third type of input data is the Post Office Box (PO Box) address. These types of addresses represent a rented, dedicated box within a postal delivery location such as a post office. The main challenge with these types of addresses is that, by definition, they do not represent the residential location of an individual. This is a serious challenge because in most health science scenarios research investigators are interested in the geographic contexts in which the person in question lives and works, such as the location of his/her residence, workplace, recreation facilities, food outlets and commuting route. PO Box data provide health science researchers with little geographic context or utility because the person in question does not live or work at the location represented by the PO Box.

A fourth type of address data encountered in health science settings is a named place such as a nursing home, apartment building or prison. Here, instead of reporting the postal address associated with a person's residence, treatment facility or other location, the data instead describe the name of a place. While a postal delivery service can often use local knowledge to determine where a package addressed to such a location should be delivered, these types of data are often difficult for geocoding systems to process automatically without some form of alias tables that translate names of known places into valid street addresses.

A fifth and final type of input address data that arises in health science research is relative directional data. These data take the form '1 mile east of Bakersfield'; this example contains a distance '1 mile', a direction 'East of' and a referent 'Bakersfield'. Such data are most commonly encountered in field reports, such as police reports stating that a crime took place 'near the entrance of the park' or on the '500 block of Vermont Avenue'. In these cases, the exact address is not provided because one simply may not be available, or the report is intentionally vague to protect the privacy of those involved. These types of data are challenging for geocoding systems because they often blend named places along with imprecise descriptions that can be interpreted in multiple ways, thus resulting in a set of potential output locations.

4.3.2 Reference data

The reference data used by a geocoding system contain the geographic objects used by the geocoder to place an input data item into a geographic context. Typically, the reference data sets included in a geocoding system represent all of the knowledge that the system has about the world. This means that if a geographic reference object is absent for a particular input address, the system may be incapable of producing an output. The types of reference data sets employed by geocoding systems can be classified into three categories based on the type of geographic objects they represent: points, lines and polygons (see Chapter 1).

As the name describes, point-based reference data sets include geographic reference features (i.e. individual geographic objects) that are points having an *x*- and *y*-coordinate, often in geographic coordinates (latitude and longitude), but they may be defined in a different geographic projection and/or coordinate system, such as the Universal Transverse Mercator (UTM) coordinate system. Point-based reference data sets are often among the most costly to produce when they represent highly accurate geographic features such as building centroids that have been digitized from imagery. Global positioning system (GPS) locations that have been ground truthed in the field are often even more costly. Because of these high costs, point-based geographic reference data sets are generally not widely available for large areas, although the initiatives described earlier are helping to bridge this gap. The goal of the E-911 programme, for example, is to derive a point location for every address (Vieira *et al.*, 2008).

Line-based reference data sets represent geographic reference features composed of lines with a start and end point and, in most cases one, or more interior points that describe the geometry (i.e. the curvature) of the line. Street segments fall into this category and are by far the most common type of reference data sets used in US geocoding systems. Many versions of these types of data are readily available at a range of prices. These vary from the free versions made available by federal agencies, such as the TIGER/Line files created and provided by the United States Census Bureau (2012), to more expensive commercial versions – which may be derivatives of free versions, completely new versions created from scratch, or a combination of both. Commercially available versions usually have two improvements over free versions. The first is that there are enhancements to the geographies of the line segments, typically in the form of higher precision centre lines, road widths and interior curvature points that capture a more realistic representation of the street segment. The second improvement in commercial versions is that there are additional attributes in the form of alias names that capture official, colloquial and abbreviated names for street segments and the city and zip code within which they are contained. The attributes associated with street segments that facilitate geocoding include the postal address attributes that name the street (name, pre- or post-directional suffix, etc.) along with the valid address ranges that are contained along the segment. Most street segments have an even and an odd side, though anomalies do exist.

The final type of reference data set that can be found within geocoding systems is the polygon reference data set. These data sets contain geographic reference data features which are boundaries that encompass one or more internal areas. These types of reference data sets span the full range of polygon data types, from highly accurate building outlines, to property boundaries, to postal boundaries, and all the way to state boundaries. As should be clear, the type of data object contained within a polygon reference data set will indicate the level of utility that one can expect from a geocoder using that data set. Even though using a building centroid data set would result in geocodes of high spatial accuracy (assuming the file was complete and accurate), the level of usefulness decreases rapidly as one moves to larger geographic features.

4.3.3 Address parsing and normalization

While the wide variety of input data types and heterogeneous reference data sources supported by modern geocoding systems means that a larger amount of data may be successfully processed, it also presents unique challenges to geocoder users and developers. Specifically, a common vocabulary of terms is required in order to successfully match an input data item to one or more reference objects in the reference data sets. The input data must be transformed into the form and format used by the reference data sets. In geocoding systems, this process is normally accomplished in two steps: address parsing and address normalization.

Address parsing identifies which terms in the input address correspond to specific address components. For example, the address parser used by a geocoding system would be able to separate the example address '3616 Trousdale Pkwy, B55, Los Angeles CA 90089-0374' into the set of attributes Number = '3616', Name = 'Trousdale', Suffix = 'Pkwy', SuiteType = '' (blank, missing, or null), SuiteNumber = 'B55', City = 'Los Angeles', State = 'CA', ZIP = '90089', ZIP + 4 = '0374'. Address parsing thus separates the terms found in the input address into individual components and associates one or more data types with each. This is usually based on synonym tables that identify alternative forms for the same word, such as like 'STREET', 'ST', and 'STR', all mapping to the same suffix 'ST'. However, it is often the case that one term could potentially be mapped to two attribute types. For example, the address '1 E Ave N' could be represented by Number = '1', Name = 'E', Suffix = 'Ave', Post-Directional = 'North', as well as Number = '1', Pre-directional = 'E', Pre-Type = 'Avenue', Name = 'N'. In these instances, the terms in the input address are assigned all possible attribute types and an empirical approach, a heuristic (rule-of-thumb) or a probabilistic approach is used to determine which is the most likely scenario given the data available for the region of interest.

Once the type (or types) of each input address component have been identified, a normalization algorithm transforms the format and values of the input address components into the version used by a particular reference data set. Several address formats exist, including the USPS Publication 28 Standard (USPS, 2012), the format used by the United States Census Bureau (2012) in the TIGER/Line files and versions used by jurisdictions around the country, such as the format used by the Los Angeles County Assessor's office as of 2012. The differences between these address formats are twofold. First, the granularity of the address components maintained may vary. This means that in one address standard, several terms may be considered as a single one, as in 'Route 22' being the name of the street in one format and 'Route' being the pre-type and '22' being the name in another. The second difference between address formats is the value used for standardized terms, such as all suffixes that equate to 'Street' being stored as the abbreviation 'ST' in one reference data set and being spelled out as the full term 'STREET' in another.

The role of the normalization process is to perform both of these tasks, i.e. to transform both the format and the values. The address normalizer receives the parsed input address which contains one or more attribute associations for each term of the input query along with a target address format for a given reference data set. The normalization process then splits or merges the terms of the input address into the correct grouping, as defined for the address format of the reference data set. Once split (or merged), the values of the input data attributes are determined using lookup tables containing the standardized values for a particular reference data set address format. In this way, the normalization algorithm can map between multiple reference data sets, each of which may rely on different address standards.

4.3.4 Matching algorithms

The matching algorithms used by a geocoding system attempt to identify candidate geographic features to use in generating an output from the reference data sets. One or more query approaches can be used to manipulate the attributes of the standardized and normalized input address data to locate a likely match. These approaches can result in zero, one or multiple candidate reference features being selected by the feature matching algorithm. Of these, the best case is when the matching algorithm produces a single unique match in which all of the address attributes of the input address are present on the candidate reference features returned and the values for each attribute are exactly the same.

When there are zero matches, this means that a candidate reference feature could not be found within the reference data sets using the attribute values as defined on the input address. Here, alternative matching strategies can be used to try to identify a likely match. These approaches usually include the use of phonetic algorithms, such as Soundex, which encode the way that a word sounds and issue a query for that representation instead of the full text in the hope of rectifying common misspellings stemming from heterography (words that are spelled differently but sound the same) and other transcription errors. Other techniques that attempt to find a match where none could be found will iteratively remove attributes of the input address and reattempt a query with a subset of the original attributes. This process, known as address relaxation, removes attributes one by one and then in combination, typically in a specific order. This approach attempts to account for input data or reference data items that are missing or have incorrect attribute values that would prevent an otherwise successful match. All of these approaches return approximate matches and necessarily assume that either the input data or the reference data were incompletely or incorrectly defined.

The final case, where multiple candidates are returned, indicates a scenario where ambiguous results have been obtained from the reference data sets. This is likely to mean that one of two things occurred: either an error in the underlying reference data sets or an error in the input submitted for processing. In the first instance, an error is the likely explanation as there should not be multiple reference features with the same attributes. Exceptions are possible, though, such as in areas where efforts such as the E-911 improvements have not yet been made (more on these efforts below) and local knowledge is relied upon to distinguish between duplicated addresses. The second instance indicates a case where the input data have been under-specified, meaning that not all possible attributes for the input data item have been defined. This scenario results in multiple matches by the feature matching algorithm because more than one reference object has values fulfilling the attribute values requested. The missing attribute(s) that were not supplied for the input address could have discriminated between the candidate features, but without these being supplied, the query yielded an ambiguous result. Examples of this kind often result when pre- or post-directionals are omitted from a query, as in the case of '123 Hill Street, Los Angeles, CA'. As with many cities, Los Angeles is divided along a semi-grid pattern with streets divided into North and South versions, each with the same city name and often with the same zip code when they are in relatively close spatial proximity. The address in this example, '123 Hill Street', exists in both of these ranges: '123 North Hill Street' and '123 South Hill Street'. So without the user supplying the pre-directional address attribute, the geocoding system cannot determine which should be the correct address. Under-specification is also a problem with apartment and condominium complexes, where the owner name or unit number is needed to distinguish between buildings.

In matching algorithm output where all potential candidates are returned, the matching algorithm results in one or more than one candidate feature. Each of these candidates has a match score assigned that captures the level of similarity between the attributes of the input address and the attributes of the candidate feature that was selected; this describes the likelihood that the candidate returned is in fact the input address that was requested (Boscoe, 2008). When computing a match score, a geocoding system will look to see whether all address attributes present on the input address are present and equivalent on the matched reference feature. If this condition is met, a 100% match score is typically assigned, meaning that the probability of the match being correct is 100% (as far as the geocoding system is concerned).

Where a 100% match is not the case, a partial match score is computed in some fashion. Several methods can be used to compute these match scores. They can be based on empirical data observations, frequency distributions of terms occurring and co-occurring in specific sequences in the reference data sets, or other heuristics. Some methods are probabilistic, meaning that they may return different results depending on the distribution of addresses in the reference data files (Jaro, 1984), while others are deterministic, meaning that they will always give the same result regardless of the distribution of the data (Goldberg, 2008). In all cases, if the score computed is below a minimum match score set by the user, the candidate is thrown out as a non-match.

In the majority of geocoding systems, a deterministic weighting scheme is used. Here, each attribute of the input address is assigned a proportional weight characterizing its importance to the overall match score. The sum of all attribute weights adds up to one. For example, the street number, street name, postal boundary code and city may each have a weight of 20%, with the remaining 20% of the score being distributed to the pre-directional, post-directional and street suffix equally. To compute the match score for a particular input data–reference feature match, a level of discrepancy (i.e. penalty) is first computed between each attribute of the input address and each corresponding attribute of the reference feature. In the case of a perfect match, a penalty of zero would apply. In non-perfect matches, these penalties are often computed based on text comparison heuristics. One example is Levenshtein distance, also known as edit distance, which is described as the number of character additions, removals or changes that would need to take place to make two words equivalent. One alternative penalty method is to use keyboard distance in addition to Levenshtein distance. Here, the edit distance penalty of a particular mismatched character between the input and reference is weighted by the distance between keys on a keyboard. Once each per-attribute penalty is computed, they are multiplied by the weight associated with the appropriate attribute and used to compute an overall match score by subtracting each attribute's penalty from a total score of 100% (a perfect match).

4.3.5 Feature interpolation

If a matching algorithm is successful in finding a relevant and sufficiently similar geographic feature in the reference data sets available to the geocoding system, feature interpolation is used in the next step to produce the geographic output that is returned to the user. The type of feature interpolation performed by the geocoding system primarily depends on the type of reference feature selected by the matching algorithm. For example, point-based features such as building centroids do not require feature interpolation because they are already in a form suitable for return to the end user if he is only expecting a geographic point as output (more on the shortcomings of this expectation follows below). As such, these reference features can be returned directly to the user without performing any other computations. In the case of linear and polygon reference data sets, the geocoding system will need to determine a suitable point along the line or within the polygon to return because the software and analysis techniques in use by most geocoding consumers cannot handle linear or areal units as the result of geocoding.

Linear interpolation

Linear interpolation calculates an appropriate output coordinate from a reference linear street segment determined to be a suitable match by the feature matching algorithm. To accomplish this, the linear interpolation algorithm uses the street address house number requested by the input query along with information about the valid street segments on both sides of the reference street segment (in the case of reference features that have one address range for each side of the street) to compute where the requested house number should fall.

In the simplest approach, a proportional distance between the lower and upper numbers of the address range is computed simply by dividing the address number requested by the numeric distance between the upper and lower numbers. For example, if the address requested is '123 Main Street' and the reference feature selected represents the 101–199 and 100–198 address ranges (even and odd sides of the street), the feature interpolation algorithm would place the output point 23/50 of the way down the street, starting from the end with the lower number (101) moving towards the upper (199). Note that the divisor would be 50 instead of 100 because it is assumed that numbers on each side of the street are either even or odd, not both. This approach is termed address range interpolation because it uses the address range associated with the reference feature to compute the output location (Bakshi *et al.*, 2004). However, it is naive for several reasons.

One shortcoming is that, in most instances, it would place the output directly in the centre of the street segment, rather than placing it off to one side of the street or the other. To address this issue, a drop back distance is generally applied to the interpolated output to move the output point away from the centre line of the street toward the side of the street with the appropriate parity (even or odd) (Cayo and Talbot, 2003). The distance and direction used to compute the drop back location may vary between geocoding systems, but typically the direction chosen is orthogonal (at 90°) to the direction of the street line and the distance is 10 or 15 m. The values of these parameters are generally arbitrarily chosen and may not be an optimal choice in every scenario, especially as one moves from urban to rural areas and parcel size increases. The end user of a geocoding system may or may not be able to set these parameters while geocoding, but they are almost never definable on a per record basis. Fortunately, research has shown that using reasonable alternatives has little overall impact on the spatial accuracy of geocoding when processing large data sets (Cayo and Talbot, 2003).

A second shortcoming of this approach is that it assumes that all possible addresses along the referenced street segment exist. In our '123 Main Street' example, 50 addresses matching to the 100–198 and to the 101–199 street segment are assumed to exist. This limitation, known as the parcel existence assumption, is typically a gross overestimation of the true number of properties along a street segment and results in the use of an incorrect denominator in the division calculation used to produce the interpolated output. This, in combination with the fact that most street numbering schemes assign house numbers starting at the low end of the range, typically results in geocode output clumping at the low end of the street segment (see Fig. 4.3). To address this issue, researchers have developed methods to introduce information about the true number of properties on the street so that a more realistic denominator can be used, resulting in geocode output with higher degrees of spatial accuracy (Bakshi *et al.*, 2004).

Areal unit interpolation

Areal unit interpolation is the process of computing an output geocode location from an areal unit (polygon reference geographic feature). In this case, the interpolation algorithm must compute a location somewhere within the boundaries of the reference data feature. Several different methods can be used to do perform this function. These include bounding box centroids, centre of mass and weighted centroids, each of which has their strengths and weaknesses (Goldberg and Cockburn, 2012) (Fig. 4.4).

As the name implies, the bounding box centroid approach first computes the bounding box of the reference areal unit. As described in Section 1.5, this is constructed by determining the

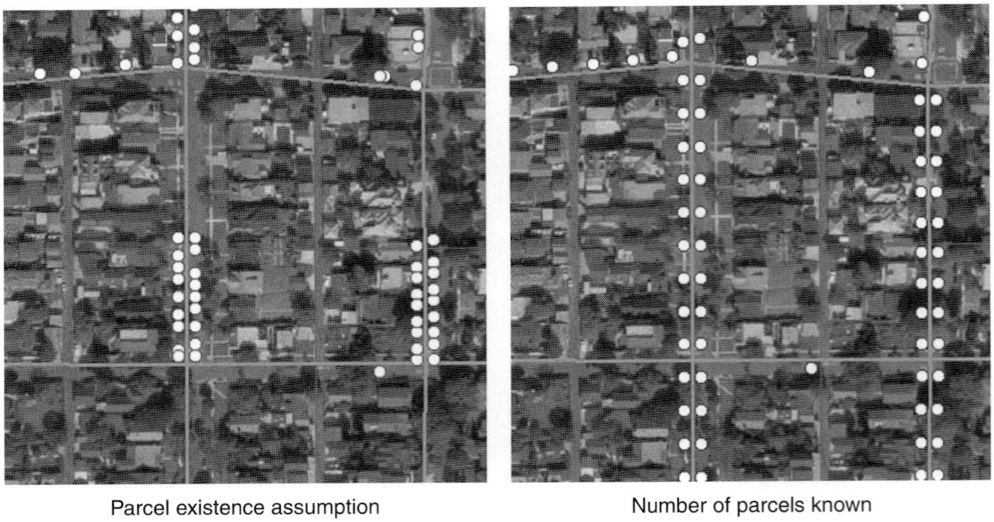

Fig. 4.3. Linear interpolation with and without the number of parcels known.

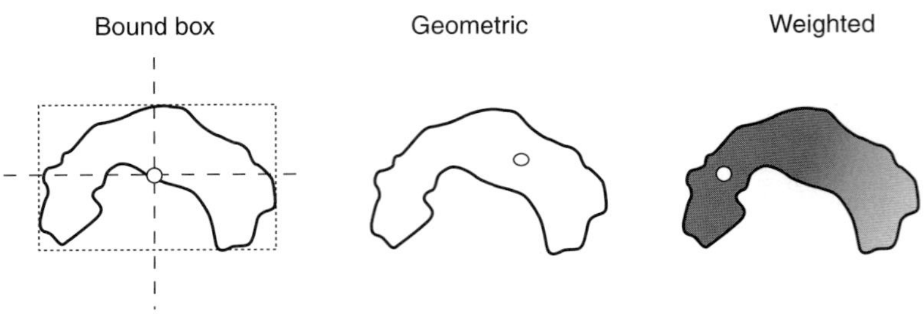

Fig. 4.4. Methods for computing areal unit centroids: bound (or bounding) box; geometric (or centre of mass); and weighted.

minimum and maximum extents of the geographic object in the four cardinal directions (north, south, east, west or top, bottom, right, left). These coordinates are used to construct a box whose centre is then derived by simple division with the output coordinate in the x direction being the average of the left and right edges, and the output coordinate in the y direction being the average of the top and bottom edges. This approach has the advantage that it is extremely fast to compute, but has the drawback that the output location may not be contained within the original boundaries of the reference data feature if it was of an awkward shape.

The second method, the centre of mass computation, uses physics-based calculations to produce the location within the reference data feature where the object would balance perfectly. This approach is more computationally expensive than the bounding box approach and often guarantees that the output will be within the boundaries of the original object, although specific cases exist where this may not be so, including shapes such as 'C', 'L' and 'O'. Another benefit of this approach is that it minimizes the maximum for potential error because, by definition of being the centroid, the output point is the closest to all other points than any other point and thus has the least chance of being more erroneous than any other point.

The third method, the weighted centroid approach, is similar to the centre of mass approach in that the output will usually be within the boundaries of the reference features. However, the weighted centroid uses ancillary information relevant to the data being geocoded to bias the location of the output towards where it is most likely to be, given the characteristics of the input data item and the distribution of the ancillary information. The most common use of weighted centroid geocoding is when population distribution data is used to bias the output of a geocode towards areas that have higher population density. The rationale for this practice is that when geocoding information about people, placing the output closer to the population centre will result in a higher likelihood that the geocode representing the person is placed correctly. The ancillary data used to bias the output will depend on the characteristics of the data being geocoded. As more contextual information about the input data is included, the additional ancillary reference information can result in more accurate geocodes (Beyer *et al.*, 2008).

4.3.6 Output data

As noted throughout this chapter, the most common form of output data that geocoding systems return is a simple latitude/longitude pair of coordinates. This information alone is sufficient to spatially enable the data and directly supports a variety of mapping, visualization and analysis functions. In addition, consumers of geocoding systems prefer to receive information describing the accuracy of geocoded data returned so they can evaluate whether data quality requirements have been achieved. The four criteria that are most commonly used to measure the quality of geocoded data are match rates, match types, match scores and spatial accuracy. The first of these describes accuracy at the holistic geocoder level, whereas the last three describe accuracy at the record level.

Match rates

Match rates describe the percentage of total data records that a geocoding system was capable of processing. This metric is computed simply by dividing the number of successfully geocoded records in a set by the total number of records in a set and multiplying by 100. For example, if a user attempted to process a database file with 100 records and the geocoding system produced a geocode for 98 of them, the match rate would be 98%. While match rates describe a general measure of geocoding completeness, they are not very useful for quantifying anything about the quality of an individual record. In fact, match rates may be somewhat deceptive if the geocoding system permits a minimum match score that is too low. This would result in some proportion of false positives, i.e. records that should not have been matched but were reported as so, thereby erroneously inflating the computed match rate. Similarly, if the minimum match score is set too high, some number of records that should have been matched may not have been, i.e. they are false negatives, which could unnecessarily reduce the match rate.

Match types

Because many reference data sets may be included within a geocoder to improve the chances of finding a match, a geocode may be drawn from any of the reference data sets available to the system. Typically, a geocoding system will start searching with the most accurate reference data sets and only move to the less accurate files if a match is not found in the more accurate versions. For example, a geocoding system may first search a building centroid data set, then a parcel data set, then a street segment data set, then a zip code data set, then a city data set. The match type of a geocoded record is an indication of the geographic reference data set that was ultimately used to compute a geocode output and is often used as a heuristic to evaluate the suitability of geocoded data for a particular purpose. This metric is one way that geocoding systems allow an end user to determine whether the quality of any particular geocode is sufficient for the purpose at hand.

In many instances, a set hierarchy is used to determine whether data are of sufficient quality. One such example is the North American Association of Central Cancer Registries (NAACCR; see http://naaccr.org) GIS Coordinate Quality Code data item. This cancer registry data item is constructed as a set of geographic match types and is often used to rank data as having better or worse quality depending on what level in the hierarchy it maps to. However, recent research has shown that owing to the non-stationary nature of the size, shape and distribution associated with administrative units across space (cities, zip codes, etc.), a static hierarchy or ranking of reference data sets may not be the best approach to determining which geocoded data are of higher quality (Goldberg and Cockburn, 2010).

For example, in urban areas, zip codes are small and cities are large, primarily because zip codes are defined based on the density of mail delivery sites: as the number goes up the size of the zip code shrinks. In contrast, in rural areas zip codes are large and cities are small because fewer people live in the region and thus the mail delivery density is less and the zip code must get larger to capture the same level of demand. Assuming that matching to a smaller region produces less spatial uncertainty in geocoder output than does matching to a larger area, because the number of possible places is smaller, a geocoding system should dynamically choose which output to use (city or zip) based on the rural/urban classification of the region in which the geocode is being placed in order to ensure the highest level of accuracy. This type of approach to reducing uncertainty is not captured in the match type metric when it is implied that one level of geographic match is always better than another (Goldberg *et al.*, 2010). Users of geocoded data must take care when determining the fitness for use of geocoded data by match score alone (as described in the next section). It is, instead, advisable to use match scores in conjunction with match type (which is not relevant if only one reference data set is used) to determine which data are of sufficient quality.

Match score

As described above (in Section 4.3.4), the match score quality metric represents the likelihood that the reference feature that was selected and used for feature interpolation was the correct one. This can be deterministically based, as when using the attribute weighting scheme presented earlier, or it can be probabilistically based, as is the case when the match score is dependent on the characteristics drawn from the distribution of the input and reference data themselves (Boscoe, 2008). In either case, it must be recognized by geocode data consumers that this quality metric does not describe anything about the spatial accuracy of the output geocode; this is important when geocoded data are to be used in spatially based research and practice. For example, even though a geocoded record may have a match score of 100%, this certainty of match at the state level of geography would not generally be considered a high-quality geocode output. Match score simply informs the user of the confidence that he/she should have about the matching process that was used to select a reference feature for output.

In the case when two geocode matches have exactly the same match score, most geocoding systems will report an ambiguous result and allow the user to choose how to handle the situation, such as interactively prompting the user to rematch, picking one or the other using a heuristic to decide (e.g. chance determined), or reverting to a lower level of geographic match. However, when multiple potential matches have slightly differently match scores, it becomes clear that the match score metric by itself has a second weakness in that it is used to determine just a single output geocode, regardless of how close the scores are to multiple candidate reference features. For example, it could be the case that one candidate match has a score of 97% and another has a match score of 96%. In this instance, it would be useful to alert the end user that there are two exceptionally close matches and permit her to review each and decide what to do, and potentially even to include information on what impact this choice would have on the subsequent work (Goldberg *et al.*, 2010) (Fig. 4.5). Users need to be aware that there could have been multiple candidate matches which were almost as equally likely. Most geocoding systems allow the review of geocoded data, including the full set of candidate matches, which should be consulted to determine whether this issue is relevant for a particular geocode.

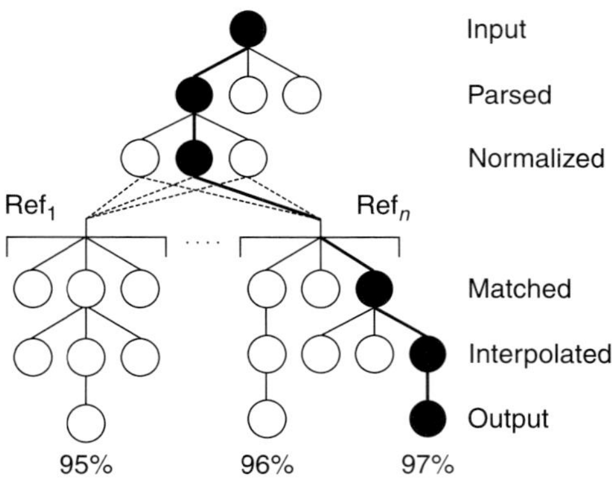

Fig. 4.5. Example of multiple potential outputs with similar match scores.

Spatial accuracy

The spatial accuracy of geocoded data can be described as the spatial distance between the output location of a geocoding system and the true location of where that geocode should have been placed in the real world (Bonner *et al.*, 2003). In most health research and application scenarios, this is often considered to be the most important quality metric that geocode data consumers should be concerned with. Unfortunately, while this quality metric is by many accounts the most important, it is also the most difficult to quantify, derive and/or obtain because it requires the existence of ground truth data for comparison with the computed results (Strickland *et al.*, 2007). These ground truth data simply do not exist for any large-scale regions. For this reason, the majority of geocoding systems available to the health community do not provide true quantitative spatial accuracy measures as metadata along with geocode results. Geocode consumers must be aware that although all of the quality metrics described so far in this chapter are useful in their own respect – match rates, match types and match scores – none are true quantitative spatial accuracy measures from which one can estimate how far any particular geocode is from the real location it is supposed to represent (Goldberg *et al.*, 2010).

As discussed above, the cost of obtaining high-resolution ground truth data for structures (building centroids) is most often too prohibitive to be performed for large-scale, regional or national studies. This is because obtaining these data most commonly requires digitization processes on remotely sensed imagery (satellite or aerial photography) or a site visit with a GPS device to record the data, both of which are manual processes that require high levels of time and effort (Goldberg *et al.*, 2008). However, efforts at the national level, such as the E-911 programme, are creating some of the data necessary for geocoding system developers and end users to evaluate the spatial accuracy of their geocoded data (Vieira *et al.*, 2008). Similarly, efforts at the local level by cities and communities across the USA and other counties who are investing in their digital geographic base data sets are also contributing data that would be helpful in this process. In both cases, though, one could argue that if these efforts result in point-based data sets that can be used for geocoding reference files, they should be used directly as such, instead of simply as a resource for evaluating the spatial accuracy of other geocoding techniques. Valid and correct as this may be, it might be the case that licensing arrangements and confidentiality concerns could prohibit the use of these data in publicly available geocoding services, but possibly allow their use in comparative geocode accuracy studies.

Because of these difficulties inherent to computing spatial accuracy measures for geocoded data, recent research has begun to push for the quantification, derivation, representation and use of spatial uncertainty boundaries for geocoded data to fill this gap (Goldberg *et al.*, 2010; Goldberg, 2011b). This approach to representing geocode spatial accuracy provides an estimate of the size of the geographic area within which a geocode is believed to fall. This information is calculated from the process that computes the geocode and primarily relies on the geographic bounds of the reference feature/s matched and used to interpolate the geocode output. The intent is for the geocoding system to return the area of the geographic reference feature used for interpolation as an indication of how large an area the region of uncertainty around the geocoded output might be. For example, if a geocode is produced by matching to a parcel in an urban area, the area of uncertainty would be the size of the parcel. Although a centroid method is used to compute a single point as output, the real point could be anywhere within the parcel's boundaries, and thus one quantification of spatial uncertainty is a measure of the number of other locations where the real location might actually be found. Because the earth can be divided into an infinite number of smaller and smaller pieces, using the area of the geographic feature provides a useful first estimate of spatial uncertainty that can guide the selection, comparison and use of geocoded data in health science.

This method of spatial uncertainty estimation fills a needed gap in geocode uncertainty representation, but it is in fact just the first step towards true geocode uncertainty estimation. All components of the geocoding process have an impact on spatial uncertainty, not just the reference feature selected. Each component introduces its own amount of uncertainty (both spatial and non-spatial) as it computes its particular output, and then propagates this error through all subsequent components (see Fig. 4.1). Recent research has begun to develop models for quantifying spatial and non-spatial uncertainty at each step, as well as the error propagation models necessary for transferring the error through the whole chain of events responsible for producing a geocode output (Goldberg *et al.*, 2010). This work is in its early stages, and more research is required before tools and techniques that affect the ways an end user can quantify the nature of the spatial uncertainty of his data become commonplace.

4.4 The Landscape of Geocoding Research and Practice

Historically, there has been a disconnect between the communities who develop geocoding tools and techniques, and those who are the end users of the data created by these systems. This gap in communication has been particularly wide for the health science community, and has often resulted in users who felt that their concerns about system functionality, performance and output accuracy were not being heard or addressed. While the health science community has been responsible for a large portion of the work that has helped to evaluate the effectiveness and accuracy of geocoding tools to date – see the literature reviews by Rushton *et al.* (2006), Goldberg *et al.* (2007) and Zandbergen (2009) for examples – little interaction has taken place to allow system developers and health sciences users to communicate on priorities for future geocoding research and development. Because of this, many in the health science community remain naive about geocoding accuracy and its implications for health science research, even though this trend is changing.

Recent efforts by the geocoding developer and health science user community have begun to address this void. One example is the *First International Geospatial Geocoding Conference* (IGCC) (see http://geocodingconference.com), which was held in Redlands, California in December 2011. This conference, organized by participants from industry, government and academic institutions, brought together a large group of geocoding developers and users to spark discussion about the priorities for where geocoding technology needs to go in the future, how the community should get there and how geocoded data could and should be used to facilitate impactful research, applications and policy making. This conference resulted in two special issues of peer-reviewed academic journals: an issue of *Transactions in GIS* focused around geocoding technology (Goldberg, 2011a) and an issue of *Spatial and Spatio-Temporal Epidemiology* focused around the use of geocoded data in health science research (Goldberg and Jacquez, 2012). These types of efforts need to continue and accelerate for the geocoding and health science communities to drive the next generation of geocoding tools and for the successful and appropriate use of geocoded data in health science research.

The article by Jacquez (2012) presented at the IGCC provides a concise road map of the current research challenges at the intersection of geocoding and health science research. This work presents five research areas where future works should be focused to drive the development and use of geocoded tools and data in meaningful and appropriate ways: standardized open access geocoding resources; validation data sets; spatially explicit error models; spatial analysis sensitivity; and policy implications. These issues are addressed in Sections 4.4.1–4.4.5.

4.4.1 Standardized open access geocoding resources

With few exceptions, there are no national or international standards for computing geocoded data, even though there are numerous academic and industry publications that detail the inner workings of the process. It is typical that each individual researcher, group or agency chooses to use the geocoding system that best meets their requirements. These requirements could be based on performance, cost, expertise and/or many other factors. Because they will vary by group, it is not uncommon for researchers to use one or more geocoding systems at a time, and it is more the rule than the exception for different geocoding systems to be used in different parts of an organization.

There has historically been little to no coordination of the geocoding systems utilized in health science research or the configurations employed – the reference data sets used, minimum match scores selected, etc. One of the primary reasons for the lack of coordination is the confidential nature of the health input data sets, which has encouraged agencies to deploy unique systems. Additionally, configuration information about the geocoder used to produce the geocoded data is not typically provided along with these data, so in many cases it is not even clear what geocoding system was used for even base-level comparisons of geocoded data! The health science community is remarkable in the number and variety of systems used to perform the same basic function. The result of this scenario is that geocoded data may not be comparable when researchers, agencies or policy makers wish to use data from multiple sources in large studies.

The cancer registry community, led by the NAACCR GIS Committee, has taken a leadership role in attempting to address many of the gaps in geocoding standardization. In 2007, this group published *A Geocoding Best Practices Guide* (Goldberg, 2008), a handbook tailored to the cancer registry community which attempts to take the first steps towards the standardization of geocoding vocabulary and processes, as well as to provide guidance on how geocoding should be done to achieve the goals of the cancer registry community under the particular constraints relevant to these organizations.

A second major undertaking by the NAACCR is to provide an open access geocoding system to the cancer registry community. This system, hosted at NAACCR facilities, provides cancer registries with the ability to use a low to no cost production quality geocoding system on demand at any time via a web interface. The goals of hosting this system are twofold. The first is to begin to standardize the tools used to produce geocoded data so that data from across the country can be compared on an equal footing and reliably used in studies where data are aggregated to regional or national levels. The second is to provide a platform for increasing the number of registries that perform geocoding as part of their operational function, as well as boosting the volume of spatially enabled health studies that use geocoded cancer registry data.

4.4.2 Validation data sets

As mentioned above, it is difficult, if not impossible, to assess the spatial accuracy of geocoded data without the existence of validation data sets for comparison. Ground truthed and/or standardized test files are necessary for geocoding developers to test the effectiveness of new algorithms and data sources in terms of improving all of the quality metrics described above – match rates, match types, match scores and spatial accuracy. Similarly, the users of geocoding systems need to have standardized and available test data files if they wish to compare the quality of two geocoding systems. Of course, real data could be used to do so but it is difficult to assess the quality of output unless the true quality that should have been returned is known.

The health science research community invests an extraordinary amount of time and effort in collecting these data for small-scale studies, as do local governments in order to facilitate more effective public services and protection. A coordinated effort is needed to begin to gather, assemble and manage these disparate resources so that they can be used by geocoding developers and users to evaluate the quality of geocoded data and geocoding systems. One of the main challenges in assembling such a resource is getting permission to use these data. Health data, by their very nature, are particularly sensitive and subject to intense confidentiality and privacy restrictions that limit their acceptable use and distribution. Government-derived data may be less restricted by jurisdiction, but concerns can arise for these data as well.

One solution to this problem is to begin to assemble synthetic data sets that can be made publicly available at no cost for the evaluation of geocoding techniques and tools. Another would be to use existing publicly available data files, such as electoral roll data, national lists of health providers or land ownership data. It is up to the geocoding developer and user communities to begin to make use of consistent standardized test files when evaluating geocoding systems. Yet another solution would be to allow the general public to contribute authoritative and/or validated data through volunteered geographic information (VGI) type approaches (Goodchild, 2007). An alternative to this could be to mine social media data for location information (Davis *et al.*, 2011). Without such coordinated efforts to generate validation data sets and make them available in a standardized format to all interested parties who seek to develop and evaluate geocoding systems and results, fair comparisons cannot be made and the quality of one geocoding system versus another cannot be quantified.

4.4.3 Spatially explicit error models

Producers and consumers are necessarily interested in the spatial accuracy of geocoded data because the use of inaccurate data in scientific or policy making scenarios can lead to incorrect, inconsistent and potentially invalid results and policy actions. However, as noted above, the spatial accuracy quality metric of geocoded data is currently the weakest defined and implemented of all the metrics used to assess geocode quality, and typically is only available for small-scale studies covering constrained geographic areas and populations.

Research into methods for computing spatial accuracy measures for routine provision to end users is desperately needed (Bonner *et al.*, 2003). Geocode data consumers, particularly those in the health science and policy making arena, must have methods to determine the suitability of the data for their intended use (Whitsel *et al.*, 2006; Zandbergen, 2008). These end users often work with high-resolution data (in both space and time) describing individuals or populations of interest, and employ geocoding to add a geographic context in which to assess the effects of one's environment on health outcomes. The spatial phenomena that these researchers investigate may operate over very small spatial scales, such as exposure to particulate matter from freeways (Lin *et al.*, 2002; Gauderman *et al.*, 2007), neighbourhood level access to healthy food or recreation resources (Sharkey and Horel, 2008; Rundle *et al.*, 2009), or exposure to light and sound and mental health (Kent *et al.*, 2009). As such, it may be possible that spatial error in geocoded data can have an impact on study outcomes because the environmental characteristic being investigated has been misclassified or incorrectly quantified. This is even more of an issue when particular segments of a population have systematic errors associated with their geocodes, as this can introduce geographic bias into an investigation (Oliver *et al.*, 2005; Bichler and Balchak, 2007; Zandbergen and Green, 2007; Wey *et al.*, 2009).

Developing spatially explicit error models for geocoded data is a challenge for the reasons described above – lack of ground truth data with which to compare, and the multifaceted way in which the components of the geocoding process interoperate and propagate error; none the less, progress must be made on this front. The uncertainty-based measures described above (Goldberg and Cockburn, 2010; Goldberg *et al.*, 2010) are a good start, but other avenues of research must be explored to complement these approaches. One area of such research could include developing locally based spatial error models for identifiable regions that have similar geocoding error behaviour. In this scenario, reasonably homogeneous regions (from the standpoint of geocoding accuracy) could be defined where the quality of geocoded output data is known to follow a particular distribution (Zandbergen, 2008). These distributions could then be applied on a region-by-region basis to associate upper and lower bounds of error for output geocodes based on where the output is computed. Other interesting areas of research could employ information from VGI and social media sources as ground truth data for developing spatial error models.

4.4.4 Spatial analysis sensitivity

Health scientists use geocoded data in spatial analysis, and it is of the upmost importance for health science researchers to understand how sensitive their methods of spatial analysis are to various amounts of error in geocoded data. At present, it is an unfortunate reality that this information is largely unknown for most spatial analysis techniques. Some techniques of analysis may be highly sensitive to minor changes in the quality of geocoded data, resulting in exceptionally variable results. Others, by contrast, may not be sensitive at all. At present, there is little guidance in the literature aside from the work of Zandbergen (2012).

The geocoding developer and user communities must address this knowledge gap by performing sensitivity studies on spatial analysis techniques. To accomplish this task, researchers must run and rerun the same experiments while holding everything constant other than the quality of the geocoded data to see what effect this has on the results of a given spatial analysis technique, both in isolation and when used in conjunction with other tools. The challenging part of this research is generating geocoded data with known levels of quality, in particular because most geocoding systems do not allow users to change internal processing parameters that would affect the quality of the output. However, exceptions do exist. For example, a researcher could increase and decrease the match score setting to observe impacts on spatial analysis results as differing amounts of false negatives and positives are included in a study. Similarly, researchers could include or exclude reference data sets to assess the variability in study results due to the inclusion of higher quality reference data sets (Gatrell, 1989; Ratcliffe, 2001).

These lines of research are extremely valuable to the health science community because they can serve as guidance on acceptable levels of accuracy for specific types of analysis techniques. Once completed, other researchers working on similar problems with similar data and methods can look to (and cite) this body of literature on the strengths and limitations of their study design, given the quality of their data. Of course, this assumes that the quality of geocode data can be quantified in advance and placed in context on the spectrum of geocode quality for a particular analysis technique. In the future, the standardized geocoding systems, validation data sets and spatially explicit error models described above will provide some means of providing this information. In the near term, classifying a data set simply by the available metrics – match rate, match type and match score – are a first step down this road.

4.4.5 Policy implications

In many respects, the goal of the majority of health science research is to improve human health and well-being. Typically, this is accomplished through rigorous scientific research at academic institutions, government agencies and for- and non-profit organizations around the world. These groups seek to apply the scientific method to investigate a hypothesis of interest in ways that are repeatable and valid, using methods that are appropriate to the question at hand. If successful in these endeavours, the research results may lead to some form of action, intervention or treatment that will have an impact on the health and well-being of real people. This may occur through health policy changes at the local, regional or national level that are taken in response to the findings of one or more studies that have been thoroughly reviewed. For example, where the health of a population is being adversely affected by a lack of safe recreation space, a city council may approve the construction of a new park to improve equitable access to such a facility for its citizens (Wolch *et al.*, 2005). Another example is when environmental contaminants resulting from various industry applications are found to have an association with substantial negative health outcomes, then the use or production of the chemical concerned may be banned nationwide, as in the case of the pesticide dichlorodiphenyltrichloroethane (DDT).

Geocoding plays a fundamental role in the health science research pipeline – from data collection to analysis to the conclusions that are drawn to the policy decisions that are made – because it provides the geographic data that enable spatially based investigations. As emphasized in this chapter, the quality of geocoded data may affect the results of these studies. In the most innocuous case, this may only reduce the power of a study's analyses without having substantial impacts on the results and conclusions. However, significant, non-random variation in geocode quality may have substantial effects on the decisions made, even when these decisions are based on the results of numerous studies, if all are subject to the same systematic geocoding errors.

It is our hope that policy makers make the best decisions they can, given the best data available at the time of the decision. Geocoding tools have progressed rapidly in recent years as new algorithms and data sources have become readily available. In this changing light, there is a need to revisit policy decisions that were based in part on the use of geocoded data to better understand whether the correct policy decisions were taken. The types of sensitivity analysis for spatial analysis techniques described previously are a good starting place for this type of research, which would shed light on whether policy decisions may have been made based on flawed data, and whether corrective action is warranted.

4.4.6 Geocoding resources

Last in this section, we summarize some of the many commercial and other geocoding platforms that exist and can fit every operational need from desktop to online application programmer interfaces (APIs) to cloud-based solutions. These are widely available from a number of spatial companies, such as Esri (http://www.esri.com), Google (https://maps.google.com), MapQuest (http://www.mapquest.com), Pitney Bowes (http://www.pb.com), TomTom (http://geocode.com), and Yahoo (http://maps.yahoo.com), just to name a few. These commercial systems typically work well for most regions of the world, though their licensing costs may be prohibitive for certain groups or agencies with few resources to dedicate to geocoding because it is not the primary mission of the organization concerned. Other low to no cost solutions do exist, such as the Texas A&M University (TAMU) Geoservices System (http://geoservices.tamu.edu). TAMU maintains a list of other geocoding resources, including those for countries other than the USA, on its TAMU Geoservices web site. US cancer registries should consult the NAACCR web site to obtain information about the free use of the version of the TAMU Geoservices System hosted by NAACCR. This is a copy of the service offered at TAMU and is provided to the cancer community at no cost through a partnership with the NAAACR, National Cancer Institute (NCI) and TAMU.

4.7 Conclusion

This chapter has introduced the reader to why geocoding is an important topic in health science research. A detailed explanation of the internal workings of the geocoding process and its constituent components provides health science researchers with the knowledge necessary to understand where their data come from and how the issues involved in their production and use may affect study design and outcomes. In addition, this chapter has detailed and expanded upon the recent research agenda offered by Jacquez (2012) in the hope that the next generation of geocode developers and users will be able to make important contributions to the enhancement of geocoding tools, the spatially based investigations they are used within and the larger efforts of health scientists to improve the health and well-being of human populations around the globe.

Despite the limitations of geocoding systems and the geocoded data they produce, these data are a fundamental part of the health science research pathway. They provide the underlying spatial context for numerous studies and will continue to do so well into the future. While not all-encompassing – as it focuses primarily on US data – the information in this chapter should provide the basic knowledge that health scientists need to work with geocoding systems in an informed manner.

Acknowledgements

Dr Goldberg's contribution was supported in part by award number 5P30ES007048 from the US Department of Health and Human Services (DHHS) National Institute of Environmental Health Sciences (NIEHS), by contract numbers N01-PC-35139 and HHSN261200900015C/ADB N02PC-2009-00015 from the US DHHS National Cancer Institute (NCI) and by cooperative agreement number 1H13EH000793-01 from the US Centers for Disease Control and Prevention (CDC). Dr Jacquez's contribution was supported in part by grant number R21LM011132-01A1 from the National Library of Medicine (NLM). Ms Mullan's contribution was supported in part by the Health Program within the Australian Cooperative Research Centre for Spatial Information. The contents of this work are solely the responsibility of the authors and do not necessarily reflect the official views of any of these sponsors.

References

Bakshi, R., Knoblock, C.A. and Thakkar, S. (2004) Exploiting online sources to accurately geocode addresses. In: Cruz, I.F. and Pfoser, D. (eds) *Proceedings of the 12th Annual ACM International Workshop on Geographic Information Systems, GIS '04, Washington DC, USA, November 12–13, 2004*. ACM Press, Washington, DC, pp. 194–203.

Beyer, K.M.M., Schultz, A.F. and Rushton, G. (2008) Using ZIP codes as geocodes in cancer research. In: Rushton, G., Armstrong, M.P., Gittler, J., Greene, B.R., Pavlik, C.E., West, M.M. and Zimmerman, D.L. (eds) *Geocoding Health Data – The Use of Geographic Codes in Cancer Prevention and Control, Research, and Practice*. CRC Press, Boca Raton, Florida, pp. 37–68.

Bichler, G. and Balchak, S. (2007) Address matching bias: ignorance is not bliss. *PIJPSM* (*Policing: An International Journal of Police Strategies and Management*) 30, 32–60.

Bonner, M.R., Han, D., Nie, J., Rogerson, P., Vena, J.E. and Freudenheim, J.L. (2003) Positional accuracy of geocoded addresses in epidemiologic research. *Epidemiology* 14, 408–411.

Boscoe, F.P. (2008) The science and art of geocoding. In: Rushton, G., Armstrong, M.P., Gittler, J., Greene, B.R., Pavlik, C.E., West, M.M. and Zimmerman, D.L. (eds) *Geocoding Health Data – The Use of Geographic Codes in Cancer Prevention and Control, Research, and Practice*. CRC Press, Boca Raton, Florida, pp. 95–109.

Boscoe, F.P., Johnson, C.J., Henry, K.A., Goldberg, D.W., Shahabi, K., Elkin, E.B., Ballas, L.K. and Cockburn, M. (2011) Geographic proximity to treatment for early stage breast cancer and likelihood of mastectomy. *The Breast* 20, 324–328.

Brody, J.G., Vorhees, D.J., Melly, S.J., Swedis, S.R., Drivas, P.J. and Rudel, R.A. (2002) Using GIS and historical records to reconstruct residential exposure to large-scale pesticide application. *Journal of Exposure Analysis and Environmental Epidemiology* 12, 64–80.

Brody, J.G., Aschengrau, A., McKelvey, W., Rudel, R., Swartz, C. and Kennedy, T. (2004) Breast cancer risk and historical exposure to pesticides from wide-area applications assessed with GIS. *Environmental Health Perspectives* 112, 889–897.

Cayo, M.R. and Talbot, T.O. (2003) Positional error in automated geocoding of residential addresses. *International Journal of Health Geographics* 2:10. Available at: http://www.ij-healthgeographics.com/content/2/1/10 (accessed 14 March 2013).

Cockburn, M., Mills, P., Zhang, X., Goldberg, D. and Ritz, B. (2011) Prostate cancer and ambient pesticide exposure in agriculturally intensive areas in California. *American Journal of Epidemiology* 173, 1280–1288.

Davis, C.A. Jr, Pappa, G.L., de Oliveira, D.R.R. and Arcanjo, F. de L. (2011) Inferring the location of Twitter messages based on user relationships. *Transactions in GIS* 15, 735–751.

Gatrell, A.C. (1989) On the spatial representation and accuracy of address-based data in the United Kingdom. *International Journal of Geographical Information Science* 3, 335–348.

Gauderman, W.J., Vora, H., McConnell, R., Berhane, K., Gilliland, F., Thomas, D., Lurmann, F., Avol, E., Kunzli, N., Jerrett, M. and Peters, J. (2007) Effect of exposure to traffic on lung development from 10 to 18 years of age: a cohort study. *The Lancet* 368, 571–577.

Goldberg, D.W. (2008) *A Geocoding Best Practices Guide*. North American Association of Central Cancer Registries, Springfield, Illinois.

Goldberg, D.W. (2011a) Advances in geocoding research and practice. *Transactions in GIS* 15, 727–733.

Goldberg, D.W. (2011b) Improving geocoding match rates with spatially-varying block metrics. *Transactions in GIS* 15, 829–850.

Goldberg, D.W. and Cockburn, M.G. (2010) Improving geocode accuracy with candidate selection criteria. *Transactions in GIS* 14 (Supplement s1),149–176.

Goldberg, D.W. and Cockburn, M.G. (2012) The effect of administrative boundaries and geocoding error on cancer rates in California. *Spatial and Spatio-Temporal Epidemiology* 3, 39–54.

Goldberg, D.W. and Jacquez, G.M. (2012) Advances in geocoding for the health sciences. *Spatial and Spatio-Temporal Epidemiology* 3, 1–5.

Goldberg, D.W., Wilson, J.P. and Knoblock, C.A. (2007) From text to geographic coordinates: the current state of geocoding. *URISA Journal (Journal of the Urban and Regional Information Association*) 19, 33–47.

Goldberg, D.W., Wilson, J.P., Knoblock, C.A., Ritz, B. and Cockburn, M.G. (2008) An effective and efficient approach for manually improving geocoded data. *International Journal of Health Geographics* 7:60. Available at: http://www.ij-healthgeographics.com/content/7/1/60 (accessed 14 March 2013).

Goldberg, D.W., Wilson, J.P. and Cockburn, M.G. (2010) Toward quantitative geocode accuracy metrics. In: Tate, N.J. and Fisher, P.F. (eds) *Accuracy 2010, Leicester, UK, 20–23 July. Proceedings of the Ninth International Symposium on Spatial Accuracy Assessment in Natural Resources and Environmental Sciences*. International Spatial Accuracy Research Association (ISARA), pp. 329–332. Available at: http://www.spatial-accuracy.org/system/files/img-X07133402_0.pdf (accessed 14 March 2013).

Goodchild, M.F (2007) Citizens as sensors: the world of volunteered geography. *GeoJournal* 69, 211–221.

Gordon-Larsen, P., Nelson, M.C., Page, P. and Popkin, B.M. (2006) Inequality in the built environment underlies key health disparities in physical activity and obesity. *Pediatrics* 117, 417–424.

Grumbach, K., Hart, L.G., Mertz, E., Coffman, J. and Palazzo, L. (2003) Who is caring for the underserved? A comparison of primary care physicians and nonphysician clinicians in California and Washington. *The Annals of Family Medicine* 1, 97–104.

Henry, K.A., Boscoe, F.P., Johnson, C.J., Goldberg, D.W., Sherman, R. and Cockburn, M. (2011) Breast cancer stage at diagnosis: is travel time important? *Journal of Community Health* 36, 933–942.

Jacquez, G.M. (1998) GIS as an enabling technology. In: Gatrell, A.C. and Löytönen, M. (eds) *GIS and Health*. Taylor and Francis, London, pp. 17–28.

Jacquez, G.M. (2012) A research agenda: does geocoding positional error matter in health GIS studies? *Spatial and Spatio-Temporal Epidemiology* 3, 7–16.

Jaro, M. (1984) *Record Linkage Research and the Calibration of Record Linkage Algorithms*. SRD Research Report No. CENSUS/SRD/RR-84/27, Bureau of the Census Statistical Research Division Report Series, United States Bureau of the Census, Washington, DC.

Jerrett, M. *et al.* (2008) Traffic-related air pollution and asthma onset in children: a prospective cohort study with individual exposure measurement. *Environmental Health Perspectives* 116, 1433–1438.

Kent, S.T., McClure, L.A., Crosson, W.L., Arnett, D.K., Wadley, V.G. and Sathiakumar, N. (2009) Effect of sunlight exposure on cognitive function among depressed and non-depressed participants: a REGARDS cross-sectional study. *Environmental Health* 8:34. Available at: http://www.ehjournal.net/content/8/1/34 (accessed 14 March 2013).

Kruger, D.J., Reischl, T.M. and Gee, G.C. (2007) Neighborhood social conditions mediate the association between physical deterioration and mental health. *American Journal of Community Psychology* 40, 261–271.

Lin, S., Munsie, J.P., Hwang, S.A., Fitzgerald, E. and Cayo, M.R. (2002) Childhood asthma hospitalization and residential exposure to state route traffic. *Environmental Research* 88, 73–81.

Meliker, J.R., Slotnick, M.J., AvRuskin, G.A., Kaufmann, A., Jacquez, G.M and Nriagu, J.O. (2005) Improving exposure assessment in environmental epidemiology: application of spatio-temporal visualization tools. *Journal of Geographical Systems* 7, 49–66.

Morgenstern, V., Zutavern, A., Cyrys, J., Brockow, I., Gehring, U., Koletzko, S., Bauer, C.P., Reinhardt, D., Wichmann, H.E. and Heinrich, J. (2007) Respiratory health and individual estimated exposure to traffic-related air pollutants in a cohort of young children. *Occupational and Environmental Medicine* 64, 8–16.

Myers, W.P., Westenhouse, J.L., Flood, J. and Riley, L.W. (2006) An ecological study of tuberculosis transmission in California. *American Journal of Public Health* 96, 685–690.

Nuckols, J., Gunier, R., Riggs, P., Miller, R., Reynolds, P. and Ward, M. (2007) Linkage of the California Pesticide Use Reporting Database with spatial land use data for exposure assessment. *Environmental Health Perspectives* 115, 684–689.

Oliver, M.N., Matthews, K.A., Siadaty, M., Hauck, F.R. and Pickle, L.W. (2005) Geographic bias related to geocoding in epidemiologic studies. *International Journal of Health Geographics* 4:29. Available at: http://www.ij-healthgeographics.com/content/4/1/29 (accessed 14 March 2013).

Ratcliffe, J.H (2001) On the accuracy of TIGER-type geocoded address data in relation to cadastral and census areal units. *International Journal of Geographical Information Science* 15, 473–485.

Reynolds, P. *et al.* (2004) Residential proximity to agricultural pesticide use and incidence of breast cancer in the California Teachers Study cohort. *Environmental Research* 96, 206–218.

Ritz, B. and Rull, R.P. (2008) Assessment of environmental exposures from agricultural pesticides in childhood leukaemia studies: challenges and opportunities. *Radiation Protection Dosimetry* 132, 148–155.

Rose, R.I. (2001) Pesticides and public health: integrated methods of mosquito management. *Emerging Infectious Diseases* 7, 17–23.

Rull, R., Ritz, B. and Shaw, G. (2006) Neural tube defects and maternal residential proximity to agricultural pesticide applications. *American Journal of Epidemiology* 163, 743–753.

Rundle, A., Neckerman, K.M., Freeman, L., Lovasi, G.S., Purciel, M., Quinn, J., Richards, C., Sircar, N. and Weiss, C. (2009) Neighborhood food environment and walkability predict obesity in New York City. *Environmental Health Perspectives* 117, 442–447.

Rushton, G. (2003) Public health, GIS, and spatial analytic tools. *Annual Review of Public Health* 24, 43–56.

Rushton, G., Armstrong, M.P., Gittler, J., Greene, B.R., Pavlik, C.E., West, M.M. and Zimmerman, D.L. (2006) Geocoding in cancer research: a review. *American Journal of Preventive Medicine* 30, S16–S24.

Sharkey, J.R. and Horel, S. (2008) Neighborhood socioeconomic deprivation and minority composition are associated with better potential spatial access to the ground-truthed food environment in a large rural area. *The Journal of Nutrition* 138, 620–627.

Strickland, M.J., Siffel, C., Gardner, B.R., Berzen, A.K. and Correa, A. (2007) Quantifying geocode location error using GIS methods. *Environmental Health* 6:10. Available at: http://www.ehjournal.net/content/6/1/10 (accessed 14 March 2013).

Turabelidze, G., Zhu, B.P., Schootman, M., Malone, J.L., Horowitz, S., Weidinger, J., Williamson, D. and Simoes, E. (2008) An epidemiologic investigation of amyotrophic lateral sclerosis in Jefferson County, Missouri, 1998–2002. *Neurotoxicology* 29, 81–86.

United States Census Bureau (2012) TIGER/Line Shapefiles. United States Census Bureau, Washington, DC. Available at: http://www.census.gov/geo/www/tiger (accessed 13 March 2013).

USPS (2012) Mailing Standards of the United States Postal Service, Publication 28 – Postal Addressing Standards. USPS, Washington, DC.

Vieira, V., Fraser, A., Webster, T., Howard, G.J. and Bartell, S. (2008) Accuracy of automated and E911 geocoding methods for rural addresses. In: *Abstracts: ISEE 20th Annual Conference, Pasadena, California, October 12–16, 2008: Contributed Abstracts. Epidemiology* 19, S352.

Wey, C.L., Griesse, J., Kightlinger, L. and Wimberly, M.C. (2009) Geographic variability in geocoding success for West Nile virus cases in South Dakota. *Health and Place* 15, 1108–1114.

Whitsel, E.A., Quibrera, P.M., Smith, R.L., Catellier, D.J., Liao, D., Henley, A.C. and Heiss, G. (2006) Accuracy of commercial geocoding: Assessment and implications. *Epidemiologic Perspectives and Innovations* 3:8. Available at: http://www.epi-perspectives.com/content/3/1/8 (accessed 14 March 2013).

Wolch, J., Wilson, J.P. and Fehrenbach, J. (2005) Parks and park funding in Los Angeles: an equity-mapping analysis. *Urban Geography* 26, 4–35.

Zandbergen, P.A. (2008) Positional accuracy of spatial data: non-normal distributions and a critique of the National Standard for Data Accuracy. *Transactions in GIS* 12, 103–130.

Zandbergen, P.A. (2009) Geocoding quality and implications for spatial analysis. *Geography Compass* 3, 647–680.

Zandbergen, P.A. (2012) Error propagation models to examine the effects of geocoding quality on spatial analysis of individual-level datasets. *Spatial and Spatio-Temporal Epidemiology* 3, 69–82.

Zandbergen, P.A. and Green, J.W. (2007) Error and bias in determining exposure potential of children at school locations using proximity-based GIS techniques. *Environmental Health Perspectives* 115, 1363–1370.

5 Visualization and Cartography

Aldo Aviña[1]* and Chetan Tiwari[2]
[1]*University of North Texas Health Science Center, Fort Worth, Texas, USA;*
[2]*University of North Texas, Denton, Texas, USA*

5.1 Introduction

The drive for discovery and exploration of new lands and resources led to ancient people's need for geographical maps. Many ancient maps, thousands of years old, have been found in cave dwellings and on rocks in Europe, depicting the surrounding geography of that region (Utrilla *et al.*, 2009). Indigenous cultures used sand, sticks and stones to create reliefs of island chains and lands. Babylon, Egypt and Greece were among the first empires to use maps as a means for economic trade, civil information or military advantage (Bagrow and Skelton, 1985). The ancient Greeks are the most renowned for their initial work in cartography. Ptolemy's work in his book *Geographica* (published in AD 150) provided instructional guides on making maps. He was the first to use a system of longitude and latitude lines derived from celestial measurements. In the 8th century AD, the Spanish monk Beatus of Liébana took a different approach to cartography. He created the *Beatine* map – which is one of the most significant cartographic works of the European High Middle ages – using religious literary work with Ptolemaic influences. Also known as the *T and O* map (*orbis terrarium* – an orb or circle of the lands with the letter T inside an O), this map was a religious interpretation of the world (Bagrow and Skelton, 1985; Williams, 1997). Jerusalem was at the centre of the map. Asia was in the top half, Africa in the bottom right quarter, and Europe in the bottom left quarter. The *T and O* map was seen in different forms, including a more detailed form known as the *Mappa Mundi* which was published in AD 1300.

Beginning in the 15th century, nautical exploration of the unknown world increased in intensity. For this type of exploration, better maps with improved details of coastlines and river systems were developed. Cartography became more scientific and this led to improvements in accurate measurements of locations, map projection systems and forms of representation such as atlases of political and other thematic boundaries. Advancements in surveying techniques, data collection and mapping technologies consistently enhanced the accuracy, quality and cartographic design of maps.

As a consequence of these improvements in cartographic methods and technology, geographers began to question the validity and also the utility of traditional map representations. It was argued that knowledge obtained through empirical data acquisition and statistical measurement must also be represented

* E-mail: aldo.avina@unt.edu

objectively (Smith, 1999). In other words, maps should be created without the intentional addition, removal or withholding of integral information. At the same time, it was recognized that maps provide a partial and selective view of reality, given the complexities of real world phenomena. Kitchin and Dodge (2007) have argued that cartography should be viewed as a process-oriented science rather than a representational science – in that maps are created and embedded in a specific moment in time and within a specific social and technical context.

Maps are constantly evolving and informing the spatial processes in play, and thereby influencing how maps are used by people to understand and solve spatial problems and what conscious and unconscious decisions are made by map readers in their use and interpretation of maps. Further, with developments in computational capabilities, GIS (geographical information system) software, and the availability of large volumes of spatially indexed data, maps are no longer a static snapshot of what is where, but a tool for understanding spatial relationships between objects on the surface of the earth and possibly also the processes that are contributing to those observations. Expressed in another way, maps are an abstraction of real world processes that occur at a certain time and spatial scale, and within a particular social and technical context.

The visualization of spatially indexed data collected through field studies, remote sensing or secondary data sources serves two primary purposes: (i) exploratory analysis, which aids hypothesis generation or knowledge construction by uncovering previously unknown relationships in the data; and (ii) communication about geographic features and processes through static maps and other interactive GIS tools. The choice of visualization or mapping technique must be driven by the purpose of the mapping effort. MacEachren and Kraak (1997) generalize the utility of maps (and geographic visualization more generally) using the concept of a *Cartography Cube*. The three axes of this cube represent map audiences (public versus private), level of interactivity (high versus low) and data relationships (known versus unknown). Geovisualization and related analytical techniques, which are often called exploratory spatial data analysis techniques, are associated with the corner of the cube that represents the intersection of high map interaction, private audiences and unknown data relations. Cartographic standards and map-making techniques for appropriately conveying information in a map are associated with the opposite corner, which represents low interaction, public audiences and known data relationships. Different positions within the cube represent different levels of data analysis, synthesis and presentation.

GIS software including Esri ArcGIS (commercial software; available at www.esri.com/software/arcgis) and Quantum GIS (or QGIS; free and open source GIS software; available from www.qgis.org) provide analytical and cartographic capabilities to address the needs of audiences at the two extreme corners of the cartographic cube (i.e. data analysis and data representation). Increasingly, specialized GIS software packages and software development frameworks, available both in the open source domain and commercially, are being developed to provide focused exploratory data analysis and geovisualization capabilities. The open source software includes OpenGeoDa (https://geodacenter.asu.edu/ogeoda), Geovista Studio (www.geovistastudio.psu.edu/), System for Automated Geoscientific Analysis (www.saga-gis.org/), NASA's World Wind (http://worldwind.arc.nasa.gov/java/) and Google Earth (http://earth.google.com). The commercially available software includes SpaceStat (www.biomedware.com/?module=Page&sID=spacestat), among others.

Although the development and availability of easy-to-use GIS software provides many opportunities for geospatial data analysis and mapping, it is important to caution readers of this book against viewing the process of constructing a map as a software-driven production process. Instead, think of the map as a representation of observations and unknown processes that are contextualized by geographic space, time, sociocultural setting and the objectives of the map reader. The *analysis* and *presentation* of these contextualized processes is not just a picture, but also a mechanism that informs public health practitioners, decision makers and the public about their underlying factors.

5.2 Exploratory Spatial Data Analysis Using GIS and Visualization Tools

Building on the ideas of exploratory data analysis (EDA), which uses a variety of graphical techniques to understand patterns in large and complex data sets (Tukey, 1977), Anselin (1994) defines exploratory *spatial* data analysis (ESDA) as a set of techniques and tools that focus on uncovering *spatial* relationships in data. The availability of increased computational power, as well as that of large, multivariate spatio-temporal data sets, has led to new challenges in research and software development for ESDA (Andrienko *et al.*, 2003). ESDA methods and software typically include: interactive mapping techniques in which map features are linked to statistical charts and to attribute information in a table; multivariate plots such as scatter plots, conditional plots and parallel coordinate plots; statistical procedures such as cluster analysis and spatial regression; and spatial data transformation functions (Anselin *et al.*, 2006). ESDA is typically seen as a first step to understanding and analysing large and complex data sets.

The generation of summary statistics and basic graphs prior to any data analysis is useful for understanding data distributions and for identifying any outliers and obvious errors/biases that may be present in the data. OpenGeoDa is free GIS software that implements several methods for EDA and ESDA. It includes tools to create basic statistical summaries and graphs, a variety of smoothed and unsmoothed thematic maps (a discussion of smoothing can be found in Chapter 8), spatial autocorrelation statistics, spatial regression, as well as several advanced visualization techniques that include cartograms, map animations, parallel coordinate plots and conditional plots.

Figure 5.1 uses malaria incidence and population data from Colombia (a sample data

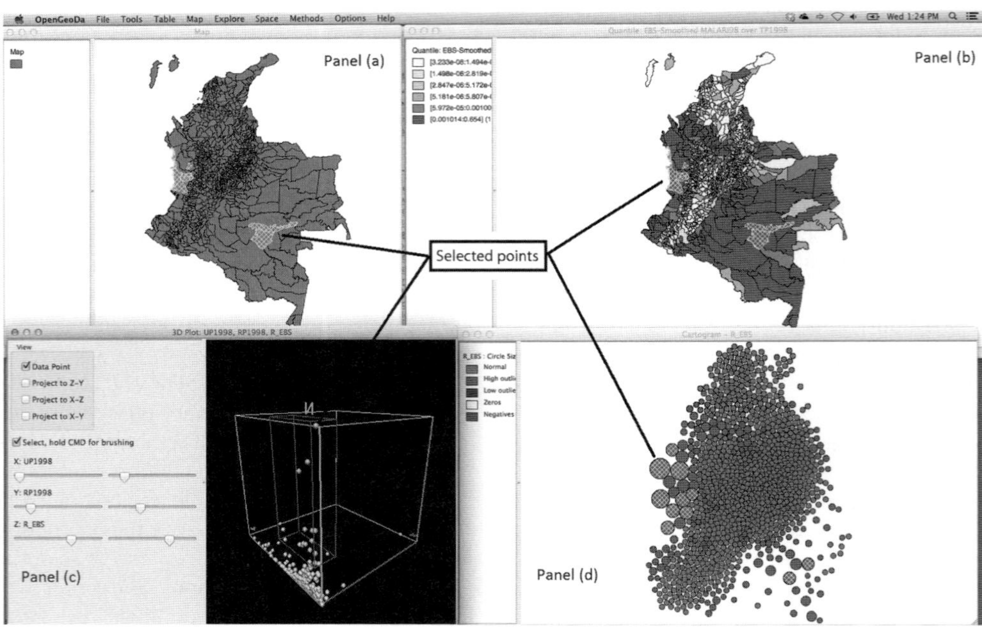

Fig. 5.1. Examples of exploratory spatial data analysis (ESDA) tools in OpenGeoDa software using a sample data set from OpenGeoDa on malaria incidence and population data from Colombia. Panel (a), base map of municipalities. Panel (b), smoothed map of malaria incidence; darker grey indicates higher malaria risk. Panel (c), 3-D scatter plot of relationship between malaria incidence and the urban and rural context; *x*-, *y*- and *z*-axes (given as X, Y and Z) are urban populations, rural populations and malaria incidence; the smaller box is a sub-selection of the population with the highest malaria rates. Panel (d), malaria rates indicated using exaggerated sized symbols (a cartogram).

set obtained from OpenGeoDa and available at http://geodacenter.org/downloads/data-files/malariacolomb.zip) to demonstrate an example of ESDA using OpenGeoDa. The map in panel (a) is a base map of municipalities in Colombia. Panel (b) shows a smoothed map of malaria incidence with the darker shades of grey indicating higher levels of malaria risk. The 3-D scatter plot in panel (c) represents the relationship between malaria incidence and the urban and rural context. The *x*-, *y*- and *z*-axes represent urban populations, rural populations and malaria incidence rates. Each observation in the scatter plot represents a municipality in Colombia. The smaller box inside the 3-D scatter plot represents a sub-selection of the population that has the highest observed malaria rates. The scatter plot suggests that these areas are likely to be more rural than urban. The hatched areas on the maps (in panels a, b and d) represent this sub-selection of data values. The ability to link observations in multiple views of the data (such as maps and plots) is known as *brushing*. Panel (d) represents malaria rates using symbols that are exaggerated in size based on the observed rate. Such maps are known as *cartograms*, where land area is intentionally distorted based on the value of some thematic mapping variable.

Other forms of commonly used geovisualization techniques include parallel coordinate plots (PCP), conditional maps and space–time animations. PCPs are particularly useful for visualizing multivariate data (Inselberg, 1985). This technique uses a series of vertical axes to define *n* variables. Each data observation is represented as a continuous series of line segments that intersect each vertical axis (or variable) at locations that are scaled according to the data range for that variable. Data observations that share similar attributes across all *n* variables will appear as a cluster of line segments. In OpenGeoDa, the PCP is also linked to all other active graphs and plots in the current project, thereby enabling identification of the level of association between multivariate data clusters and spatial clusters.

Conditional plots are useful for plotting the relationship between two variables that is conditional on the value of a third variable. The third variable – or the conditional variable – must be one that can be divided into some *n* groups.

Visualizing change in geographic patterns over time can be effectively accomplished using animated maps. The use of animated weather maps is a common example that showcases the utility of mapping a certain attribute (e.g. rainfall) and its change over space and time. One of the earliest and most well-known examples of computer map animations is Tobler's (1970) visualization of population growth in Detroit, Michigan, USA. Map animations are generally categorized into three categories: (i) animations that emphasize change in position (e.g. the movement of a ship near a port); (ii) animations that emphasize location (e.g. an animation that shows the positions of major earthquakes over time); and (iii) animations that emphasize an attribute (e.g. the change in population demographics in a city over time). OpenGeoDa provides limited map animation capabilities. A comprehensive tutorial on these three and other ESDA methods, as well as sample data sets can be found on the OpenGeoDa web site (https://geodacenter.asu.edu/learning/tutorials).

Software such as Google Earth and NASA World Wind provide a virtual, interactive globe that allows users to navigate to different locations on the earth's surface and selectively observe from a large collection of thematic and satellite-derived data available at different spatial scales (see Chapter 3). These data include satellite imagery, physical infrastructure such as roads and railway lines, demographic data obtained from national census data sets or international agencies, and user-contributed photographs, among others. Geographic data layers produced using most standard GIS software can easily be converted into file formats that are compatible with Google Earth or NASA World Wind. Google Earth uses an Extensible Markup Language (XML) variant called Keyhole Markup Language (KML). KML files can be generated using Esri ArcGIS, Quantum GIS or other free utility programs such as shp2kml 2 from Zonum Solutions (www.zonums.com) or ogr2ogr from GDAL –the Geospatial Data Abstraction Library (available at www.gdal.org/ogr2ogr.html). In Fig. 5.2, the map overlay, along with the symbolization that uses shades of grey to represent different levels of malaria incidence in Colombia (using the same data set as for Fig. 5.1), was generated using shp2kml.

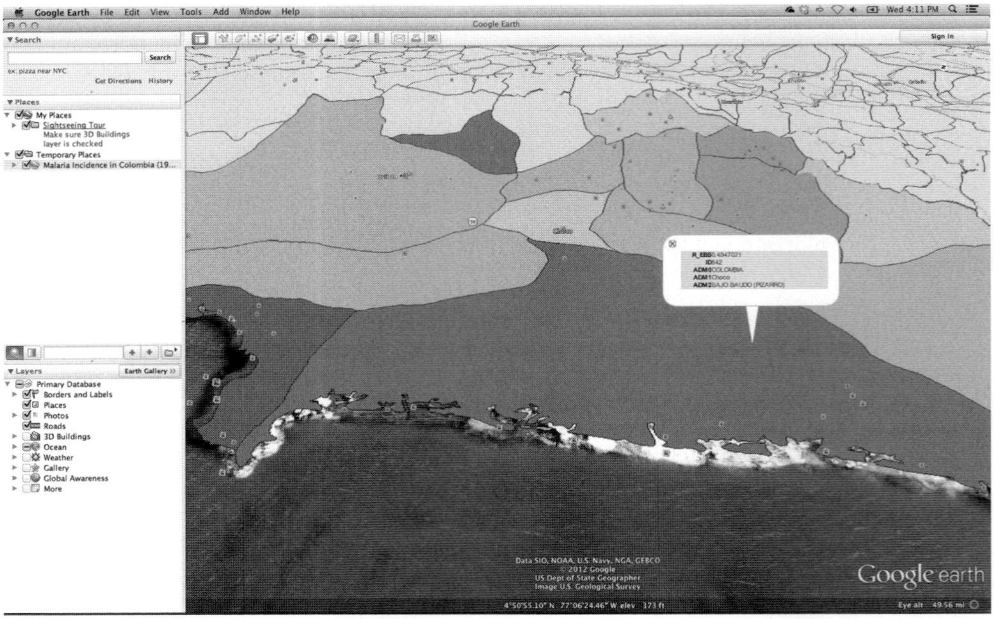

Fig. 5.2. Interactive exploration of data using Google Earth. The map overlay and differing shades of grey represent different levels of malaria incidence in Colombia, and were generated by converting the data set used in Fig. 5.1 to KML format.

5.3 Map Construction and Cartographic Design

The *cartographic process* described by Jensen and Jensen (2012) provides a generalized sequence of steps needed for communicating information in a map to its readers:

1. A conceptualization is needed of the geographic process being mapped. For example, creating a map of cancer deaths in relation to the population in a particular geographic region and time period may be a useful representation of the risk of cancer mortality.

2. A clear definition of the primary purpose and audience of the map is required. The choice of descriptive text, technical details and symbology used in the map must reflect its purpose and intended audience. Information that is relevant to one audience may be irrelevant to another. For example, a public health professional may understand terminology such as 'directly age adjusted' or 'cumulative incidence', while a GIS professional may understand details about 'spatial accuracy' and 'map projections'. The map-maker must be careful about the information that is contained and communicated in the map.

3. Data collection and analysis are needed to create the map defined in the previous step. The data can be primary data collected through surveys and remote sensing techniques, or secondary data that is obtained from data sources such as public health agencies, censuses, etc. Privacy and confidentiality concerns often dictate that secondary health data be made available in an aggregated form (for example, as postal code-level counts of a disease). Generally, the representation of such data must be consistent with its scale. Analysis techniques such as kernel density estimation methods may be used to convert area-level data into surface representations. Supplemental data needed for map design must also be collected at this stage. For example, highway data is sometimes used to provide spatial context in a map.

4. The design and construction of the map must be driven by standard cartographic design principles. These principles dictate the use of cartographic feature types (point, line or polygon),

their symbolization and other map elements in order to convey the intended information as accurately as possible to the map reader. For example, line symbols of varying thicknesses may be used to represent different levels of a road hierarchy. Further details of these principles are discussed in detail later in the chapter.
5. An evaluation of the map in relation to its intended purpose must be conducted. This can be accomplished through a process of feedback and map revision, and this step may require the collection of additional data or changes in the design of the map.

Although GIS software can be used to process data (step 3) and generate maps (step 4), when used incorrectly, it can also result in maps that are misleading owing to inadequate technical knowledge surrounding the storage and analysis of spatial data in a GIS, the presentation of incomplete or biased information, and bad map design (Monmonier, 1996). The cartographic principles outlined in the remainder of this chapter provide a basic set of guidelines that will help map-makers to present data in a manner that is unbiased and consistent with standard cartographic practices.

5.3.1 Projections and coordinate systems

The earth is an ellipsoidal, three-dimensional object with a complex surface (Snyder, 1987). Our goal is to represent information collected on or near the surface of such an object into a two-dimensional plane on a sheet of paper or computer screen. We start the process of 2-D representation by fitting our data to some predefined model of the earth, which is usually a spheroid (also known as an ellipsoid), although a simplified view such as a sphere is sometimes used for mathematical ease. Local variability on the surface of the earth has resulted in many different spheroid definitions. The latest definitions are based on satellite measurements and are able to accurately capture deformities in the shape of the earth due to gravitational forces. For reasons of mapping accuracy, localized spheroids that are specific to smaller geographic areas are also commonly used.

The different models of the earth are defined using several parameters. These include a datum, which defines the position of the spheroid relative to the centre of the earth. In other words, the datum is a fixed point that defines the point of origin for a specific model of the earth. The process of projecting information from 3-D to 2-D is dependent on the map-maker's choice of model and datum. For example, in the USA, the 1927 North American Datum (NAD27) defines the geographic centre (or the datum) of the USA as a point located on a hog farm near Lebanon, Kansas. Other systems may use the centre of the earth as the datum; these include the North American Datum 1983 (NAD83), and the World Geodetic System 1984 (WGS84). Note that it is possible and common that geographic data are collected using the same model of the earth, but different datums. Because each datum uses a different starting point, the actual shape of the model earth will vary between such data sets. Any analysis conducted using inconsistent datum definitions is likely to result in offset errors between data sets. In some cases, these offsets may be so small that they are easy to miss, thereby resulting in incorrect analysis. These are of particular concern in public health research when fine-scaled measurements of exposure are made on the basis of two or more well-defined sets of points on the earth's surface (e.g. school locations and some industrial activity). Even though current GIS software is capable of automatically fixing such errors, it is strongly advised that the data be made consistent before the start of any mapping exercise.

The process of projecting data from the assumed model of the earth to a planar representation is best explained by the following example. Imagine a transparent and spherical glass ball floating in the centre of a dark room. Painted on the ball is the outline of the continents and inside the ball is a light bulb. When you switch on this light, the image of the earth on the glass ball is projected on to all the walls, the floor and the ceiling of the room. This is the basic principle behind projecting geographic data. In the centre of each wall (the same occurs with the floor and ceiling), you notice that you see a projection of part of the earth that looks close to reality. But as you look closer to the edges of the wall, you notice that the projection of the Earth becomes distorted. These distortions can be minimized for certain geographic regions by moving and reorienting the walls in the room, thereby resulting in different projected images of the continents. There are three basic types of orientations that are commonly used: cylindrical, conic and azimuthal. A cylindrical projection is one in which the walls of the room are wrapped around the earth as a cylinder that makes a single line of contact with the earth's surface at the equator or other location. Cylindrical projections preserve directions and angles, but distort shape and area. Conic projections are those in which the walls are shaped into the form of a cone, which is then placed on top of the earth. These projections are useful for mapping areas in the upper latitudes. Finally, azimuthal or planar projections are those in which the wall is a single surface that is tangential to the earth's surface. These types of projections are often used to map areas near the poles.

For example, consider the map of the world illustrated in Fig. 5.3. This map was constructed using an oblate spheroid (also called ellipsoid) model of the earth based on the work of Alexander Ross Clarke in 1866, and is referenced to the NAD27 datum. Note that the general shape of the central USA and other areas close to the equator look normal, while areas near the poles are severely distorted, thus affecting area calculations and shape. All projections distort data, and the type and properties of the projection system used will dictate the kind of distortion (area, shape, scale, etc.) and the geographic areas most affected by it. Depending on the type of distortion, projection systems are generally classified into three major types:

1. Equivalent projections or equal-area projections are those that represent the sizes of all areas in a map in correct proportion to one another. However, these projections will distort shape. They are useful in applications where the depiction of areas is important. Common examples include the Lambert Azimuthal Equal-Area projection and the Albers Equal-Area Conic projection.

2. Conformal projections are those that maintain correct angles around every point on the map. Consequently, these types of projections maintain accurate shapes but distort area. They are useful in navigation applications. A commonly used example is the Universal Transverse Mercator (UTM) projection that is described in Section 1.2.

3. Equidistant projections are those that maintain accurate distances along given lines (such as a meridian) from any point on the earth's surface. It is important to configure this projection such that the selected point is tangential to

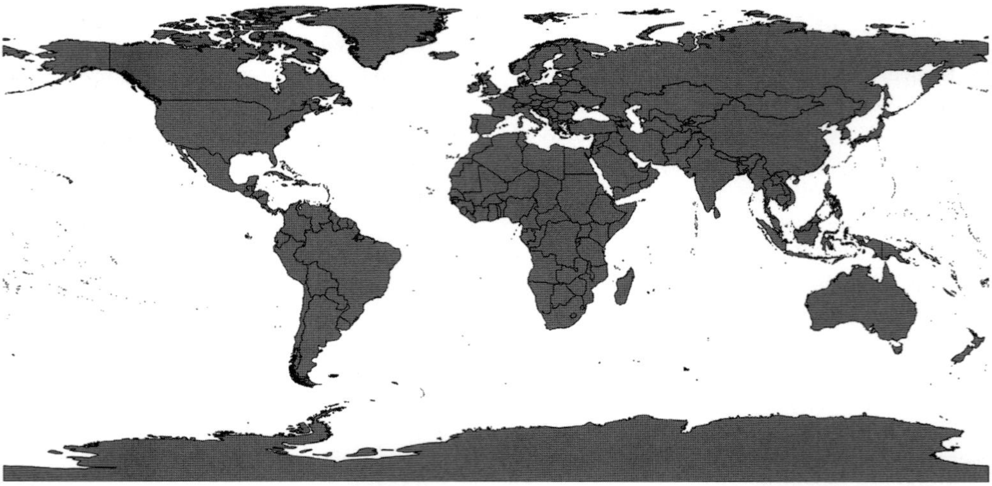

Fig. 5.3. Map of the world produced using an oblate spheroid model of the earth based on Clarke (1866).

the earth's surface. In other words, the selected point must be at the centre of the map. These projections are known as Azimuthal Equidistant projections and are useful for applications where distances measurements are important (e.g. aeronautical charts). A commonly used example is the Lambert Azimuthal Equal-Area projection.

The choice of an appropriate projection system is best determined by the intended purpose of the map. Although there is no specific criterion that defines the best choice of a projection system for a specific purpose, the generalized principles discussed above can help to guide the map-maker to make an informed decision about the trade-offs that are associated with different types of projections. It is sometimes helpful to examine regional standards when deciding which projection system to use. For example, GIS departments of many local governments in the USA provide their data in the State Plane Coordinate System.

Conversions between different projection systems can be easily done in most GIS software. In fact, both Esri ArcGIS and Quantum GIS provide 'on the fly' projection capabilities – meaning that the software would automatically re-project the data to meet the projection definition of other data sets that are currently loaded in the software. Quantum GIS provides a large library of predefined projection definitions that have been compiled from various sources including the European Petroleum Survey Group (EPSG), Institut national de l'information géographique et forestière (IGN, the French National Institute of Geographic and Forest Information), and the Open Source Geospatial Foundation (OSGeo). An excellent reference guide for technical information on different projection systems is SpatialReference.org (available at http://spatialreference.org). A final note of caution: although many GIS software packages will automatically re-project your data for you, it is always better to ensure that all your spatial data are projected into a consistent format when conducting any kind of spatial analysis. Conducting analysis on data that is in two different projected coordinate systems is like comparing apples and oranges. An in-depth technical discussion of projections and coordinate systems can be found in Snyder's *Map Projections: A Working Manual* (1987).

5.3.2 GIS data structures

Raster and vector are the two most commonly used data structures for storing geographic information in a computer. The vector data model uses points, lines and polygons to represent objects on the surface of the earth while the raster data model uses a matrix of pixels in which each pixel contains a value that represents the magnitude of a certain observation (e.g. elevation). Vector representation is useful for identifying discrete objects on the surface of the earth, while raster data is appropriate for representing large areas of continuous measurements.

Within the vector model, data can be further classified into the three basic feature types of points, lines and polygons (see Chapter 1). Point features use a single *x*-, *y*-coordinate pair (such as latitude and longitude) to represent features that occur as discrete points on the surface of the earth. Linear features include roads and streams and these are represented using a linked set of locations that are connected to each other in between a starting and an ending location. Polygons are used to represent features that occupy some area, such as a lake or administrative unit. In the simplest case, polygons are represented using a closed sequence of lines. The type of geographic data (point, line or area) influences the map-maker's choice of mapping style. For example, dot density maps use an arrangement of identical point symbols to represent the density distribution of some geographic phenomena. Flow maps can be used to represent the flow of populations or natural resources from one place to another. The thickness of the lines used in these maps can be changed to represent the amount of resources that flow from one place to another. Finally, polygon data can be represented using different colours or shades of colour to represent different magnitudes of a quantitative variable. Such maps are known as choropleth maps.

The raster data model is used to represent continuous data observations that are typically made for large geographic regions. Raster data consists of equal-sized cells that are organized into rows and columns. The cell size may vary and is defined using *x* and *y* dimensions for each pixel. For example, a raster cell of size 5 km × 5 km encompasses a geographic area of

25 km². A common example of this type of data is a remotely sensed image that consists of a regular array of similarly sized cells. Each cell can contain one or more values that can be mapped using GIS software. Vector data structures (i.e. points, lines or polygons) can be converted into a raster format and vice versa. Depending on the cell size, this conversion may result in severe distortion. Generally, point features will appear similar to how they would in a vector representation, while linear and polygon features tend to get distorted. Line features and polygons constructed using lines appear jagged and blocky. The jagged light grey blocks in Fig. 5.4 represent a rasterized version of the polygon represented by the black line.

Vector and raster data can be used together in a GIS. For example, it is possible to determine land use type (stored as raster data) for a city boundary (stored as vector polygons). Concepts of projections and coordinate systems, as well as recommendations for map design, are applicable to representations of all geospatial data regardless of their data structure.

5.3.3 Cartographic elements and map design

This section describes the elements of a map that a cartographer should keep in mind. In order to best present a map, additional information is sometimes needed to explain the map to the user. We will use maps from the Iowa Cancer Maps web site (www.uiowa.edu/iowacancermaps) as examples. The following map elements are commonly used:

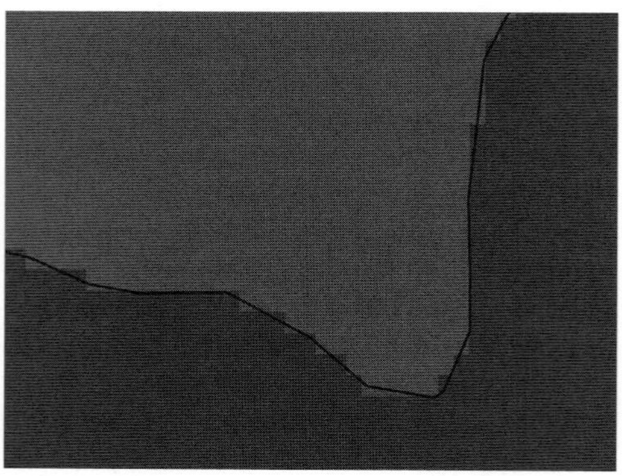

Fig. 5.4. Comparison between the representation of raster and vector data.

Figure–ground

The key idea behind this method of organizing content on a map is to enable the map reader to easily separate the most important element/s on the map from background information. *Figure* refers to the primary thematic content, while *ground* refers to the background information. On close examination of the high-resolution map images for breast cancer incidence on the Iowa Cancer Maps web site (www.uiowa.edu/iowacancermaps/images/Breast_Incidence_00_05.jpg), notice that the surface of breast cancer incidence (*Figure*) is overlaid on top of a topographic image of the state (*Ground*). The intent behind the map design is to focus the reader's attention first on the spatial patterns of breast cancer incidence, while also providing several pieces of information in the background (including the topographic map, legend, scale bar, north arrow and explanatory text).

Title

The title provides information about the map contents. It must be concise and should contain information about the thematic content of the map, the location (or place) and time. The title should have the largest font on the map. Subtitles may be used to provide additional information; however, they are not necessary. For example, maps of cancer burdens in Iowa are titled using a *Place, Thematic Content, Time* style (e.g. Iowa, Breast Cancer, Incidence Rate, 2000–2005; see www.uiowa.edu/iowacancermaps/breast_incidence.html).

Legend

A legend describes the symbology used on a map. It provides vital information that allows the map reader to understand the information and patterns seen on the map. There are many different kinds of legends that can be constructed using standard GIS software. In general, we recommend that the legend be appropriately titled. It can contain multiple entries – one for each data layer in the map, or a single entry that describes the primary content. The legend on the breast cancer incidence map only provides information on the primary thematic content of the map, i.e. the burden of breast cancer incidence in Iowa expressed as a ratio of observed cases to expected cases. Legends may be oriented horizontally or vertically and must be placed on the map in a manner that balances the different cartographic elements, including scale bars, north arrows and other supplemental information.

Scale bar or scale text

A scale enables the map reader to determine the distance between two points on a map. It is generally a ratio of the distance on a map to the actual distance it represents on the surface of the earth. The term *large scale* map is used to refer to a map that shows small geographic area with high levels of detail. Conversely, the term *small scale* map is used to show large geographic areas within limited detail. Small scale maps typically use some generalization methods to limit the amount of detail that is shown in a map. For example, line generalization methods may be used to smooth out a winding road. Information about the scale informs the map reader about the level of detail that is present in the map and is therefore an important component of the map output. Unless the target group is completely familiar with the map product, or is mapping large geographical areas, it is necessary to provide appropriate scale information.

There are several different scale options available in most GIS software. These include representative fraction (e.g. a US Geological Survey topographic map of 1/24000), a text description of relationship based on measurable units (e.g. 1 inch = 500 ft), and a graphical scale bar that is automatically constructed based on the current zoom level of the map. It is important to choose measurement units that will not distract the map reader with a large and unmanageable numbers on the scale bar, e.g. using 'Feet' instead of 'Miles' on the Iowa Cancer map example. It is important to pay attention to the scale bar as software may sometimes add one in the default map units which, for unprojected data, are decimal degrees. Such scale bars are generally meaningless as they are hard to interpret. Note that it is incorrect to include a scale bar when large areas are mapped using projection systems that do not have a constant scale. Additionally, the map reader must be cautioned against using the scale bar when an inset map of different scale is included along with the primary map. For example, inset maps are commonly used to provide a larger geographic context to a focused study area.

Symbols

Symbols are used to differentiate between different types of objects on the map. They are generally identified using six visual dimensions: size (e.g. a graduated symbol map uses symbols of different sizes to represent the magnitude of a quantitative variable), shape (e.g. locations of schools in relation to polluting industries can be represented using two different symbol types, thus allowing the map reader to quickly identify that there is an important difference between the two objects), value (this is the relative lightness or darkness of colour and is often used for creating graduated colour ramps), texture (e.g. hatch patterns are sometimes used to delineate different areas on a map), orientation (e.g. arrows that change direction to show wind flow patterns) and hue (e.g. different colours can be used to represent nominal data categories). While graduated symbols may be used to represent some quantitative variable, such maps tend to get busy and confusing when a large number of overlapping symbols of different sizes are used.

Classification methods and colouring schemes

Quantitative data such as disease rates are typically represented using colours that are grouped into different classes based on a number of different classification methods. Typically, data are grouped into three to seven classes arranged in ascending or descending order. Each group or class is then assigned a unique colour. There are several different classification methods that can be used. It is important to note that the spatial patterns observed on a map will be different depending on the type of method used.

Common methods include natural breaks, equal interval and quantiles (Cromley and McLafferty, 2002). The natural breaks method automatically generates a pre-specified number of classes with varying ranges that are derived by examining naturally occurring breaks in the statistical distribution of the data. Jenk's optimization methods, which are designed to maximize between-class variance and minimize within-class variance, are commonly used for implementing this classification method (Brewer and Pickle, 2002). The equal interval method divides the data into equal ranges, depending on the number of classes chosen. The quantiles classification method orders the observed data and then places an equal number of observations in each class. Different names are sometimes used to represent the different number of classes (e.g. quartiles when four classes are used and quintiles when five classes are used). Note that the actual data ranges will vary depending on the distribution of the data.

A number of different colouring schemes can be used to represent the classified data. Sequential colouring is appropriate for mapping ordered data. These colouring schemes are usually generated by varying value (i.e. the relative lightness or darkness of a colour) in combination with hue (i.e. a primary colour). Lighter colours are assigned to lower data values while darker colours are assigned to higher data values. Diverging colour schemes are used when the data being mapped have a central, usually neutral, value. This data point is typically represented using a light (or transparent) colour. Sequential colour schemes may be used on either side of this central value. For example, the breast cancer incidence maps use a sequential colouring scheme based on warm colours (such as shades of red and orange) to classify rates that are greater than the state rate (the transparent central data value), and cool colours such as shades of blues are used to classify rates that are lower. Qualitative data are typically represented using colours with no progression. An excellent web resource for colouring choices, developed by Cynthia Brewer, can be accessed at http://colorbrewer2.org/. This web site provides colour ramps for the three types of colouring schemes (sequential, diverging and qualitative) along with details of their suitability for colour-blind individuals, printing, photocopying or computer display purposes. Colour Brewer styles can easily be imported into QGIS software.

North arrow

A north arrow helps to orient the map. The use of north arrows is a convention that has stayed steadfast in map-making. They are particularly useful when small areas are being mapped. Current GIS software packages provide several north arrow styles. However, care must be exercised when deciding their size and placement in a map. When a north arrow is absent, north can be assumed to be in the upward direction.

Labels

Labels allow the map reader to identify and relate to unfamiliar features on the map. Cities, counties, rivers and states are features that are commonly labelled. Labels must be positioned in a manner that makes it easy for the map reader to associate the label with its intended object. Additionally, the placement of labels is further restricted by the presence of other objects (as well as their labels) on a map. The process of labelling features on a map can be a tedious process, and to aid this, most GIS software provides optimization algorithms that automate the placement of labels in a manner that results in the least overlap between objects and labels on the map. Such algorithms are also useful for online mapping services, including Google Maps and Bing Maps. A formal description of labelling algorithms can be found in Tamassia (2012).

Supplemental information

Typically this includes the cartographer's name and/or organization, date, copyright information and disclaimers. Technical information on the map projection and data sources can also be included. In the Iowa cancer map example, the map-makers provide information about the analysis method in a brief paragraph on the map. Such information can be useful in explaining the assumptions and parameters that were used in the construction of the map.

Background and borders

These elements are not essential and are based on the map-maker's preference. A background colour could be used to soften a stark, white map. It also fills empty space, keeping the eyes from becoming distracted by that space. A simple, decorative border may be used to provide a container for all the different map elements. A reference grid or graticule containing information on location coordinates is sometimes added to the map border.

5.4 Making a Map in Quantum GIS (QGIS)

In this mapping example, we will produce a choropleth map of urban population in municipalities in Colombia. Recall that choropleth maps are a kind of thematic map in which polygons or areas (Colombia municipalities in this case) use a sequential colour scheme to represent different magnitudes of a quantitative variable (urban population). We use QGIS software to create the final map output, although the cartographic principles used are generally applicable to other GIS software, including Esri's ArcMap. The data set used in this example is a shapefile of Colombia municipalities (colmunic.shp) obtained from the previously mentioned file of malaria incidence and population data from Colombia (malariacolomb.zip file; see Section 5.2).

Vector data can be added in QGIS by clicking on 'Layer > Add Vector Data'. Add the data layer 'columic', representing municipalities in Colombia. The layer properties menu (right-click on colmunic and select *Properties → Style*) provides several symbolization options, including *Single Symbol*, *Categorized*, and *Graduated*. The *Graduated* style option should be used for representing ordinal data such as population or disease rates. Choose this option and set the *Column* value to 'UP2005' and number of *Classes* to '5'. Choose any diverging colour ramp (e.g. greys) and set the *Mode* to 'Quantile'. Click on 'Apply' and 'OK'. The darkest coloured areas on the map are those with highest urban population counts. When producing choropleth maps, count data is usually normalized using area or population. However, care must be taken to ensure that small population counts are not used in such calculations as they can result in maps that are subject to the small numbers problem, which is discussed further in Sect on 8.3.2. As the primary purpose of this exercise is to demonstrate the application of the cartographic principles discussed in Section 5.3, we will continue to use the map of urban population counts for this illustration.

The next step is to verify the projection being used and to re-project the data to a different system if necessary. Clicking on the CRS Status icon on the bottom right corner of the screen brings up the Coordinate Reference System (CRS) dialogue box. Note that the data is currently unprojected and uses an ellipsoidal model of the earth referenced to the WGS84 datum. We will re-project this data to the MAGNA-SIRGAS/Colombia Bogota zone projection (EPSG:3116). Search for EPSG ID 3116 and select the projection entry. Ensure that the option to 'Enable on the fly CRS transformation' is enabled before clicking OK. You may have to reset your zoom to full extent to see the re-projected data. Note that the location coordinates are now in metres rather than latitude and longitude values.

The various cartographic elements that are shown in the map in Fig. 5.5 can be added using the following procedure:

1. Right click the colmunic data layer and select 'Rename'. Rename the layer 'Urban Population (2005)'.
2. On the menu bar, click 'File > New Print Composer'.
3. Select the desired paper size on the right menu.
4. Check 'Snap to grid' and set the spacing as desired.
5. Select 'Layout > Add Map'. In order to place the map on the page, drag a square to a desired size. You can move the map frame to a different location on the page.
6. If the map data do not fit into your frame, click on the 'Item Properties' tab on the right, and select the map dialogue, increase the scale value and click 'Update Preview'. Experiment with the frame size and the map scale to find a desirable fit.

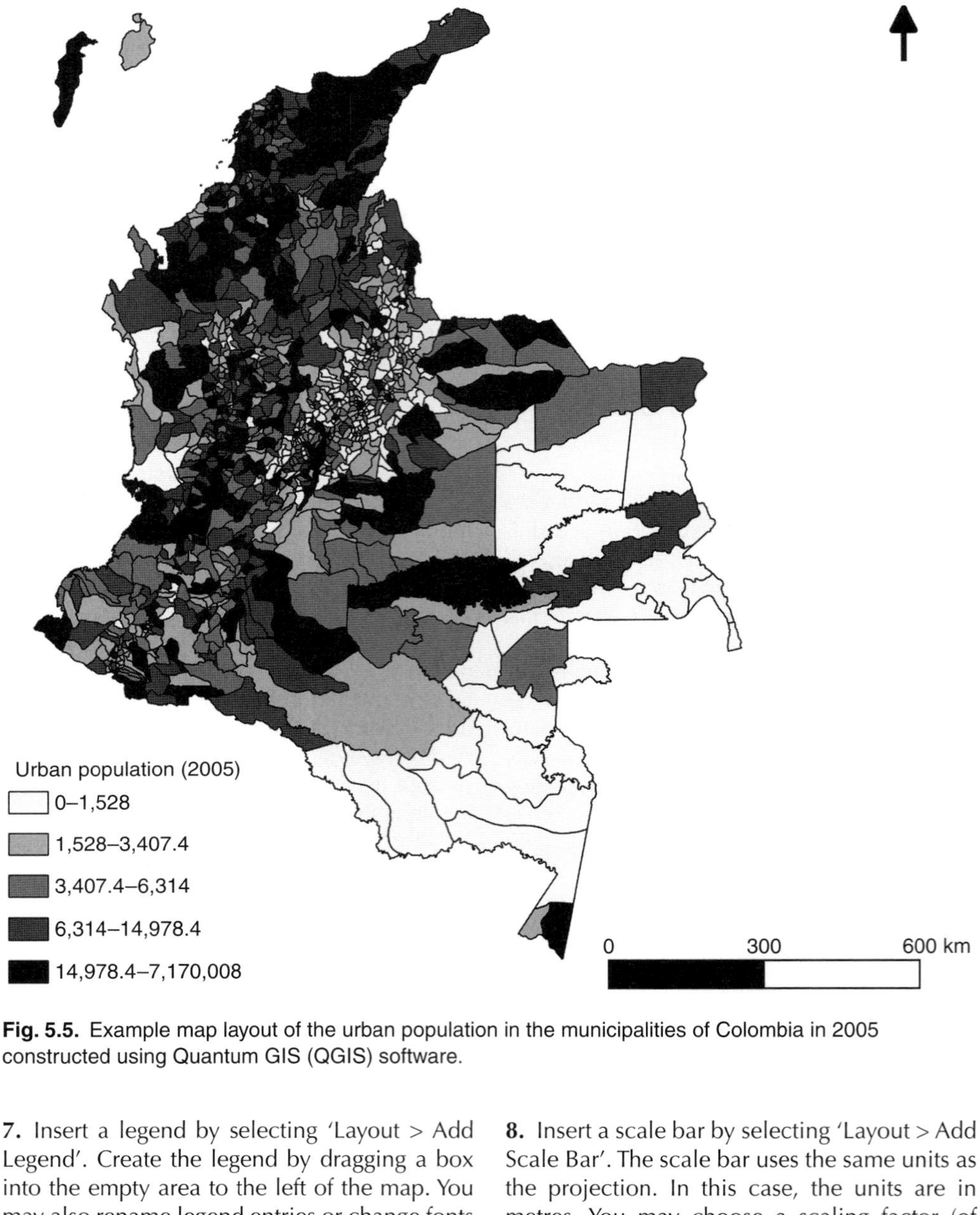

Fig. 5.5. Example map layout of the urban population in the municipalities of Colombia in 2005 constructed using Quantum GIS (QGIS) software.

7. Insert a legend by selecting 'Layout > Add Legend'. Create the legend by dragging a box into the empty area to the left of the map. You may also rename legend entries or change fonts by selecting the legend item in the map composer window and then modifying its general properties (options window on the right side of the screen). Click on the 'Legend Items' tab to reposition, add, delete or modify each legend entry. For example, you can manually change the number of significant digits on each legend item by clicking on the item and then selecting Edit (the icon that looks like a pencil and paper).

8. Insert a scale bar by selecting 'Layout > Add Scale Bar'. The scale bar uses the same units as the projection. In this case, the units are in metres. You may choose a scaling factor (of 1000 in this case) under 'Map units per bar unit' to change from metres to kilometres. The 'Unit Label' option may be used to correctly display the measurement unit on the map.

9. Add a north arrow by clicking on 'Layout > Add Arrow'. Position the north arrow in the top right corner of the screen.

10. Background information such as highways or the locations of major cities may also be added to the map to serve as additional reference points.

11. Finally, add a title to the map using the 'Layout > Add Label' option. Position the title at the top left corner of the map.

12. Position the different elements so that they are generally balanced on both sides of the map figure.

13. The map layout can then be printed or exported into a variety of other data formats, including JPG images and PDF documents.

5.5 Conclusion

The goal of this chapter has been to showcase the two primary goals of spatial data representation and mapping: (i) to visualize information to aid data exploration and hypothesis generation through exploratory spatial data analysis; and (ii) to present information to a map audience using appropriate cartographic principles. Both these objectives require different approaches that can be accomplished using specialized and often free GIS software.

However, the procedure of abstracting real world processes into a map requires many assumptions. Some of these assumptions influence the technical nature of the map (such as the choice of projection system or data classification method), while others influence its ability to convey information in an unbiased manner (such as the choice of symbols, colours and map elements).

It is important to remember that map audiences perceive maps as an accurate representation of unknown processes and often use them in decision making processes. The ability of modern GIS software to automate many of the map-making processes can often result in maps that are biased and, in some cases, incorrect. Therefore, proper judgement must be exercised in using the various features of software when producing maps. Similarly, the spatial analyses tools available in GIS software can sometime lead to improper decisions if adequate care is not taken in selecting the appropriate method of analysis and interpreting its outcomes. The general principles outlined in this chapter are important considerations that need meticulous attention before a map is produced, disseminated, or used in decision making processes.

References

Andrienko, N., Andrienko, G. and Gatalsky, P. (2003) Exploratory spatio-temporal visualization: an analytical review. *Journal of Visual Languages and Computing* 14, 503–541.

Anselin, L. (1994) Exploratory spatial data analysis and geographic information systems. In: Painho, M. (ed.) *New Tools for Spatial Analysis*. Eurostat, Luxembourg, pp. 45–54.

Anselin, L., Syabri, I. and Kho, Y. (2006) *GeoDa*: an introduction to spatial data analysis. *Geographical Analysis* 38, 5–22.

Bagrow, L. and Skelton, R.A. (eds) (1985) *History of Cartography*, 2nd edn. Precedent, Chicago, Illinois.

Brewer, C.A. and Pickle, L. (2002) Evaluation of methods for classifying epidemiological data on choropleth maps in series. *Annals of the Association of American Geographers* 92, 662–681.

Cromley, E.K. and McLafferty, S.L. (2002) *GIS and Public Health*. Guilford Press, New York.

Inselberg, A. (1985) The plane with parallel coordinates. *The Visual Computer* 1, 69–91.

Jensen, J.R. and Jensen, R.R. (2012) *Introductory Geographic Information Systems,* Prentice Hall, Boston, Massachusetts.

Kitchin, R. and Dodge, M. (2007) Rethinking maps. *Progress in Human Geography* 31, 331–344.

MacEachren, A.M. and Kraak, M.J. (1997) Exploratory cartographic visualization: advancing the agenda. *Computers and Geosciences* 23, 335–343.

Monmonier, M.S. (1996) *How to Lie with Maps,* University of Chicago Press, Chicago, Illinois.

Smith, P. (1999) Drawing new maps: a radical cartography of developmental disabilities. *Review of Educational Research* 69, 117–144.

Snyder, J.P. (1987) *Map Projections: A Working Manual.* U.S. Geological Survey Professional Paper 1395, United States Government Printing Office, Washington, DC.

Tamassia, R. (2012) *Handbook of Graph Drawing and Visualization*. CRC Press, Boca Raton, Florida.

Tobler, W.R. (1970) A computer movie simulating urban growth in the Detroit region. *Economic Geography* 46, 234–240.

Tukey, J.W. (1977) *Exploratory Data Analysis,* Addison-Wesley, Reading, Massachusetts.

Utrilla, P., Mazo, C., Sopena, M.C., Martinez-Bea, M. and Domingo, R. (2009) A paleolithic map from 13,660 calBP: engraved stone blocks from the Late Magdalenian in Abauntz Cave (Navarra, Spain). *Journal of Human Evolution* 57, 99–111.

Williams, J. (1997) Isidore, Orosius and the Beatus Map. *The International Journal for the History of Cartography* 49, 7–32.

6 Spatial Overlays

Daniel W. Goldberg,[1]* Myles G. Cockburn[2] and Adam T. Naito[1]
[1]*Department of Geography, Texas A&M University, College Station, Texas, USA;*
[2]*University of Southern California, Los Angeles, California, USA*

6.1 Introduction

One of the most powerful capabilities that a geographic information system (GIS) provides is the ability to manage, view and manipulate large amounts of disparate spatial information within a single interface. These systems remove many of the challenging aspects of data storage away from the user and allow him/her to focus on several other tasks: creatively combining and analysing spatial information to pose and answer spatially based questions; creating predictive spatio-temporal models; and developing an understanding of the role that spatial relationships play in all manner of health-related phenomena and processes. One of the major benefits that the last 40–50 years of development has brought to modern GIS products is the ability to rapidly access, display and analyse multiple GIS data sets simultaneously. The graphical user interfaces (GUIs) provided by these tools allow GIS users to add multiple GIS data sets, turn specific data sets on and off, and create any number of map designs that are useful for their end goals through manipulating map symbology and data set transparency, and by employing other fundamental cartographic and design principles.

Most commonly, however, simply displaying multiple sets of data at the same time is seldom the end goal of GIS users. This statement is particularly true when considering the community of health science researchers who regularly utilize GIS tools for research, practice and policy making. Many in this community (and others) would argue that the real power that GIS provides is found in the analytical capabilities that are built into these systems. The rich set of spatial and spatio-temporal analysis tools available within modern GIS systems put high-quality analysis techniques at the fingertips of end users in all fields. Spatial overlay operations are one of these classes of tools, and they are fundamental to GIS analysis within the health sciences. These tools, which include operations such as intersection and spatial join, among others, often comprise some of the first steps taken by health science researchers when they need to relate information contained within two or more geographic data sets to each other in order to create or derive analytical products upon which they can conduct further research.

The primary purpose of the set of spatial operations that are collectively known as spatial overlay operations is to utilize the geographic location of objects within one data set to perform some geographic process on another data set. All of these operations affect

* E-mail: daniel.goldberg@tamu.edu

the geographic boundaries and/or attributes associated with geographic objects in at least one of the data sets, meaning that new data are created each time one of these processes is applied. Some operations, such as erase, strictly affect the shape of geographic objects within the target data set, i.e. portions are removed, whereas others, such as spatial join, strictly affect the attribute data associated with the target data set, i.e. the attributes from one data set are appended to those in another.

The fundamental idea behind spatial overlays is to leverage the spatial relationships between geographic objects in different geographic data sets to accomplish some task. To achieve this goal, spatial analysis techniques employ a set of topological spatial primitives, i.e. the 4- and/or 9-intersection model (Egenhofer, 1991; Chen *et al.*, 2001), to determine relationships between the boundaries (or locations in the case of a point or line, because these do not have interior areas) of geographic features within two or more geographic data sets. These primitives include operators such as Contains, Intersects, Overlaps and Disjoint, and characterize the spatial relationships between two or more geographic objects. Storing these topological relationships between objects allows a GIS to identify objects that are spatially related to each other very quickly, rather than searching the entire set of objects in a reference data set each time a user issues the query 'Identify all geographic objects whose boundaries overlap the boundaries of this object of interest', for example. Depending on the specific operation, different primitives may be used to determine which portions of the geometries to retain/disregard in the output and/or which features in corresponding data sets should be merged together, split or associated by transferring the attributes from objects in one data set to another.

The next section of this chapter describes several common spatial overlay operations. After defining these operations, several instances in which spatial overlay can be a useful analysis technique in health science research are presented. Next, a case study which utilizes spatial overlay operations in the context of environmental health research is provided. The chapter concludes with final remarks and recommendations for successfully employing spatial overlay operations in health science research and practice.

6.2 Spatial Overlay Operations

The most common spatial overlay operations available in modern GIS platforms consist of: (i) erase; (ii) identify; (iii) intersect; (iv) symmetrical difference; (v) union; (vi) update; and (vii) spatial join. These are described below in Sections 6.2.1–6.2.7, and depicted in Figs 6.1 and 6.2. Each of these tools plays a unique role in the use of spatially based analysis techniques for health science. In all cases, each spatial operation requires at least two separate geographic data sets. The first, which we will define as the target data set, is the one that will have the operation applied to it. The second, which we will refer to as the operation data set, is the one whose geometry will be used to perform an action. The following sections describe the details of these operations along with example cases as to when and why they might be used in an analysis framework. The erase, identify and intersect operations are displayed in Fig. 6.1a; symmetrical difference, union and update operations are shown in Fig. 6.1b. The spatial join operation is discussed after the other six (and displayed in Fig. 6.2).

6.2.1 Erase

The erase spatial overlay operation uses the geographic boundaries of features within the operation data set to remove, or to erase, portions of the geographic shapes associated with features in the target data set. In Fig. 6.1a (left), this process is depicted by the circular areas being erased from the polygon areas.

6.2.2 Identity

The identity spatial overlay operation uses the geographic boundaries of the features within the operation data set to split the geographic

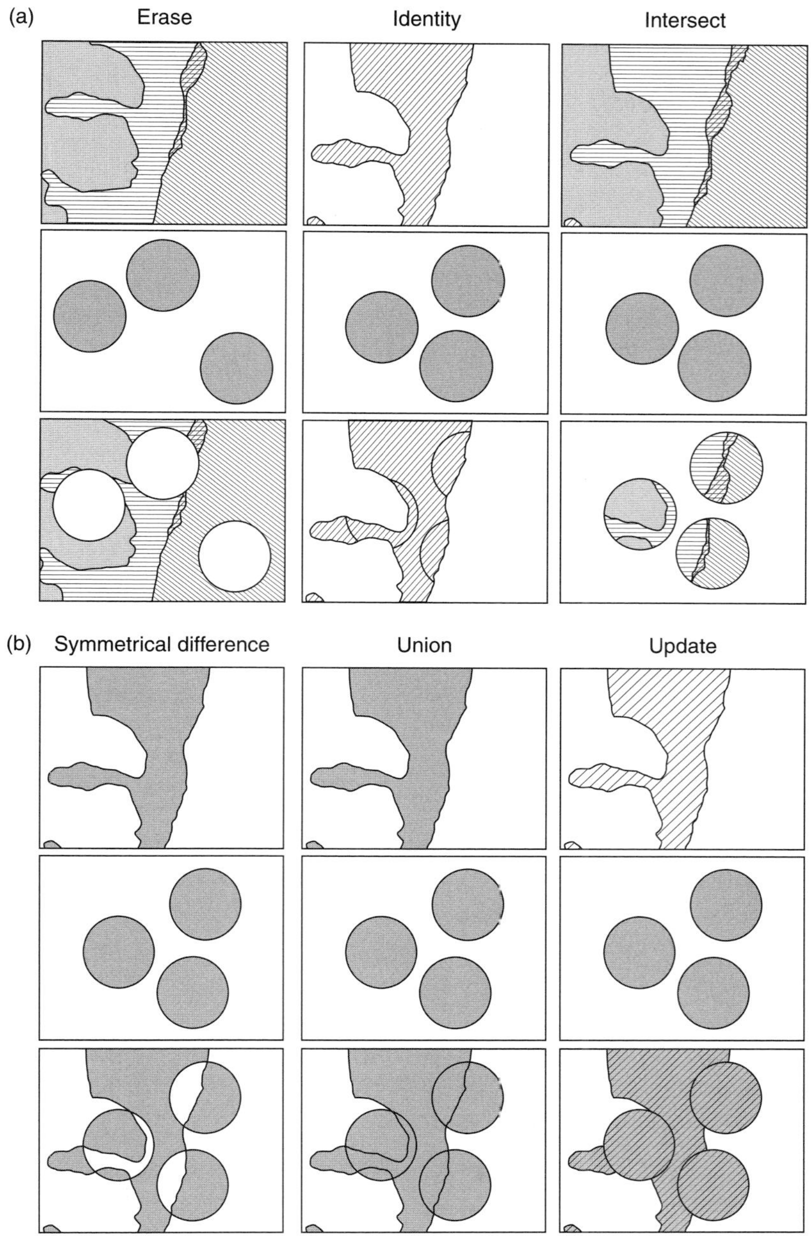

Fig. 6.1. (a) Hypothetical examples of erase, identify and intersect spatial overlays; (b) hypothetical examples of symmetrical difference, union and update spatial overlays.

shapes associated with features in the target data set. In this case, only the portion of the geography of the operation features that are completely contained within the boundaries of the target geographies are retained in the output. The output features in the target adopt the attributes of the operation features. The output feature boundary is the same as the target, but it also includes the area intersected by the operation features.

The effect of running this operation is to clip the geographic extents of the geographies contained in the target data set by those of the operation data set, and to split the resulting geographies into smaller pieces using the boundaries of the features contained within the operation data set. This operation can be seen in Fig. 6.1a (middle) where the circular regions are used to create slices in the polygon layer. The areas where the circular areas overlap with the polygons are split from the main (original) polygon area into separate polygons of their own. Note that the entire circular shape is not kept, just the area that overlapped with the polygon.

6.2.3 Intersection

The intersection (intersect) spatial overlay operation uses the geographic boundaries of features within the operation data set to extract portions of the target data set geographic features where the two overlap spatially. In this case, only the portions of the target features that are covered by the geographic shape of the operation features are retained, while the remainder of the target feature is discarded. This can be seen in Fig. 6.1a (right) where just the areas of the polygons that are covered by the circular areas are kept.

6.2.4 Symmetrical difference

The symmetrical difference spatial overlay operation determines areas that are common to geographic boundaries of the features within the operation data set and those in the target data set. This operation removes the common areas, resulting in a new geography that represents the merged features that are not common to either operation or target features. The output layer has an extent that is identical to the target and operation layer combined (as if it were a union), but the area overlapped by the operation layer has been removed. This operation is shown in Fig. 6.1b (left) where the areas that are common to both the circular regions and the polygons have been removed. Note that this could be considered as a special case of the erase operation.

6.2.5 Union

The union spatial overlay operation is similar to the identity spatial overlay operation. However, in the case of the union operation, the full geographies of both the operation and target data sets are retained, whereas in the identity operation the portion that was not contained within the target data set is discarded. As in the result of the identity spatial operation, the original geographies of the features within the target data set are split by the boundaries of the features within the operation data set. The output features adopt the attributes of the target features. An example of this operation is seen in Fig. 6.1b (middle) where the full geometries of the polygon and the circular layers are both kept. Note that the areas where the circular regions and the polygon intersect result in independent polygons whose boundaries are created by the original boundaries of both layers.

6.2.6 Update

The update spatial overlay operation is similar to the union spatial overlay operation. However, while the full geographies of the features in the operation data set are retained, features in the target data set overlapped by features in the operation data set are discarded. The output features are identical to the union of the two features, but the features of the operation data set are preserved. This operation updates the attributes of the target layer, but means that both the operation and the target layers must have the same attribute fields in order to work. The results of such an operation can be seen in Fig. 6.1b (right) where the target layer (polygon) is updated to include new features from the operation layer (circular). Areas in the polygon layer that were covered by the circular regions are removed from the geometry of the original polygon and included in the polygon output layer as independent shapes.

6.2.7 Spatial join

The spatial join spatial overlay operation uses the geographic boundaries of features within the operation data set to associate attributes of these features on to features of the target data set where the corresponding features in the two are within a specified spatial distance threshold of each other and obey specific topological relationship conditions. In this case, the geometry of the target data set is not altered. Instead the attributes of the operation data set are copied to the target data set for each feature that meets a specific topological relation constraint. Most GISs that support spatial join allow the user to specify whether the topological relation between features in each data set should be one of the following: (i) intersect; (ii) contain; (iii) within; or (iv) closest.

The spatial join operation is arguably the most commonly used spatial overlay operation. In many instances, features in the target data set may not be related to those in the operation data set and vice versa. As a result, users typically have the option of specifying an appropriate behaviour. For example, a user can specify that: (i) all attribute records are kept regardless of whether a match can be found; or (ii) records are eliminated if an attribute match does not exist. In the parlance of traditional relational database management systems (RDBMS), these are known as left or right joins for case (i), and outer joins for case (ii).

Additionally, the spatial join operation is unique in that it permits one-to-one and many-to-one relationships. Users can typically choose how they wish the operation to handle these cases. The particular decision chosen by a user will be dependent on the goal of the project, the context of the data being processed and the logical schema of the phenomena represented in both data sets.

A graphical depiction of the spatial join operation is displayed in Fig. 6.2. In this case, the source tables displaying the attributes of two county data sets are shown. The left hand table contains county-level population counts, along with number of deaths. The right hand table displays county-level information for age adjusted cancer mortality. The spatial join operation is applied using the population count geographic data as the target data set and the age adjusted cancer mortality table as the operation data set. The result of this operation is that the attributes of the age adjusted cancer mortality table are appended to the corresponding rows in the population table. This particular case involves a one-to-one relationship, meaning that the spatial footprint of each individual geographic feature (i.e. county) in the population table matched exactly to one spatial footprint in the age adjusted cancer mortality table.

6.3 Applications of Spatial Overlays in Health Science

Fundamental to many environmental epidemiology studies is the assignment of environmental exposure values from up-to-date and accurate databases to an individual, and their subsequent use in spatial analysis. This information is typically obtained by intersecting the location of the individual and the geographic pattern of the environmental factor to be measured. These intersections are performed using one or more of the spatial overlay operations described above.

The types, amounts and time periods of such environmental factors being estimated and investigated by a study can vary greatly – from hour-by-hour ultraviolet (UV) exposure (e.g. Rigel *et al.*, 2003; Thieden *et al.*, 2004), to daily exposure to smoke from a wild fire (e.g. Bowman and Johnston 2005; Frankenberg *et al.*, 2005; Johnston *et al.*, 2006; Viswanathan *et al.*, 2006), to yearly exposure to smog emissions (e.g. Künzli *et al.*, 2000; Nafstad *et al.*, 2004; Bayer-Oglesby *et al.*, 2005), to lifetime exposure to particulate matter resulting from living next to an airport (e.g. Steinmaus *et al.*, 2004). Even though each of these studies requires the investigation of multiple time periods, spatial areas and environmental dosages, they all share one common aspect: the need to link exposure estimates drawn from one or more geographic data sets to individuals represented by some other spatial representation. Spatial overlay operations allow health science researchers to achieve these goals.

In these scenarios, the existence and usability of accurate data describing the environmental factor under investigation upon which spatial overlay operations can be applied are critical. However, having data at hand that is completely accurate and designed, a priori, to be usable is the exception, not the rule.

Spatial join

COUNTY	CENSUS POPULATION	DEATHS
Galveston County	291,309	567
Lubbock County	278,831	566
Jefferson County	252,273	605
Webb County	250,304	289
McLennan County	234,906	475
Smith County	209,714	489
Brazos County	194,851	190
Hays County	157,107	192
Johnson County	150,934	269
Ellis County	149,610	234
Ector County	137,130	286
Midland County	136,872	227
Guadalupe County	131,533	198
Taylor County	131,506	300
Wichita County	131,500	287

+

COUNTY	AGE ADJUSTED CANCER MORTALITY
Galveston County	64
Lubbock County	50.6
Jefferson County	58.2
Webb County	23.2
McLennan County	62.5
Smith County	53.5
Brazos County	49.8
Hays County	40.8
Johnson County	63
Ellis County	60.1
Ector County	62.2
Midland County	47.4
Guadalupe County	46
Taylor County	53.3
Wichita County	73.2

↓

COUNTY	CENSUS POPULATION	DEATHS	AGE ADJUSTED CANCER MORTALITY
Galveston County	291,309	567	64
Lubbock County	278,831	566	50.6
Jefferson County	252,273	605	58.2
Webb County	250,304	289	23.2
McLennan County	234,906	475	62.5
Smith County	209,714	489	53.5
Brazos County	194,851	190	49.8
Hays County	157,107	192	40.8
Johnson County	150,934	269	63
Ellis County	149,610	234	60.1
Ector County	137,130	286	62.2
Midland County	136,872	227	47.4
Guadalupe County	131,533	198	46
Taylor County	131,506	300	53.3
Wichita County	131,500	287	73.2

Fig. 6.2. Hypothetical example of a spatial join spatial overlay operation in the USA.

This situation stems from the many ways in which these data sources are typically created. They can be the result of scientific measurements, reported data values or calculated data values. For instance, it would be impossible to calculate potential individual UV exposure without either giving everyone a personal UV meter (which is expensive), or by having a data source that captures how much potential UV would have been in an area where that person was, at the time they were there. While the latter option is more desirable and realistic, stations that measure the full spectrum of the UV wavelength (UVA and UVB) are relatively rare. To provide insight on potential UVB dosages, recent research has shown that UVB estimates produced from UVA stations may be sufficiently accurate, and thus UVB estimates are being produced and utilized (e.g. Tatalovich *et al.*, 2006).

The types of environmental estimations described above raise a series of important questions that must be asked along and between all three axes of time, space and dose. For example: is the time period covered by the reference data relevant to the time period for which exposure is to be estimated? Is the dose described at an appropriate spatial resolution to allow the realistic determination of accurate exposure levels? Is the dose imputed from the data source relevant to the personal exposure? Is the dose described at the correct temporal resolution to realistically determine accurate exposure levels?

6.4 Spatial Overlay Methods for Pesticide Exposure Assessment in California's Central Valley

Each of these issues have come to the forefront during a series of recent research investigations into the effect of pesticide exposure in California's Central Valley (e.g. Bell *et al.*, 2001; Rull *et al.*, 2001, 2006; Rull and Ritz, 2003; Reynolds *et al.*, 2005; Marusek *et al.*, 2006; Nuckols *et al.*, 2007; Cockburn *et al.*, 2011; Wang *et al.*, 2011), as well as elsewhere in the country (e.g. Ward *et al.*, 2000; Brody *et al.*, 2002, 2004). In each case, these studies used the spatial overlay operations that have been described in this chapter to compute environmental exposure assessments. These studies will be summarized below.

The methods presented in these studies vary because each employed different levels of information to describe the distribution of pesticide over an area. As these new information sources are introduced, the ways in which spatial overlay operations are applied become increasingly sophisticated to leverage the knowledge drawn from additional data availability. In the specific research scenarios described below, investigators have focused on improving the spatial and temporal specificity of the reference data used for the spatial overlay operations. These advances have enhanced our understanding of the means by which exposure can and should be computed at an individual level.

Bell *et al.* (2001) calculated exposure estimates utilizing California's Pesticide Use Report (PUR) database (California Department of Pesticide Regulation, 2000), which links the type, amount in pounds, acreage and date applied, method of application and locations to which regulated pesticides had been applied with sections of the Public Land Survey System (PLSS). Rull *et al.* (2001) and Rull and Ritz (2003) investigated the exposure misclassification resulting from the spatial resolution of the one square mile PLSS sections (i.e. grid cells) concerned, and the likelihood that the pesticide may not disperse equally within these cells. They compared the approach of Bell *et al.* (2001) with one that used the California Land Use Reports (LU) (California Department of Water Resources, 2005). The LU data describe the actual spatial geometry of croplands in terms of which crops are grown, and from these it can be determined which pesticides were applied. This data source allows one to increase the validity of the resulting pesticide exposure estimates because it relies upon source data with a finer spatial and temporal resolution in the spatial overlay operations that ultimately compute exposures.

Nuckols *et al.* (2007) overcame a limitation of Rull *et al.* (2001) and Rull and Ritz (2003) by not aggregating seasonal crops into a single classification and assuming that each was equally likely, thus improving the temporal certainty of the data. Studies outside California have employed similar methods and examined the feasibility of calculating historical lifetime exposures by incorporating additional/ancillary data sets (e.g. Ward *et al.*, 2000; Brody *et al.*, 2002, 2004).

This progression in the use of data sources demonstrates that as new data sources become available (both current and historical) for use in spatial overlays as applied to exposure estimation, there is an opportunity to repeat the execution of exposure models, both to determine previous misclassifications and to create more accurate exposure assessments. Further, as new climatic models are developed that explain the dispersion of pesticides in relation to environmental factors, the ability to easily incorporate these data so as to improve the validity of existing exposure assessments further will need to be developed.

The following sections detail the different approaches in which spatial overlays have been utilized to compute exposure estimations in the group of studies that have investigated California's Central Valley. As the methods progress in sophistication, emphasis is now placed on how the addition of greater amounts of information into the spatial overlay process improves exposure estimation through the reduction of uncertainty associated with the source data sets.

6.4.1 PUR database definition

As already noted, the model by Bell *et al.* (2001) made use of the PUR data available from the state of California Department of Pesticide Regulation that links pesticide applications to one square mile sections of the PLSS, whereas Rull *et al.* (2001) and Rull and Ritz (2003) made use of the higher resolution LU data from the California Department of Water Resources. The PUR database can be considered as a set of n individual records, app_i, each representing a single pesticide application. The total database, or combined set of all applications, $[Apps]$, is simply the union of all individual applications. The size of this set, $|[Apps]|$, is equal to the number of application records, n.

$$[Apps] = \bigcup_{i=1}^{n} app_i \tag{6.1}$$

$$|[Apps]| = n \tag{6.2}$$

Each of the individual applications app_i, within $[Apps]$ can be represented as a vector describing the attributes of interest: t, the date and time of application; c, the chemical applied; p, the pounds of pesticide applied; a, the acreage it was applied to; and l, the location (PLSS ID) where it was applied.

$$app_i = \langle t, c, p, a, l \rangle \tag{6.3}$$

From each individual application record, app_i, the density of a particular chemical, c, applied during a particular application, i.e. $density(l, app_i(c))$, within a PLSS grid cell, l, can be computed by dividing the pounds applied, $app_i(p)$, by the application acreage, $app_i(a)$. In the case of the PUR database, $[Apps]$, each application, app_i, corresponds to the application of a single chemical within a single grid cell, l, so that $density(l, app_i(c))$ can be rewritten simply as $density(app_i)$. This should be distinguished from the case where a single application, app_i, represents the application of a set of multiple chemicals, as could be the where another PUR-like database is used that contained multiple chemicals per record. In this latter case, the equations developed and used throughout this chapter would need to be altered.

$$density(app_i(c)) = \frac{app_i(p)}{app_i(a)} \tag{6.4}$$

$$density(app_i) = density(app_i(c)) \tag{6.5}$$

It should be noted at this point that the $density(app_i)$ of the application of a chemical is associated with the entire area within the one square mile PLSS grid cell, l. From the PUR data alone, it is impossible to determine where within the cell the application occurred. The set of equations above can be used to assign pesticide application levels, per chemical, to each of the grid cells that comprise the PLSS grid cells.

6.4.2 The PUR–PLSS exposure model

The generalized workflow of the processing steps necessary to complete the Bell *et al.* (2001) model is as follows: (i) an address is turned into a spatial location by the process of geocoding; (ii) this spatial point is then intersected with a spatial data set containing geographic polygons representing the one square mile PLSS grids using the intersection spatial overlay operation; (iii) the PLSS grid cell ID of the intersected PLSS grid cell and the density of chemical application as defined in the PUR database are linked using a relational database to join with the PLSS grid cell ID of the PLSS sections from (ii) as the key.

6.4.3 The PLSS grid cell section

Because the PUR data has a maximum spatial resolution of one square mile, Bell *et al.* (2001) were forced to restrict their analyses of exposure to 'narrow' and 'broad' classifications, as shown in Fig. 6.3. In this figure, the black dot represents the location of a subject's geocoded address, 'Narrow' means the exposure levels were used from the single PLSS grid cell that a person lived in (cell with horizontal lines) and 'Broad' means this particular cell and the eight surrounding cells (with vertical lines) were used.

To formulate a notation for this phenomenon, we can first observe that the PLSS grid is essentially a raster data set, or set [*G*], composed of *p* columns and *q* rows, with each individual grid, $G_{x,y}$, being defined in terms of its relative position along the *x* and *y* axes. This is depicted graphically in Fig. 6.4, where the origin of the coordinate system has been made arbitrarily at the bottom left corner, and is shown mathematically in Eqn 6.6.

$$[C] = \bigcup_{x=0}^{p} \bigcup_{y=0}^{q} G_{x,y} \tag{6.6}$$

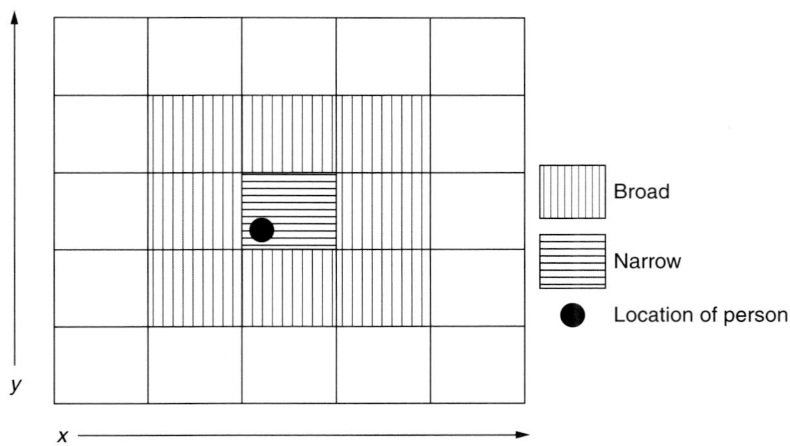

Fig. 6.3. The pesticide exposure classification used by Bell *et al.* (2001) for the analysis of California's Pesticide Use Report (PUR) database for a particular subject (person, black dot): narrow, exposure based on a single grid cell of the California Public Land Survey System (PLSS); broad, exposure based on this single grid cell and the surrounding eight grid cells.

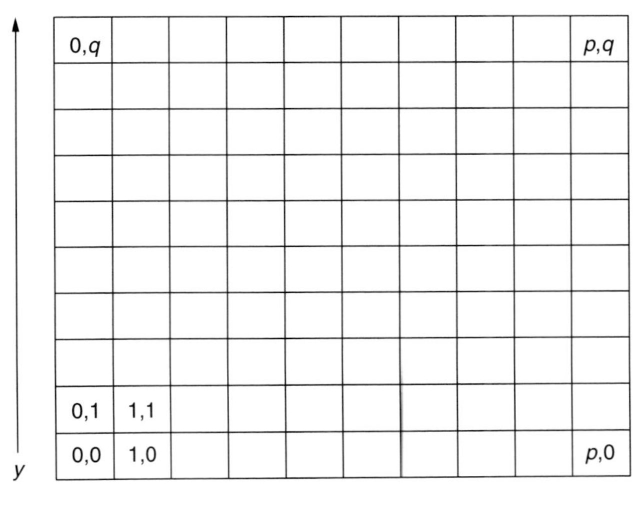

Fig. 6.4. Raster grid cell generation for the California Public Land Survey System (PLSS).

With this notation, one can define a subset of $[G]$, $[G_s]$, representing the set of PLSS grid cells to be included in the PUR PLSS exposure estimation. One can further define an iterative function (Eqn 6.7) to uniformly create $[G_s]$, for both the narrow and broad cases of exposure. This is accomplished by incorporating a scale factor, s, into the grid cell selection equation, which also takes as input the total PLSS grid, $[G]$, and the grid cell where the residence is, $G_{x,y}$, determined through the intersection spatial overlay operation applied to the geocoded address point as the operation data set and the PLSS grid data set as the target data set.

$$[G_s] = GetCells([G],\ G_{x,y,s}) \tag{6.7}$$

In the case of Bell *et al.* (2001), for the broad case, $s = 1$, i.e. one additional cell is included in every direction, and for the narrow case, $s = 0$, i.e. no additional cells are included in any direction. By defining an algorithm to select the appropriate PLSS grid cells at any scale, one can allow for different definitions of broad and narrow to be tested at different resolutions.

6.4.4 The PUR–PLSS exposure estimation

The list of PLSS grid cells, $[G_s]$, generated from Eqn 6.7, can be used to calculate $exp(c)$, the PUR–PLSS based exposure estimate, $exp(c)$, for a particular chemical, c. In Bell *et al.* (2001), this calculation is based simply on the overall density of the application of the particular chemical, c, within each of the individual grid cells in $[G_s]$, as listed in the PUR database, $density(app(c))$ because of the limitation of the PLSS resolution.

To accomplish this, one can define a relational database query, $getCellDensity(G_i,\ c)$, which takes a PLSS grid cell (PLSS ID) and chemical, and performs two tasks. The first is to select the correct individual pesticide application, *app*, from the total set of pesticide applications [*Apps*], based on its attributes $<t, c, p, a, l>$, in particular, the identifier of the PLSS grid cell (PLSS ID) in which the application took place, l, and the chemical used, c. The second task is to calculate and return the density of the chemical used in the application, $density(app(c))$. Thus, $exp(c)$, is calculated as the summation of densities, $density(app(c))$, of the applications of chemical c that took place in the each of the m PLSS grid cells in $[G_s]$.

$$\exp(c) = \sum_{i=0}^{m} getCellDensity(G_i, c) \tag{6.8}$$

It should be noted that the exposure calculated with Eqn 6.8 will overestimate the potential exposure values and is not a true representation of a person's actual exposure, notably because pesticides are aimed at fields and people do not live in fields. Pesticides are rarely dispersed evenly across an entire one square mile PLSS grid cell and the density information from the PUR database cannot describe where in the cell it was applied. This is because even though the PUR database reports the acreage that a chemical was spread over, it is impossible to tell from the PLSS data where within the one square mile it was applied, with every place being as likely as every other place.

6.4.5 Exposure calculation with buffered geographic PLSS areas

Instead of simply using a broad/narrow exposure classification scheme which assumes that an individual is exposed to the full density reported for each PLSS grid cell they are in (narrow exposure), or that cell plus each of the eight surrounding cells (broad exposure), it has become common to use one or more catchment areas (spatial buffers) around a point to derive a better exposure estimate, as depicted in Fig. 6.5, which uses buffers of radii 500, 1000 and 1500 m. This topic was not explored in Bell *et al.* (2001), but it is offered here as the next logical extension to their work.

In this case, after applying a geospatial buffer to create a circular area of a particular radius around the geocoded point as in the left hand figure in Fig. 6.6, the intersection spatial overlay operation can be used to cut the PLSS grid cells into just the sections that fall into the buffered region as depicted in the right hand image in Fig. 6.6. The result of the intersection operation is a set of m partial grid cells (spatial polygons) $[P]$ from which a more precise chemical exposure density can be calculated.

By dividing the original density returned from the PUR database from the *getCellDensity*

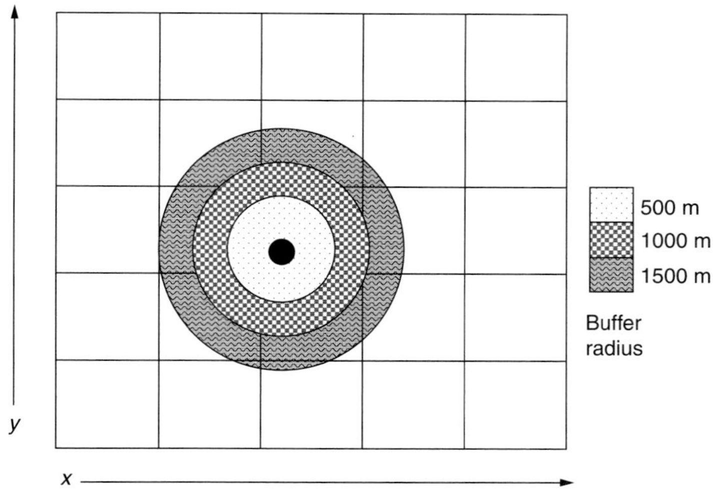

Fig. 6.5. Pesticide exposure calculation based on spatial buffers around a geocoded point among grid cells of the California Public Land Survey System (PLSS).

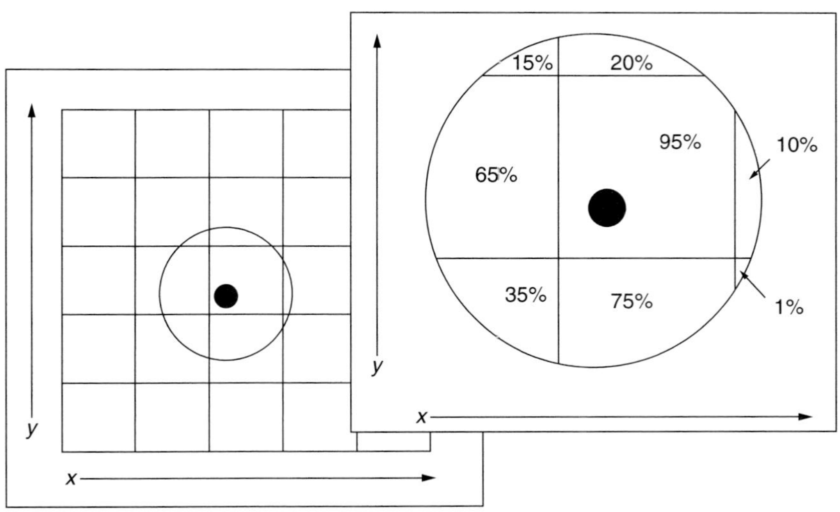

Fig. 6.6. Left, spatial buffer around a geocoded point among grid cells of the California Public Land Survey System (PLSS), and right, intersection overlay operation applied to the buffered area to determine the grid cell sections that fall into the buffered region.

(G_i, c) function, by the proportion of the area of the cell, P/m_i^2, the exposure estimate may more accurately represent the chemical application that a person might have been exposed to. This new exposure calculation is shown in Equation 6.9.

$$\exp(c) = \sum_{i=0}^{m} \frac{getCellDensity(G_i, c)}{P / mi^2} \quad (6.9)$$

It should be noted that the exposure estimates produced with this new method still assume that the pesticides were applied at a constant density throughout the entire one square mile PLSS grid cell. This new method simply tries to obtain a more accurate proportion of the pesticide that a person was exposed to by taking an exposure equal to the proportion of the area of the PLSS grid cell to which they were potentially exposed. At this point, no other information exists regarding the location of the application within the PLSS grid cell.

6.4.6 The PUR land use exposure model

Rull *et al.* (2001) and Rull and Ritz (2003) realized the assumption that the pesticide application occurs at a constant density across the PLSS grid cell is false (pesticides are not typically applied at a constant density across an entire one square mile PLSS grid cell), and inconsistent with the data in the PUR database which states the actual acreage the chemicals were applied to.

As shown in Fig. 6.7, in contrast to the low resolution of the PLSS grid cell (top left) the LU maps depict where within the one square mile PLSS grid cells the actual crop fields are located (bottom left). These LU maps contain polygons with attributes describing which crops are grown in that field from surveys conducted by the State of California on a county-by-county basis, once every 7–10 years. However, the polygons lack the PLSS grid cell IDs needed to link them directly to the PUR database. Through the use of the spatial join spatial overlay operation, these two data sets can be linked to associate these PLSS grid cell IDs with the crop field polygons (Fig. 6.7, right), as accomplished by Rull *et al.* (2001) and Rull and Ritz (2003).

Rull *et al.* (2001) and Rull and Ritz (2003) used these more accurate spatial distributions in conjunction with buffered geocoded addresses to determine individual pesticide exposure as depicted in Fig. 6.8. In this hypothetical example, the individual would be classified as exposed to chemical *a* in grid cell [1,1] and chemical *c* in grid cells [0,0] and [0,1].

This method accounts for the observation that the spatial locations of croplands from the

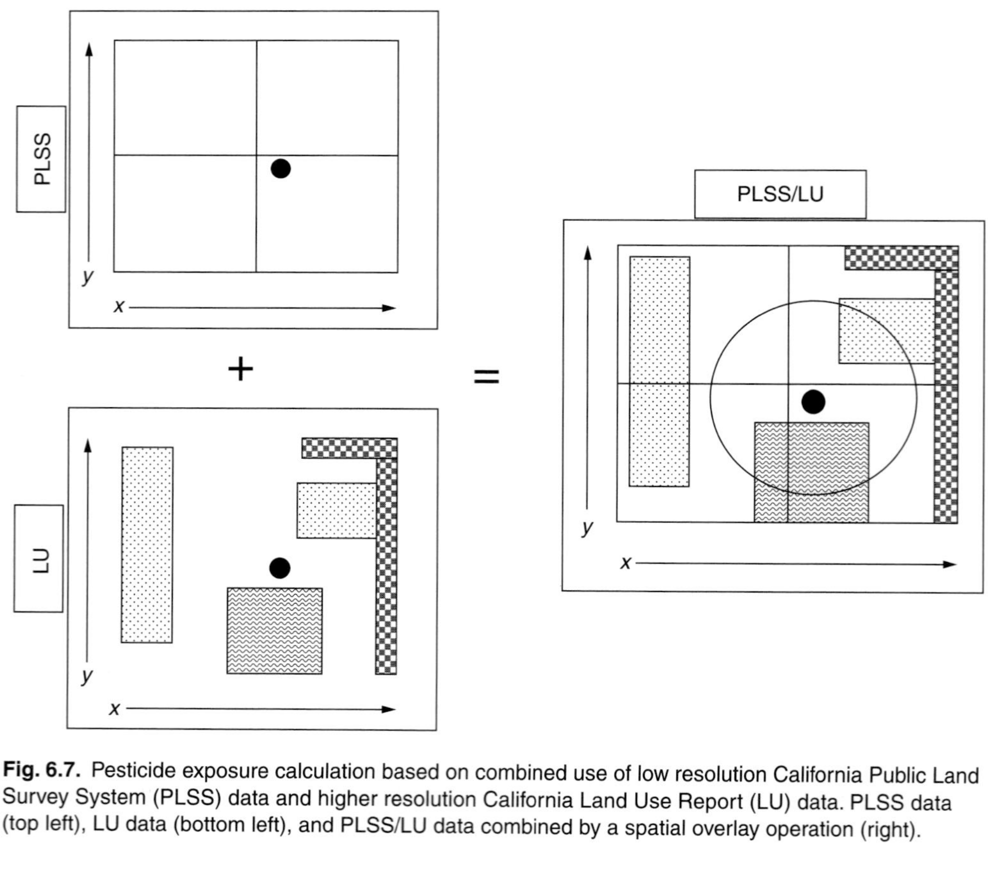

Fig. 6.7. Pesticide exposure calculation based on combined use of low resolution California Public Land Survey System (PLSS) data and higher resolution California Land Use Report (LU) data. PLSS data (top left), LU data (bottom left), and PLSS/LU data combined by a spatial overlay operation (right).

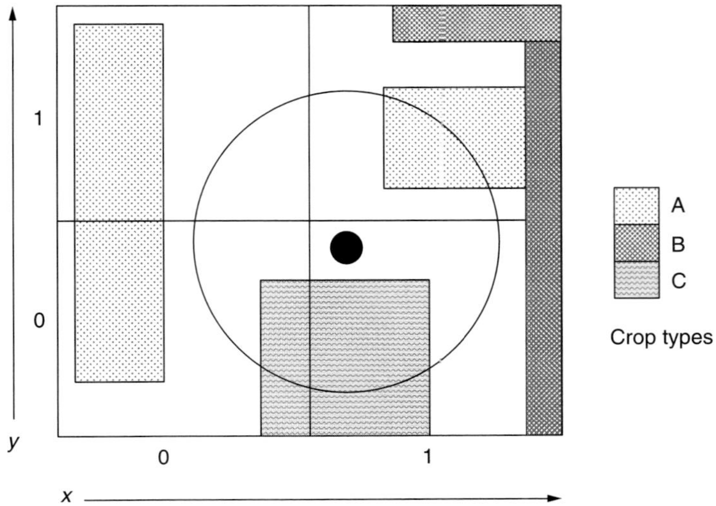

Fig. 6.8. Example pesticide exposure classification based on the PLSS/LU map shown in Fig. 6.7 (right) with a buffered geocoded address. See caption to Fig. 6.7 for more information.

LU data can be used to more accurately predict whether or not a subject should be classified as exposed to a chemical. Here, the LU data are employed via the spatial intersection overlay operation to more accurately calculate potential exposure values. Rull *et al.* (2001) and Rull and Ritz (2003) developed a hierarchical scheme to account for incorrect data within and inconsistencies between the three data sets they used: the PLSS grid cells, PUR database and LU polygons. These tiers represent level of uncertainty between the PUR data listing which chemicals were dispersed where, in what quantities and on what crops, versus what the surveyed LU assignments were and how their temporal accuracy degrades over time as land, and in particular crop fields, are repurposed over time.

A tier 1 match occurs in the case when the PUR record can be matched to a PLSS grid cell with the correct PLSS ID, and the PUR crop type exists within the PLSS/LU intersected data set. A tier 2 match occurs when the PLSS grid cell can be matched, but the PUR crop type does not exist in the PLSS/LU intersected data set. A tier 3 match occurs when the PLSS grid cell can be matched, but there are no crops within the PLSS/LU intersected data set.

For a tier 1 match, the chemical density from the PUR database is assumed to have been applied only to land from the PLSS/LU data set composed of fields of the particular crop types listed in the PUR database. For a tier 2 match, the chemical PUR density is assumed to have been applied to all of the crop fields within the PLSS/LU data set, taking into account that crop fields may have been repurposed in the years between LU surveys, and that any of the crop fields are equally likely targets for pesticide application. For a tier 3 match the density is assumed to have been applied to the entire one square mile PLSS grid cell, because there is no other information about where within the cell it could have been applied.

It should be noted that even at the highest resolution match, the spatial resolution of the PUR location (PLSS ID) and the locations of the typed crop fields (LU) are not enough to determine sub-field application areas. For instance, a pest may strike a small section of a field to which a chemical is then applied, but it is impossible to determine this from the available data. Thus, for tiers 1 and 2, if multiple fields of the same crop (tier 1) or different crops (tier 2) are within a PLSS grid cell, it is not known which one the chemical was applied to, so the most conservative assumption treats them all as equally likely. Further, the actual location within a field is not known, so again the most conservative assumption is to treat the entire area (of possibly more than one field) as an equally likely target for application. Therefore, the density calculations reflect this uncertainty by dispersing the density of the chemical from the PUR database (pounds/acres) over the whole area defined as the match area, at each of the tiers: total area of LU crop field of particular type within PLSS cell for tier 1; total area of all LU crop fields of any type within PLSS cell for tier 2; and total area of PLSS grid cell (one square mile) for tier 3.

An example LU polygon data set joined with the corresponding PLSS grid is depicted in Fig. 6.9, and illustrates the various options (i.e. tiers). Several examples from the PUR database for a few of these grid cells are shown in Table 6.1, which lists the chemical, the grid cell it was applied to, and the pounds and acres of the application. Table 6.1 also shows the tier the chemical was matched to along with the total number of fields of the particular crop type within the PLSS grid cell and the number of polygons produced of the particular crop type within the cell after the buffer around the subject has been used as the operation data set in an intersection spatial overlay operation with the LU polygons as the target data set.

For row 1 in Table 6.1, the PUR database reports that chemical *a* was distributed on crop type A in PLSS cell [1,0], but the LU lists no crops within this cell, resulting in a tier 3 match. For row 2, the PUR database reports that chemical *c* was distributed on crop type D within PLSS cell [0,0], but the LU does not report the crop type D as being within that cell, resulting in a tier 2 match. Additionally, there are three fields in PLSS cell [0,0], and the intersection with the individual's buffer results in three intersected polygons being produced as independent spatial geometric objects. In row 3, the PUR database reports that chemical *b* was applied to crop type B, which exists within the LU data for the correct PLSS cell, resulting in a tier 1 match, with a total of two crop type B fields, and one intersect being created. Row 4 is also a tier 1 match, with one crop type A field in the PLSS cell and one intersect being created.

6.4.7 Exposure calculation with LU crop polygons

The buffer-based approach outlined as an extension to the work of Bell *et al.* (2001) was applied as an extension to the work of Rull *et al.* (2001) and Rull and Ritz (2003) by Nuckols *et al.* (2007), and also by Cockburn

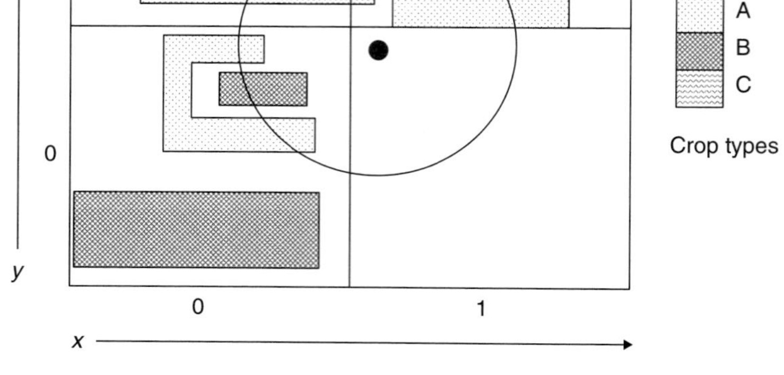

Fig. 6.9. An example LU (California Land Use Report) polygon data set of crop fields joined with the corresponding PLSS (California Public Land Survey System) grid distribution.

et al. (2011) and Wang *et al.* (2011). The densities used to calculate exposure estimates were calculated as proportions of the total LU polygon sections created through the intersection spatial overlay operation of the LU data (target data set) and the buffered geocoded address data (operation data set) as shown in Fig. 6.10, derived from the LU depicted in Fig. 6.8.

6.4.8 Generalization of the exposure estimation process

What should be clear at this point is that there are a fundamental series of data sources and operations required for any exposure assessment study. These fundamental components of the exposure estimation process are modelled in Fig. 6.11, which shows the types of processing performed. These operations are to (i) create a catchment area (b); (ii) obtain the exposure areas; (iii) calculate the exposure per area; and (iv) combine each individual exposure into a total exposure. This workflow is, of course, extremely generalized and has been specifically designed to encompass the four exposure estimation models described so far, which are (in order of increasing complexity): (i) Bell *et al.* (2001); (ii) Bell *et al.* (2001) extended; (iii) Rull *et al.* (2001) and Rull and Ritz (2003); (iv) Nuckols *et al.* (2007), Cockburn *et al.* (2011) and Wang *et al.* (2011). The spatial processes performed within a GIS, as shown in Fig. 6.12, are geocoding (Fig. 6.12a), buffering (Fig. 6.12b) and the intersection spatial overlay operation (Fig. 6.12c).

6.4.9 Flexibility

The preceding example studies illustrate one of the main benefits that spatial overlay operators bring to environmental exposure assessment: flexibility. This flexibility can be described in terms of the number and types of exposure data it can employ (i.e. exposure data sets), the variety of geographic objects that can be used within the spatial intersection operations (e.g.

Table 6.1. Example chemical application tiers of certainty for crops in California from PUR–LU–PLSS (Pesticide Use Report–Land Use Reports–Public Land Survey System) data.

Row	Chemical	Cell	Crop	Pounds	Acres	Tier	Fields	Intersects
1	*a*	[1,0]	A	25	300	3	0	0
2	c	[0,0]	D	15	30	2	3	3
3	*b*	[0,0]	B	10	100	1	2	1
4	*a*	[0,0]	A	20	60	1	1	2

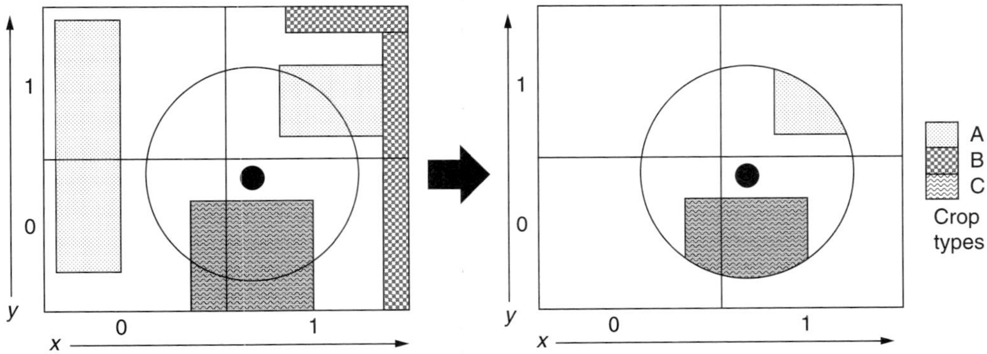

Fig. 6.10. Pesticide exposure estimation calculated as proportions of total LU polygon sections created by intersection spatial overlay of the LU target data set and the buffer-based geocoded address (operation data set), derived from the LU depicted in Fig. 6.8.

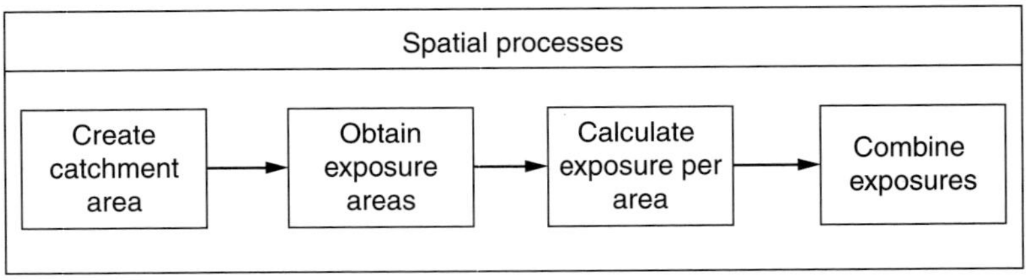

Fig. 6.11. Fundamental components of the pesticide exposure estimation process showing the types of processing performed.

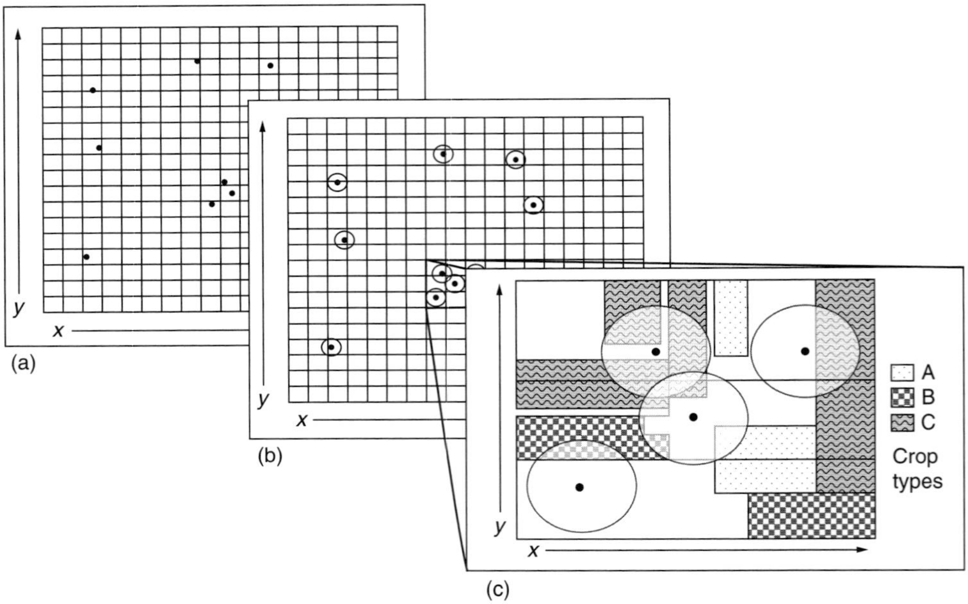

Fig. 6.12. The spatial processing components performed within a geographic information system for the estimation of pesticide exposure: (a) geocoding; (b) buffering; and (c) the intersection spatial overlay operation.

circular buffer, wind rose buffer), the mathematical operations that can be used to derive exposure estimates based on different criteria (e.g. per PLSS grid cell, per crop field, tiered), and the support for multiple methods of combining per-area spatial exposures into a single exposure for the individual.

By implementing an exposure model as a series of spatial overlay operations, new hypotheses, data sets and heuristics can easily be incorporated into that model as it is developed. For example, in the work presented by Bell *et al.* (2001) (extended), Rull *et al.* (2001) and Rull and Ritz (2003), Nuckols *et al.* (2007), Cockburn *et al.* (2011) and Wang *et al.* (2011) a circular buffer size was used. GIS and spatial overlay operations enable the buffer size to become another variable to the process. As such, each subject can have its exposure estimated by buffers of varying sizes, e.g. at constant steps, such as all buffer sizes from 10 m to 10,000 m at 10 m intervals.

6.5 Conclusion

This chapter has introduced the types of spatial overlay operations that can be performed within GIS applications and illustrated their usages within several spatially based health contexts. The case study analysis that was included explored ways in which health science researchers have utilized spatial overlays to assess environmental exposure assessment. These studies have illustrated that spatial overlay operations are flexible and capable of handling many forms of input data (points, lines and polygons). Each specific overlay operation has a role in the analytical pipeline of spatially based health research. The techniques provide analytical capabilities for developing models and generating data for subsequent epidemiological and other health-related investigations. The challenge for health science researchers is utilize these techniques in appropriate ways and to the fullest extent of their power.

Acknowledgements

This work was supported in part by the National Institute of Environmental Health Sciences (grants ES10544, U54ES12078 and P30 ES07048), the National Cancer Institute (grants CA110846 and N01-PC-35139), the Centers for Disease Control and Prevention (cooperative agreement 1H13EH000793-01), the National Institute of Neurological Disorders and Stroke (grant NS 038367) and the Department of Defense Prostate Cancer Research Program (grant 051037); in addition, initial pilot funding was provided by the American Parkinson's Disease Association. The contents of this work are solely the responsibility of the authors and do not necessarily reflect the official views of any of these sponsors.

References

Bayer-Oglesby, L., Grize, L., Gassner, M., Takken-Sahli, K., Sennhauser, F.H., Neu, U., Schindler, C. and Braun-Fahrländer, C.(2005) Decline of ambient air pollution levels and improved respiratory health in Swiss children. *Environmental Health Perspectives* 113, 1632–1637.

Bell, E.M., Hertz-Picciotto, I. and Beaumont, J.J. (2001) A case-control study of pesticides and fetal death due to congenital anomalies. *Epidemiology* 12, 148–156.

Bowman, D.M.J.S. and Johnston, F.H. (2005) Wildfire smoke, fire management, and human health. *EcoHealth* 2, 76–80.

Brody, J.G., Vorhees, D.J., Melly, S.J., Swedis, S.R., Drivas, P.J. and Rudel, R.A. (2002) Using GIS and historical records to reconstruct residential exposure to large-scale pesticide application. *Journal of Exposure Analysis and Environmental Epidemiology* 12, 64–80.

Brody, J.G., Aschengrau, A., McKelvey, W., Rudel, R.A., Swartz, C.H. and Kennedy, T. (2004) Breast cancer risk and historical exposure to pesticides from wide-area applications assessed with GIS. *Environmental Health Perspectives* 112, 889–897.

California Department of Pesticide Regulation (2000) Pesticide use reporting: an overview of California's unique full reporting system. Sacramento, California. Available at: http://www.cdpr.ca.gov/docs/pur/purovrvw/ovr52000.pdf (accessed 18 March 2013).

California Department of Water Resources (2005) Land Use Survey Overview. Division of Statewide Integrated Water Management Water Use and Efficiency, Sacramento, California. Available at: http://www.water.ca.gov/landwateruse/lusrvymain.cfm (accessed 18 March 2013).

Chen, J., Li, C., Li, Z. and Gold, C. (2001) A Voronoi-based 9-intersection model for spatial relations. *International Journal of Geographical Information Science* 15, 201–220.

Cockburn, M., Mills, P., Zhang, X.Z., Zadnick, J., Goldberg, D. and Ritz, B. (2011) Prostate cancer and ambient pesticide exposure in agriculturally intensive areas in California. *American Journal of Epidemiology* 173, 1280–1288.

Egenhofer, M. (1991) Reasoning about binary topological relations. In: Günther, O. and Schek, H. (eds) *Proceedings of the Second International Symposium on Advances in Spatial Databases (August 28–30, 1991)*. Lecture Notes in Computer Science, Vol. 525, Springer Verlag, Berlin, pp. 143–160.

Frankenberg, E., McKee, D. and Thomas, D. (2005) Health consequences of forest fires in Indonesia. *Demography* 42, 109–129.

Johnston, F.H., Webby, R.J., Pilotto, L.S., Bailie, R.S., Parry, D.L. and Halpin, S.J. (2006) Vegetation fires, particulate air pollution and asthma: a panel study in the Australian monsoon tropics. *International Journal of Environmental Health Research* 16, 391–404.

Künzli, N. *et al.* (2000) Public-health impact of outdoor and traffic-related air pollution: a European assessment. *The Lancet* 356, 795–801.

Marusek, J.C., Cockburn, M.G., Mills, P.K. and Ritz, B.R. (2006) Control selection and pesticide exposure assessment via GIS in prostate cancer studies. *American Journal of Preventive Medicine* 30, 109–116.

Nafstad, P., Haheim, L.L., Wisløff, T., Gram, F., Oftedal, B., Holme, I., Hjermann, I. and Leren, P. (2004) Urban air pollution and mortality in a cohort of Norwegian men. *Environmental Health Perspectives* 112, 610–616.

Nuckols, J., Gunier, R., Riggs, P. Miller, R., Reynolds, P. and Ward, M.H. (2007) Linkage of the California Pesticide Use Reporting Database with spatial land use data for exposure assessment. *Environmental Health Perspectives* 115, 684–689.

Reynolds, P., Hurley, S.E., Gunier, R.B., Yerabati, S., Quach, T. and Hertz, A. (2005) Residential proximity to agricultural pesticide use and incidence of breast cancer in California, 1988–1997. *Environmental Health Perspectives* 113, 993–1000.

Rigel, E.G., Lebwohl, M., Rigel, A.C. and Rigel, D.S. (2003) Daily UVB exposure levels in high-school students measured with digital dosimeters. *Journal of the American Academy of Dermatology* 49, 1112–1114.

Rull, R.P. and Ritz, B. (2003) Historical pesticide exposure in California using pesticide use reports and land-use surveys: an assessment of misclassification error and bias. *Environmental Health Perspectives* 111, 1582–1589.

Rull, R.P., Ritz, B., Krishnadasan, A. and Maglinte, G. (2001) Modeling historical exposures from residential proximity to pesticide applications. In: *Proceedings of the Twenty-First Annual ESRI User Conference, San Diego, California, July 9–13, 2001.* Esri, Redlands, California. Available at: http://proceedings.esri.com/library/userconf/proc01/professional/papers/pap401/p401.htm (accessed 15 March 2013).

Rull, R.P., Ritz, B. and Shaw, G.M. (2006) Neural tube defects and maternal residential proximity to agricultural pesticide applications. *American Journal of Epidemiology* 163, 743–753.

Steinmaus, C., Lu, M., Todd, R.L. and Smith, A.H. (2004) Probability estimates for the unique childhood leukemia cluster in Fallon, Nevada, and risks near other US military aviation facilities. *Environmental Health Perspectives* 112, 766–772.

Tatalovich, Z., Wilson, J.P. and Cockburn, M.A. (2006) A comparison of Thiessen polygon, kriging, and spline models of potential UV exposure. *Cartography and Geographic Information Science* 33, 217–231.

Thieden, E., Philipsen, P.A., Heydenreich, J. and Wulf, H.C. (2004) UV radiation exposure related to age, sex, occupation, and sun behavior based on time-stamped personal dosimeter readings. *Archives of Dermatology* 140, 197–203.

Viswanathan, S., Eria, L., Diunugala, N., Johnson, J. and Mcclean, C. (2006) An analysis of effects of San Diego wildfire on ambient air quality. *Journal of the Air and Waste Management Association* 56, 56–67.

Wang, A., Costello, S., Cockburn, M., Zhang, X., Bronstein, J. and Ritz, B. (2011) Parkinson's disease risk from ambient exposure to ziram, maneb, and paraquat at work and home. *International Journal of Epidemiology* 26, 547–555.

Ward, M.H., Nuckols, J.R., Weigel, S.J., Maxwell, S.K., Cantor, K.P. and Miller, R.S. (2000) Identifying populations potentially exposed to agricultural pesticides using remote sensing and a geographic information system. *Environmental Health Perspectives* 108, 5–12.

7 Spatial Cluster Analysis

Jin Chen*
AT&T Shannon Laboratory, Florham Park, New Jersey, USA

7.1 Introduction

Spatial cluster analysis plays an important role in many areas of public health. It can help to identify locations that have unusually high or low disease occurrence, health care availability and health care utilization. Confirmed clusters can be used to define the areas that are worthy of further investigation and possible intervention.

This chapter provides an overview of the basic concepts and techniques of spatial cluster analysis along with a novel geovisual analytics approach for enhancing the detection and interpretation of spatial clusters. Because colour is an integral part of this geovisual analytic approach, colour versions of the figures that are included in the chapter are available at www.albany.edu/fboscoe/gisbook.

7.2 Definitions

A spatial cluster is most commonly defined as a group of neighbouring objects that are more similar to each other than to objects outside the cluster (Han and Kamber, 2006). Simply put, similar objects are grouped into the same cluster. Therefore, this type of cluster is generally referred to as *similarity-based cluster*. Knox (1989) described a similarity-based disease cluster as a geographically and/or temporally bounded group of disease occurrences related to each other through some social or biological mechanism, or having a common relationship with some other event or circumstance. An example of this type of cluster is a group of neighbouring places that have significantly higher disease rates than the surrounding places; such an area may also share some distinct environmental or socio-economic characteristics that could relate to the disease.

In addition, Han *et al.* (2001) defined a *density-based cluster* as a 'density region of objects in the data space which are separated by regions of low density'. From a statistical perspective, Knox (1989) also defined a density-based cluster as 'a geographically bounded group of occurrences of sufficient size and concentration to be unlikely to have occurred by chance'. This type of cluster is in contrast to complete spatial randomness, which defines a situation where 'an event is equally likely to occur at any location within the study area' (Waller and Gotway, 2004), as illustrated in Fig. 7.1. This definition of cluster has been widely adopted in the public health literature (Cromley and McLafferty, 2002; Lawson,

* E-mail: jinchen1000@gmail.com

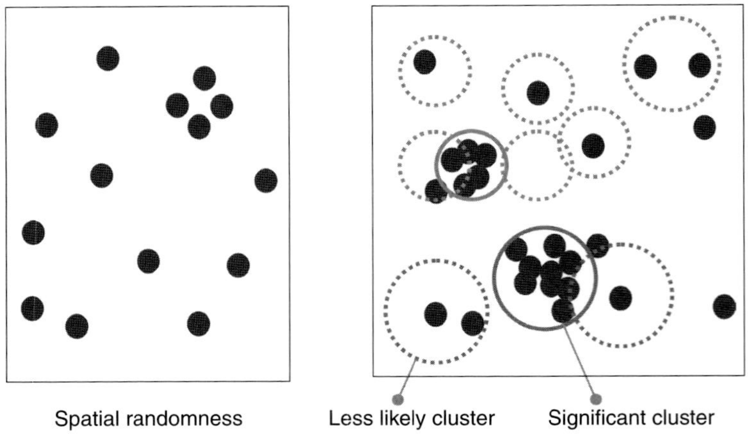

Fig. 7.1. Spatial randomness versus spatial clustering. In spatial randomness (left image), events occur at any location with an equal chance. In contrast, a significant spatial cluster (right image) contains an unusual concentration of events.

2006). Put simply, a disease cluster is any area of significant elevated risk for a disease within the study region (Lawson, 2006); this is often referred to as a hot-spot cluster. An example of this type of spatial cluster is a high-risk region for a disease; this has a significantly higher number of cases within the boundary of the cluster than in the region outside the boundary.

These two types of spatial clusters – similarity based and density based – represent different spatial entities and can be used for addressing different public health problems. In Fig. 7.2, the two types of cluster are shown illustrating disease rates. On the left, a similarity-based cluster represents a group of neighbouring places with similar mortality rates of a disease. The mortality rates within the cluster vary little, but are significantly higher than in the places outside the cluster. In contrast, the density-based cluster has an overall significantly high mortality rate within its boundary. However, the mortality rates of individual places within the cluster are not necessarily similar; put another way, the within-cluster variance can be large. Density-based clusters are often more interesting than similarity-based clusters in epidemiology research. For example, epidemiologists are interested in spatial clusters with a high concentration of disease incidence where the rates are significantly high overall, rather than in the similarity of the incidence rates within a cluster.

Figure 7.3 illustrates the application of a similarity-based clustering method (LISA) and a density-based clustering method (SaTScan) to US cervical cancer mortality data (as standardized mortality ratios) for the years 2000 to 2004. The similarity-based spatial clusters (left) and the density-based spatial clusters (right) are identified and shown on the maps. Specifically, the LISA method identifies similarity-based clusters by describing the *spatial autocorrelation* among places, i.e. the extent to which particular places are similar to, or different from, their neighbours. As a result, LISA classifies the spatial clusters into four types of association patterns: high–high, low–low, high–low, low–high. The high–high and low–low patterns (those with positive local spatial autocorrelation) are typically referred to as spatial clusters, while the high–low and low–high patterns (those with negative local spatial autocorrelation) are considered to be spatial outliers, as detailed in Anselin (2009). In this case, the high–high patterns in the map (understood as high-risk places adjacent to high-risk places), are considered to be spatial clusters of high risk for cervical cancer mortality. It should be kept in mind that the spatial clusters identified by LISA only refer to the core of the clusters. The true boundaries of the clusters are likely to extend to the neighbouring places as well. In contrast, the density-based clustering

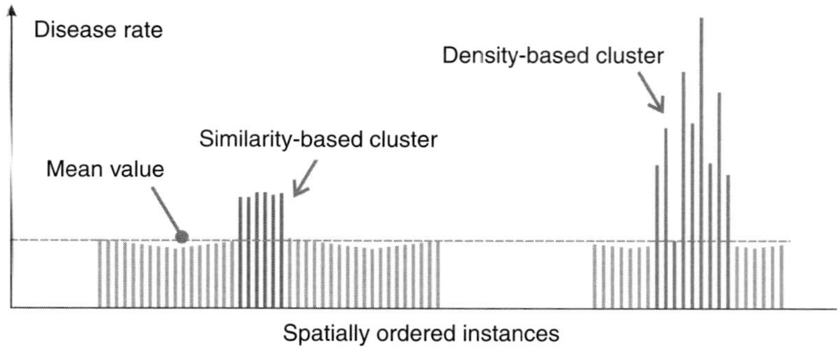

Fig. 7.2. Two types of spatial clusters: similarity-based clusters versus density-based clusters. The vertical bars represent a disease rate at a location. The similarity-based cluster (left) has locations with similar disease rates. The density-based cluster (right) has locations with high rates, but their rates are not necessarily similar (so the variance could be large).

method – SaTScan – detected high-risk spatial clusters for cervical cancer mortality that covered much broader geographic areas. Compared with these density-based clusters, the LISA method misses some important clusters that have many high-risk places, but less similarity within the clusters (as shown in Fig. 7.3).

In summary, public health researchers need to carefully consider which types of spatial clusters can represent the spatial objects/processes involved in the problems at hand, and choose appropriate spatial clustering methods accordingly. Section 7.3 (next) briefly reviews the two types of spatial clustering methods.

7.3 Clustering Methods for Geographic Data Analysis

The data mining community has developed many clustering algorithms, as detailed by Han and Kamber (2006). Some of these algorithms can be applied to geographic data analysis. These methods can be categorized as partitioning methods, hierarchical methods and density-based methods, as discussed in Han *et al.* (2009). In addition, the statistics community has also developed numerous clustering methods (Hastie *et al.*, 2001), particularly scan statistics (Glaz and Balakrishnan, 1999), which can be used to identify clustering in point data. Some of these have also been extended to aggregated data. Furthermore, the geography community has a long history of developing methods for point pattern analysis (O'Sullivan and Unwin, 2003; Smith *et al.*, 2008). In recent years, geographers have extended some classic clustering methods and applied them to the analysis of geographically referenced data. Rather than review all of these methods, here I focus only on those methods that apply to the detection of similarity-based clusters and density-based spatial clusters.

7.3.1 Similarity-based clustering

Traditional spatial statistics and exploratory spatial data analysis methods were developed to identify two types of clustering – global and local – both involving the concept of spatial autocorrelation. Spatial autocorrelation is observed when measurements made at nearby locations are more related (either similar or dissimilar) than they are at distant locations. The identification of global clustering involves testing the existence of spatial autocorrelation across geographic space, without necessarily indicating any specific clusters. Global clustering can be measured by a series of methods including Moran's I, Geary's C and G-Statistics (Anselin, 1994, 1996; Getis, 1999). The identification of local clustering involves measuring local autocorrelation or association and defining clusters in specific locations. Methods for this include Anselin's Local

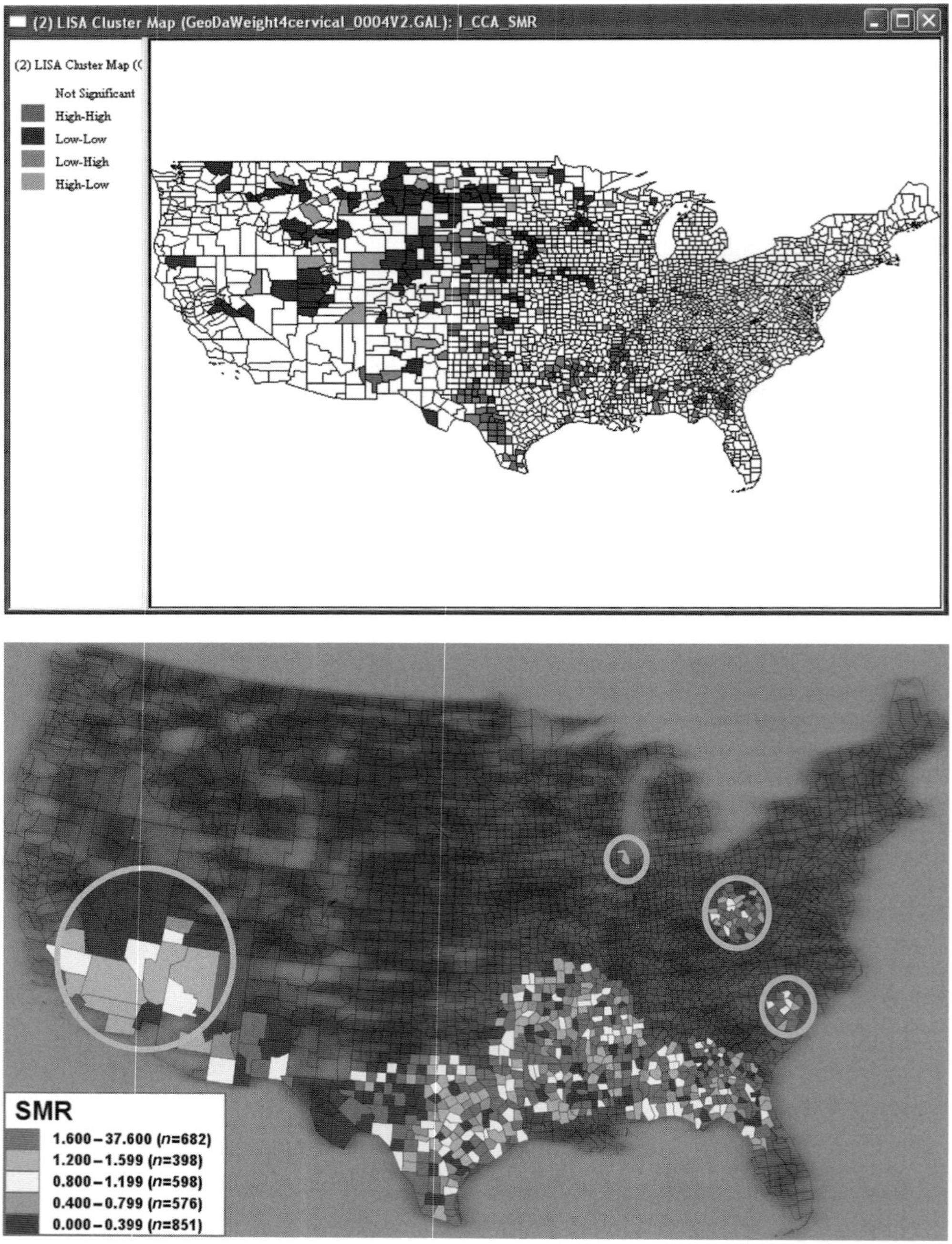

Fig. 7.3. Methods for detecting similarity-based clusters and density-based clusters of cervical cancer mortality in the USA. The maps display the standardized mortality ratio (SMR). Top: similarity-based, high-risk spatial clusters reported by the LISA (similarity-based clustering) method using GeoDa 0.9.5. Bottom: density-based spatial clusters reported by Kulldorff's spatial scan statistic using SaTScan, with results displayed in the Visual Inquiry Toolkit (VIT). The LISA method misses some important clusters reported by the spatial scan statistic, as shown in the circles in the bottom plot. Although these clusters do not have highly similar values in terms of SMR, the majority of values in them have a high SMR, and so are interesting to epidemiologists.

Indicator of Spatial Association (LISA) (Anselin, 1995), local G-Statistics (Getis and Ord, 1992; Ord and Getis, 1995) as well as their extensions, such as the AMOEBA method (Aldstadt and Getis, 2006). While these methods help to identify local hot spots and outliers, they are limited in identifying regional and national clusters in large data sets, as illustrated in Fig. 7.3. In addition, because the methods employ z-score methods and thus assume a Gaussian data distribution, they are limited in dealing with highly skewed spatial data, which includes much public health data (Conley *et al.*, 2005). Other researchers also criticize the normality and randomization assumptions employed by the methods, which 'are generally inappropriate for testing with heterogeneous count data' (Waller and Gotway, 2004; p. 230).

The similarity-based clustering methods have some further limitations when they are applied to public health data. First, many epidemiological studies are more interested in detecting density-based clusters. Secondly, many of the clustering methods are descriptive rather than inferential – the methods can describe a 'cluster' of places that are similar or associated, but do not statistically confirm their validity (i.e. with a test of significance). Finally, many of these methods do not consider the sizes of the populations at risk, and as a result suffer from the small numbers problem, where measurements made in small population areas are less reliable than are those in large population areas. The small numbers problem cannot be ignored when studying rare diseases (e.g. cervical cancer); a detailed discussion on this issue can be found in Cromley and McLafferty (2002) and Elliott and Wartenberg (2004).

7.3.2 Density-based clustering

Methods for identifying density-based clusters were initially developed for detecting clusters in point patterns, where the data are a set of locations for point objects (e.g. individual residences). A classic method for this purpose is the Geographical Analysis Machine (GAM) (Openshaw *et al.*, 1987), which was developed by the geography community. This method was later extended for the analysis of areal data. The GAM method suffers from some severe problems (Kulldorff and Nagarwalla, 1995; O'Sullivan and Unwin, 2003; p. 122; Waller and Gotway, 2004; p. 176). Most notably, it generates overlapping circles and hence identifies overlapping (and consequently redundant) clusters. Significance tests in overlapping circles are not independent of one another, thereby leading to many false 'significant' clusters. This is commonly known as the multiple testing problem. Rooted in the GAM idea, several methods (e.g. PROCLUDE) (Conley *et al.*, 2005; Duczmal *et al.*, 2007) employ a genetic algorithm to improve computational performance. However, these methods do not directly address the problem of testing cluster significance; additionally, genetic algorithms are not easy to use, requiring complex configuration. Therefore, clusters identified by GAM and its variations are usually considered only as exploratory (for identifying areas of potential concerns) rather than confirmatory (for identifying significant clusters).

Kulldorff's spatial scan statistic (Kulldorff, 1997), which was developed by the statistics community and is well known through the free SaTScan software program (www.satscan.org), substantially extended the idea of GAM and addressed the multiple testing issues that it involved by adopting a slightly different inferential framework. Instead of testing significance for each possible cluster as GAM does, Kulldorff's spatial scan statistic focuses on the single potential cluster that produces the maximum likelihood ratio, in this way adjusting for the problem of multiple testing (Waller and Gotway, 2004). So Kulldorff's spatial scan statistic is not only descriptive, but also confirmatory – it both identifies local clusters and also statistically verifies them. The method has been widely adopted in the public health and social science communities, and is perhaps the most frequently used cluster detection method in spatial epidemiology (Bhowmick *et al.*, 2008). The remainder of this chapter will focus on this method, its limitations and a novel visual analytics method designed to enhance the method and address its limitations.

7.4 The Spatial Scan Statistic

Kulldorff's spatial scan statistic method is implemented in the free software tool called SaTScan (Kulldorff and Information Management Services, 2006), which has been widely adopted for detecting disease clusters (Jemal *et al.*, 2002;

Mostashari, 2003; Sheehan *et al.*, 2004; Huang *et al.*, 2008). The first part of the name SaTScan is an abbreviation for Space and Time – the software can identify clusters in space and/or time, though this chapter is only concerned with spatial clusters. The spatial scan statistic and the SaTScan software are described in detail by Kulldorff and colleagues in a series of papers (Kulldorff and Nagarwalla, 1995; Kulldorff, 1997, 2001; Kulldorff *et al.*, 2006). The statistic is summarized here to provide context for the geovisual analytics approach that we introduce for enhancing interaction with and interpretation of the SaTScan results.

7.4.1 Description

Kulldorff's spatial scan statistic method places a circular scanning window at each of the point locations within a study area. At each of these point locations, the radius of the circle is varied from a size of zero (i.e. covering only a single point) to a user-defined maximum radius. In this manner, the method generates a large number of distinct circular windows, each including a different set of neighbouring points for the clustering test. The windows that have a significantly high concentration of events are considered to be 'spatial clusters', while the other windows – shown as dashed circles in Fig. 7.1 (right) – are discarded. The null hypothesis of the Kulldorff spatial scan statistic states that the event is randomly distributed in geographic space and that the expected event count is proportional to the population at risk (which may be adjusted by age or other covariates). The alternative hypothesis is that there is an increased number of events within an area compared with those in the outside areas. For any circular window, if the null hypothesis is statistically rejected, then the geographic area defined by the scan window can be considered as a spatial cluster.

For each circle, rejection of the null hypothesis is based on a likelihood ratio statistic. The likelihood ratio is proportional to the expression shown in Eqn 7.1:

$$\left(\frac{C}{e}\right)^{c}\left(\frac{C-c}{C-e}\right)^{C-c} I() \qquad (7.1)$$

where C is the total number of cases, c is the observed number of cases within a circle, e is the adjusted expected number of cases within the circle and $I()$ is a binary indicator that facilitates the identification of high-risk clusters ('hot spots') and/or low-risk clusters ('cold spots'). When SaTScan is set to scan for high-risk clusters, $I()$ is equal to '1' when $c>e$ and equal to '0' otherwise; for low-risk clusters, $c>e$ would change to $c<e$; and for both types of clusters, $I() = 1$ (Kulldorff, 2006). The circle with the maximum likelihood ratio among all radius sizes at all possible point locations is considered to be the most likely cluster (called the *primary cluster*). SaTScan calculates and reports a logarithm of the likelihood ratio (LLR) for each cluster. As described in the SaTScan User Guide, to evaluate the statistical significance of the primary cluster, 'a large number of random replications of the data set are generated under the null hypothesis. The p-value is obtained through Monte Carlo hypothesis testing, by comparing the rank of the maximum likelihood from the real data set with the maximum likelihoods from random data sets. If this rank is R, then the p-value = $R/(1 + \#$ simulations)' (Kulldorff, 2006; p. 16). In SaTScan, the default value for the number of simulations is 999.

SaTScan also identifies *secondary clusters* that have significantly large likelihood ratios but are not the primary cluster (Kulldorff, 1997). If the secondary clusters do not overlap the primary cluster, then they are of great interest as they are able to reject the null hypothesis on the basis of their own strength (Kulldorff, 2006); these clusters can be considered to be spatial clusters as well.

7.4.2 Detecting spatial clusters with SaTScan

This section briefly illustrates how SaTScan was used to detect the cervical cancer clusters in the USA that are used as an example in the remainder of the chapter. For the purely spatial analysis performed here, the input data consisted of three files: (i) a case file, with each record in the file containing a location ID (here, a code indicating a US county) and the number of disease events occurring in this location; (ii) a population file, with a location ID and the population at the location; and (iii) a coordinates file, with a location ID and a latitude and longitude of a central point. These files were selected using the Input tab in SaTScan. In the Analysis tab, the Poisson model was selected; the Poisson model is suitable for rare events such as cervical cancer. In order to apply the visual analytics approach described later, the Output tab was set to include the output all of the optional text files. Finally, in the Advanced Output Features dialogue page, accessible via the Output tab, there is an option to set the Maximum Reported Spatial Cluster Size. This value is the maximum radius of the scan circle specified by users, and is subsequently referred to as the *maximum size* parameter. This parameter can set an upper bound on the circle radius in one of two ways: (i) by specifying the maximum percentage of the total population at risk within the circle; or (ii) by specifying the geographic extent of the circle. The former method is the default and is used in the research reported here. When setting the maximum size based upon population at risk, the default maximum size value, as recommended in the SaTScan user guide, is set to 50% of the total population at risk. To run multiple scans (e.g. 50 scans, as suggested later), the user needs to set the parameter with various values (i.e. 50 values from 1 to 50% with steps of 1) and rename 'output file' accordingly (e.g. US_cervical_cancer_1pct.txt and US_cervical_cancer_50pct.txt).

7.4.3 Limitations

SaTScan has made the spatial scan statistic widely accessible, and has had a substantial impact on numerous domains in which spatial clusters are of interest (e.g. crime analysis, ecology, epidemiology; see http://www.satscan.org/references.html). However, two issues make the use of the method and interpretation of its results problematic: (i) the current version of SaTScan (version 9.1.1 at the time of this writing) lacks cartographic support for understanding the clusters in a geographic context; and (ii) results from the method are sensitive to the selection of scaling parameters, but the system provides no direct support for making these choices. Each of these issues is discussed below.

First, SaTScan does not provide cartographic support to view the identified clusters, nor a visual interface to explore cluster characteristics. Geographic information about the identified clusters (e.g. the centre location, the cluster radius, data entities included in each cluster) is available only as text. A sample of the SaTScan result that is obtained is listed below:

MOST LIKELY CLUSTER
1. Location IDs included: 22063, 22005, 22105, 22033, 22095, 22091, 22093, 22037, 22121, 22047 [location_ID - FIPS code of counties]

Coordinates / radius	(30.435485 N, 90.722813 W) / 660.75 km
Population	75226248
Number of cases	2627
Expected cases	1964.53
Annual cases/100000	3.7
Observed/expected	1.337
Relative risk	1.388
Log likelihood ratio	113.293401
Monte Carlo rank	1/1000
P-value	0.001

In order to visualize the geographic location and size of the clusters, a user must process this textual output and export it to geographical information system (GIS) software (e.g. ArcGIS). This is a time-consuming process and inhibits the interactive exploration of multiple parameter configurations for the interpretation of the results. Because of this limitation, researchers often simply choose default parameters or make some other arbitrary choices that do not reflect the characteristics of the geographic phenomena. Further, in published examples (Jemal *et al.*, 2002; Hsu *et al.*, 2004; Fukuda *et al.*, 2005), the data under study (e.g. aggregated disease data) and the SaTScan clusters are typically depicted on two separate maps, making the interpretation of SaTScan clusters relative to the original data set difficult. In one of the few efforts to address this problem, Boscoe *et al.* (2003) propose a single integrated map that combines the likelihood ratio with relative risk. Here, the proposed methodology builds from this core idea of integrating cluster output with relative risk information and takes advantage of both established and novel interactive geovisualization methods to enhance the understanding of SaTScan results.

Secondly, it is difficult to determine an optimal setting for SaTScan scaling parameters (Waller and Gotway, 2004; Fukuda *et al.*, 2005). Confusing and even misleading results are possible if the parameter choices are made arbitrarily. The focus of the research presented here is on the aforementioned maximum size parameter. The default maximum size setting of 50% seldom produces usable and informative results because the reported primary cluster often occupies a large proportion of the study area (Haining, 2003). The task of determining the most appropriate maximum size is challenging. This choice can be context dependent and is influenced both by the geographic scale of processes leading to clusters and by the research goals. Furthermore, too large a maximum size can hide small, homogeneous clusters within larger, heterogeneous clusters, and too small a maximum size can miss significant, regional-level clusters. SaTScan provides limited guidance for the selection of an appropriate maximum size value. Moreover, our research to address this problem prompted a broader question on the sensitivity of SaTScan results to parameter choices.

The sensitivity of SaTScan to the maximum size parameter has two components. The first is that SaTScan clusters tend to contain heterogeneous contents, particularly when using large maximum size values. Such clusters are composed not only of the high-risk locations that are of interest in epidemiological cluster detection, but also of many low-risk locations that are not of interest. The second component of sensitivity to the maximum size parameter relates to the stability of clusters in terms of location and size as the maximum size value is varied. Adjustments to the maximum size parameter by only several percentage points may cause large shifts in both the location of identified clusters and their radii.

To address these two issues with SaTScan – the lack of cartographic output and sensitivity related to both heterogeneous content and circle centre/size instability – we propose a geovisual analytics approach to enhance interpretation of SaTScan results.

7.5 Geovisual Analytics of SaTScan Results

Geovisual analytics is a sub-area of the emerging research discipline of visual analytics, with specific focus on problems involving geographic phenomena (Andrienko *et al.*, 2007). Visual analytics is defined in the research agenda as 'the science of analytical reasoning facilitated by interactive visual interfaces' (Thomas and Cook, 2005; p. 4) Geovisual analytics allows users to interactively explore visual representations of geographic information, to recognize and process patterns/outliers from a visual scene, to link these patterns and outliers to existing mental schemata and knowledge bases, and to arrive at an appropriate course of action given the visual input (Johnson *et al.*, 2006; Keim *et al.*, 2006). The discipline of geovisual analytics can be used to enhance traditional methods of scientific inquiry to the end of gaining insight into geographic phenomena, drawing conclusions about these phenomena and directing subsequent scientific investigation or policy action (Keim *et al.*, 2006). The research reported here proposes a novel geovisual analytics approach that combines the strength of advanced visualization methods with the analytical capabilities of the spatial scan statistic. The approach used is demonstrated through the analysis of a data set on cervical cancer mortality data for the continental USA, aggregated by county and for the period 2000 to 2004. The research focus is to identify high-risk clusters of cervical cancer risk. The risk is measured in terms of the standardized mortality ratio (SMR) expressed as the ratio of observed to expected cases for each of the individual enumeration units in the studied area (Chen *et al.*, 2008b). The proposed approach is implemented in the Visual Inquiry Toolkit (VIT) (Chen and MacEachren, 2008; Chen *et al.*, 2008a), which was developed by the author and is available from the GeoVISTA Center at the Department of Geography of Pennsylvania State University (GeoVISTA Center, 2010).

The remainder of this section discusses how to use VIT to analyse the SaTScan results, followed by a discussion of the sensitivity of the SaTScan results to the maximum size parameter. The sensitivity is reflected in two ways: (i) heterogeneous content of clusters;

and (ii) instability of clusters in location and size. Finally, a general method for interactively visualizing SaTScan results is introduced, together with a reliability visualization method to address the sensitivity issues.

7.5.1 Analysing SaTScan results using the Visual Analytics Toolkit (VIT)

When analysing SaTScan results with VIT, two sets of input data are required: (i) the geospatial vector data in Esri shapefile format for displaying the geographic map; and (ii) spatial clusters data in DBF (DataBase File) format reported by SaTScan.

For the US cervical cancer analysis, the shapefile consists of 3105 US counties joined with SMR data in CSV (Comma-Separated Values) format. Loading the data is easy: simply click File > Open a data file, and open the shapefile (either a shapefile – .shp, or a .dbf file). A geographic map shows up displaying some data specified in the drop-down list on top of the map. In order to display the mortality risk of the data, simply click on the drop-down list, and choose the variable name of the SMR data – i.e. CCA_SMR in the sample data. VIT displays the SMR data in a geographic map.

To better interpret SaTScan results, the SMR data are classified into five categories: high risk, intermediate high risk, normal risk, intermediate low risk and low risk. The categories are encoded in diverging colours. The classification is done on the Visual Classifier screen (Fig. 7.4), within which we choose 'Univariate' classification and set the attribute to be classified as 'CCA_SMR'. The Visual Classifier provides several typical classification methods, including Quantiles and Equal Intervals. In this case, the 'Self defined' classification method is selected to set user-specified category boundaries. Specifically, the boundaries are set as 0.0, 0.4, 0.8, 1.2, 1.6 and 37.6 (the maximum value of the SMR values), as shown in the dialogue for 'Set boundary for categories' in Fig. 7.4. This dialogue pops up on clicking the 'set values' button on the right. The five categories are then coloured in a diverging colour scheme (by clicking the 'set colors' button); for example, orange represents high risk, blue low risk and white normal risk. Once these steps are completed, the geographic map will display the SMR data in the selected colours.

Next, we consider the SaTScan output data. The output for each scan produces a list of location IDs for each identified cluster. The user can load the output files of the scans into the VIT as a batch by specifying the folder

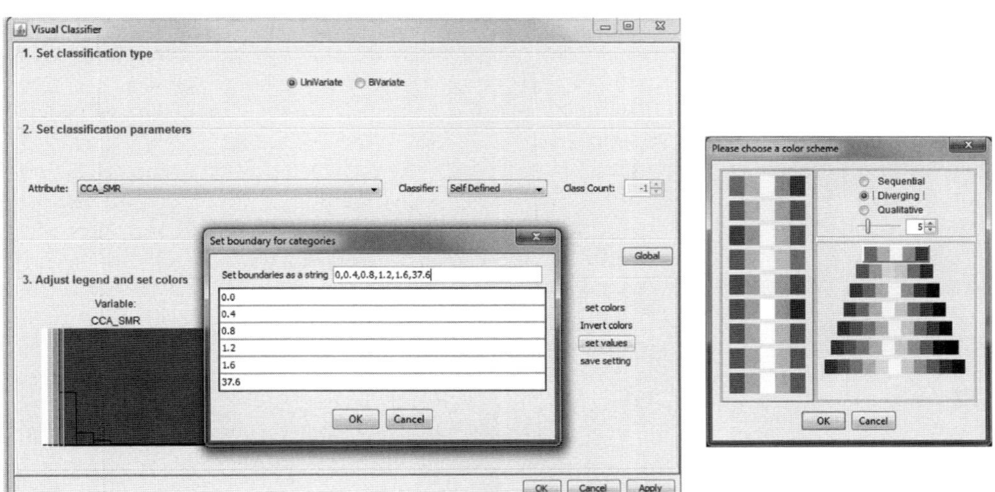

Fig. 7.4. Classification and colour-encoding of standardized mortality ratio (SMR) data for clusters of cervical cancer in the USA using the Visual Classifier.

where the files are stored in the computer. Specifically, click the menu SaTScan Tools > Import SaTScan Results, and in the popup dialogue, specify the folder. The results are then loaded into a tabular interface (shown in Fig. 7.7) and are listed under the 'SaTScan Outcomes' node on the left. This interface is linked dynamically to a choropleth map, so that clicking on a result will display the clusters on the geographic map.

7.5.2 Heterogeneous and core high-risk clusters

SaTScan often reports *heterogeneous clusters* – i.e. statistically significant clusters that contain a considerable number of low-risk places. A heterogeneous cluster usually contains smaller, homogeneous subsets that have sufficient statistical powers to reject the null hypothesis based on their own strength, as has been noted previously in the literature (Jemal *et al.*, 2002; Chen *et al.*, 2008b). The phenomenon is caused by the tendency of SaTScan 'to identify large areas with large populations but small elevations in risk, since such areas have the highest statistical power. Smaller clusters contained within these areas that have higher elevations in risk but lower, though statistically significant, likelihood ratios, are ignored' (Boscoe *et al.*, 2003; p. 274). While SaTScan identifies the larger clusters on statistical grounds, the core clusters are of more practical interest from both a research and policy perspective because a core cluster has homogeneous contents and is more stable against parameter variation (e.g. maximum size) than a heterogeneous cluster. In contrast, a heterogeneous cluster has heterogeneous contents and is unstable in terms of location and size under parameter variation. A heterogeneous cluster usually contains one or several core clusters. The existence of heterogeneous clusters is demonstrated as clusters A and C in Fig. 7.5, where the maximum size parameter is set to 40%.

To facilitate the identification of core clusters and avoid potentially misleading heterogeneous clusters, it is necessary to avoid the selection of an excessive maximum size value. For example, the core cluster B in Fig. 7.5 is

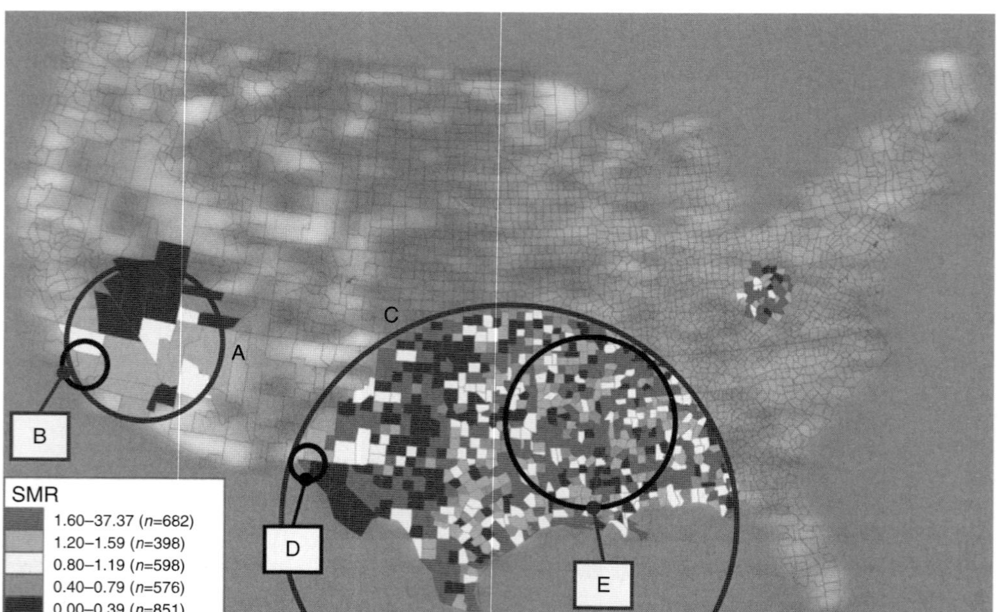

Fig. 7.5. Clusters of standardized mortality ratio (SMR) for cervical cancer in the USA: A and C, heterogeneous clusters; B, D and E, core clusters. Not all clusters in the data set are indicated in this figure.

reported as a significant cluster when the maximum size value is set to 4%. Although consisting of only Los Angeles County (in California), the cluster contains 3.4% of the US population at risk, thus has stronger statistical power than low-population places. As the maximum size is increased to more than 6%, the core cluster expands to the extent of cluster A in Fig. 7.5. Even though it is statistically valid, cluster A is a heterogeneous cluster because 52.4% of its counties (11 out of 21 counties) are not high risk. This example demonstrates that a core cluster may be a single county (as in cluster B) as long as its risk and population at risk are sufficiently larger than those in the surrounding areas. Similarly, we suggest that the heterogeneous cluster C contains core clusters D and E.

Conversely, when the maximum size parameter is too small, SaTScan may report only the smallest core clusters, missing region-level core clusters of homogeneous high-risk places. For example, this occurs when the maximum size is set to be 1%, 2% and 3%; only cluster B is reported instead of other high risk places in cluster A. In summary, the choice of an appropriate maximum size parameter is not trivial, and the proposed geovisual analytics approach can help to address this issue.

7.5.3 Instability of SaTScan clusters

In order to obtain core clusters, it is useful to run SaTScan multiple times using different maximum size values, particularly for relatively large data sets (e.g. US data aggregated by county). In the case of the US cervical cancer data being studied here, 50 scans were obtained in which the maximum size parameter increased from 1% to the default 50%, in steps of 1% increments. The results of the 50 SaTScan runs were interactively compared by using the *map matrix* (MacEachren *et al.*, 2003) component of VIT. In a map matrix, each SaTScan result is shown on a small choropleth map, allowing for side-by-side comparison. Eight of these scans (with maximum sizes set to 4%, 6%, 8%, 10%, 20%, 30%, 40% and 50%) are displayed in Fig. 7.6 to illustrate the variation in SaTScan results caused by increasing the maximum size parameter. In Fig. 7.6, it can be seen that as the maximum size parameter is increased, the primary SaTScan cluster (marked in the black circle on each small map) expands from a smaller sized core cluster at a maximum size parameter of 4% (in circle E) to its fullest extent at a maximum size parameter of 50% (in circle H). In this process, core clusters F and G, which were distinct from core cluster E at a maximum size of 4%, are encompassed by the large heterogeneous cluster H. The contents of the core, primary clusters at 4% are much more homogeneous than those in the heterogeneous, primary cluster H at 50%. So it appears that a simple solution for avoiding heterogeneity is to restrict the maximum size parameter.

However, as the maximum size is reduced, the location and size of the core clusters vary significantly, producing a new problem of core cluster instability in both location and size. For example, Fig. 7.6 shows that cluster J is reported at the maximum size parameters of 4%, 6% and 10%; it then expands into cluster J2 at a maximum size parameter of 8%, but then disappears when the maximum size parameter is above 10%. Such a finding suggests that a unique value for maximum size parameter might be necessary for identifying the correct bounds of each core cluster; there are often multiple optimal maximum size parameter values for identifying the core clusters as well. That is, cluster identification is scale dependent. Therefore, this research recommends a strategy of running multiple scans, systematically increasing the maximum size parameter with each run so that most core clusters can be identified. With this strategy, the scans will report clusters at different locations and in different sizes. Sections 7.5.4–7.5.6 discuss to how to visualize and analyse these clusters and how to obtain those that are most reliable.

7.5.4 Interactive visualization of SaTScan clusters

The geovisual analytics methods implemented in VIT directly address the lack of cartographic support for interpreting SaTScan results and the implications of the selection of scaling parameters. In this approach, a tabular interface (see Fig. 7.7) enables users to load and interactively explore multiple SaTScan results. This interface

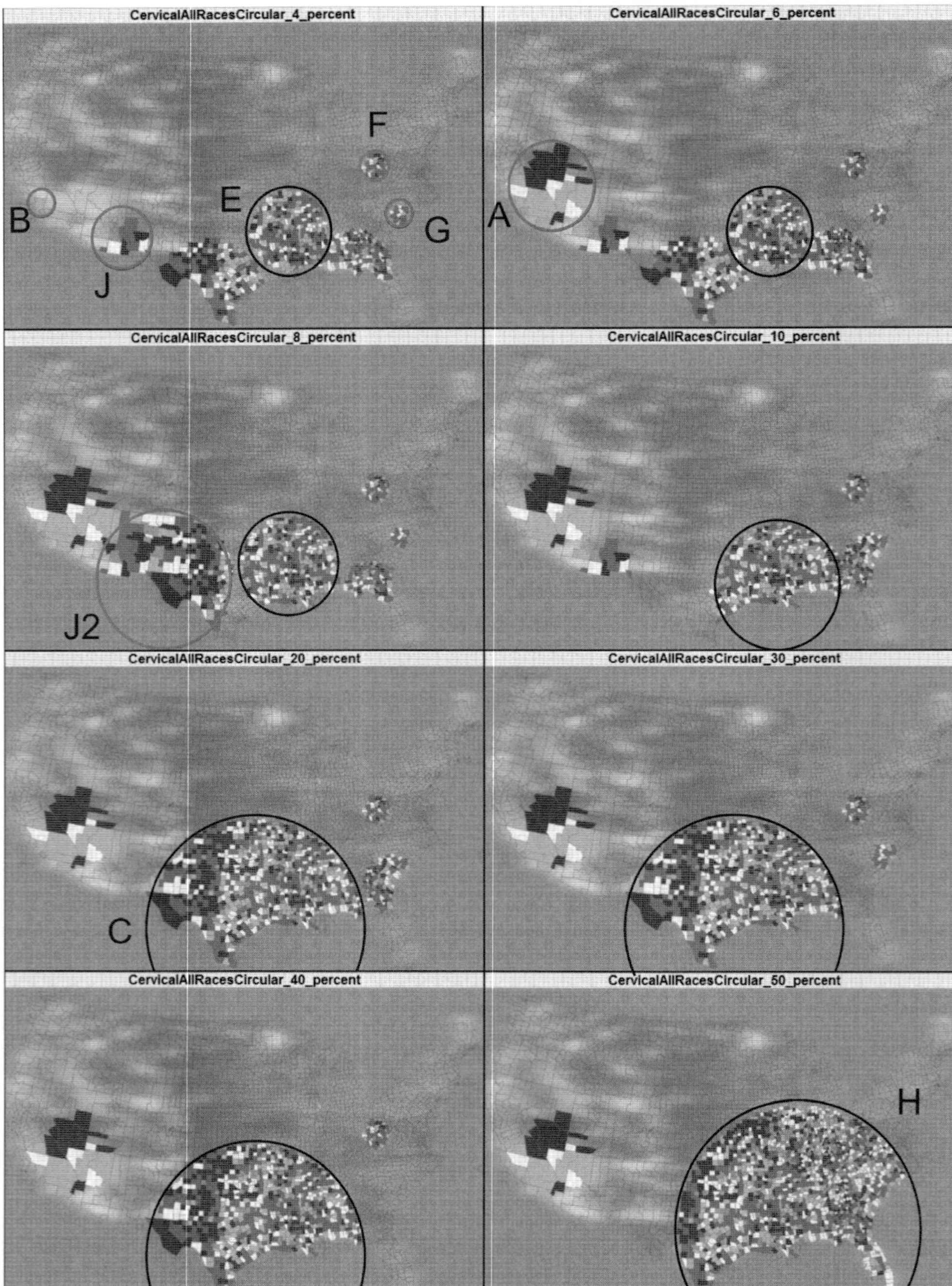

Fig. 7.6. A map matrix displaying eight runs of SaTScan (density-based clustering) using standardized mortality ratio (SMR) data for cervical cancer in the USA. The eight runs increase the maximum size parameter systematically (4%, 6%, 8%, 10%, 20%, 30%, 40%, and 50%). As the maximum size parameter is increased, the clusters reported by SaTScan vary in both location and size. Primary clusters are shown as black circles and secondary clusters as grey circles.

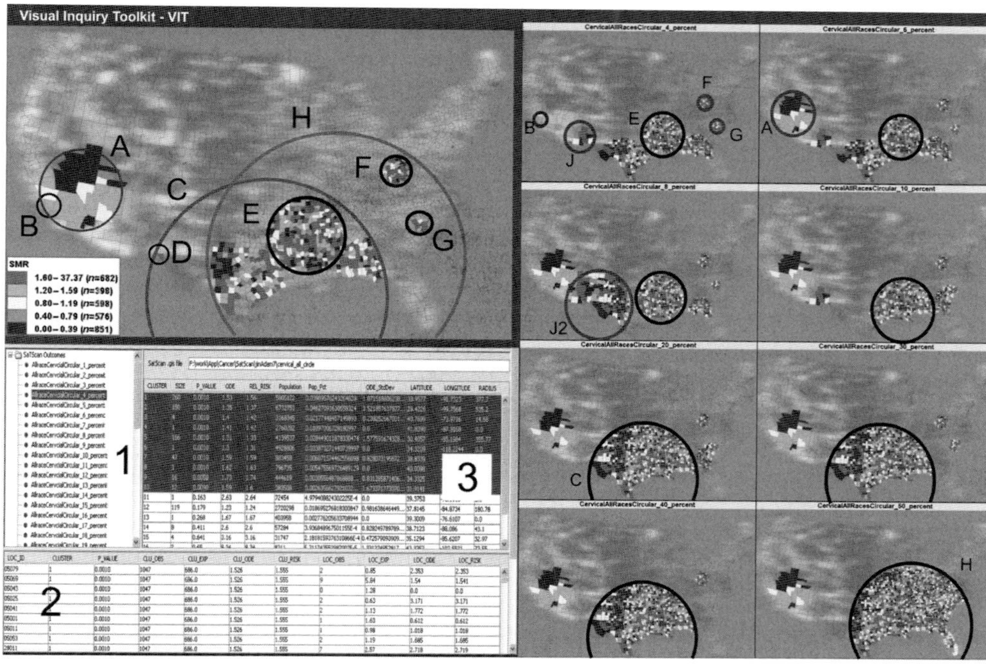

Fig. 7.7. The geovisual analytics method implemented in the Visual Inquiry Toolkit (VIT) using standardized mortality ratio (SMR) data for clusters of cervical cancer in the USA. At top left, a choropleth map. At lower left, the tabular interface. At right, a map matrix.

is linked dynamically to a choropleth map, a map matrix and related information visualization tools so that an analyst can select, visualize and compare SaTScan results produced by different maximum size parameter values.

7.5.5 Visualizing the reliability of SaTScan clusters

To discriminate stable, core clusters from heterogeneous and/or unstable ones, a method termed *reliability visualization* has been developed. This method combines the results reported by the multiple SaTScan runs into a single reliability map. Specifically, the clusters reported at each maximum size are represented in a layer, and all the layers are overlapped into a single view in which places/clusters reported by more layers have higher reliability, as illustrated in Fig. 7.8.

This method visualizes the likelihood that a county is reported within a cluster when SaTScan is run multiple times with a systematically varying maximum size parameter. In epidemiology, reliability is defined as the capacity of a test to give the same result – positive or negative – on repeated applications (Rothman and Greenland, 1998). Reliability is separated into two different types: (i) intra-observer reliability (agreement of results from the same diagnostic test given at multiple times or with multiple settings); and (ii) inter-observer reliability (agreement of multiple observers on the result of one diagnostic test). We consider reliability visualization to be of the intra-observer type of reliability because we are considering the agreement of results from multiple SaTScan runs, each with a slightly different parameter configuration. Reliability is estimated using Eqn 7.2:

$$R_i = \frac{C_i}{S} \qquad (7.2)$$

where R_i is the reliability value for location i, S is the total number of scans and C_i is the

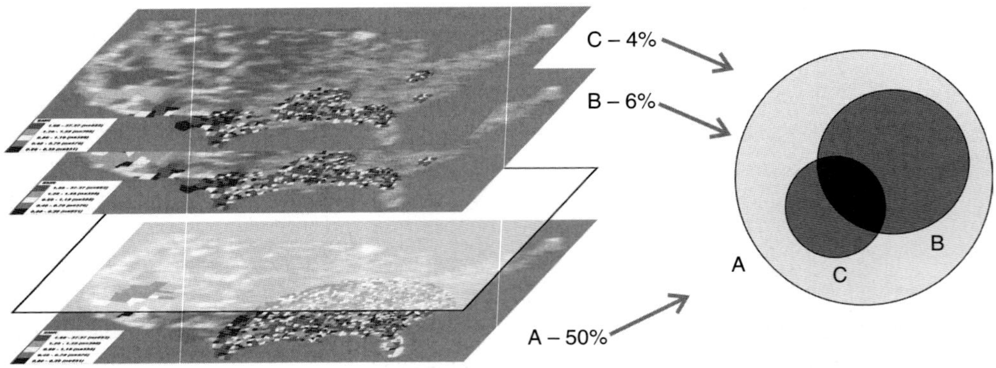

Fig. 7.8. Generating reliability visualization for clusters from SaTScan (density based) runs using standardized mortality ratio (SMR) data for cervical cancer in the USA. Clusters reported at each maximum size parameter value (here 4%, 6% and 50%) are represented in a layer, and the layers are overlaid to indicate reliability. Places/clusters reported by more layers have higher reliability.

number of scans for which that location *i* is within a significant cluster. The reliability measure has a value range from zero to one, where zero means that the location is not found in a significant cluster in any of the scans and one means that the location is within a significant cluster in all of the scans. The reliability score measures the stability of clusters reported by multiple scans. Reliability is distinct from the concept of validity, which is a measure of the probability that the cluster represents a true high-risk region. Therefore, the goal of reliability visualization is to identify stable core clusters rather than to evaluate the validity of the core clusters.

Using VIT, reliability scores for each US county were calculated using the eight scans shown in Fig. 7.6). These are visualized in Fig. 7.9 (top), which outlines the same five clusters (i.e. clusters A, B, C, D and E) as those shown in Fig. 7.5 (plus three more, F, G and H). VIT allows the user to produce such a reliability map by clicking on the menu SaTScan Tools > Add Reliability Map, and choosing the SaTScan results for calculating the reliability scores in the pop-up dialogue.

7.5.6 Evaluating the reliability visualization

While the SaTScan clusters vary considerably when using individual small maximum size parameters (as shown in Fig. 7.10), they are more stable when generated using a set of systematically chosen maximum size parameters and displayed in the reliability visualization. To evaluate the effectiveness of reliability visualization in coping with the sensitivity of SaTScan results to the choices of maximum size parameters, another reliability visualization (see Fig. 7.9 (bottom)) was generated based on a different set of eight maximum size parameter values: 5%, 7%, 9%, 11%, 19%, 29%, 39% and 49%. This set was selected systematically to have the same number of runs and similar maximum size parameter values to those of the previous set. Comparison of the top and bottom of Fig. 7.9 shows that the location and size of most core clusters (e.g. D, E, F and G) remain relatively stable, although the SaTscan clusters vary considerably when using individual maximum size parameters selected from either of the two sets. The reliability visualization 'smooths' this variation.

In addition, this research also produced a reliability map that used all 50 maximum size parameter values (from 1% to 50%) as a comparison (Fig. 7.11). This shows overall similar core clusters in the large size parameter values to those in Fig. 7.9. However, the map uses too many large maximum size values (e.g. those >20%), and so improperly puts more weight on large heterogeneous clusters than on small homogeneous clusters when calculating reliability scores. As a result, this

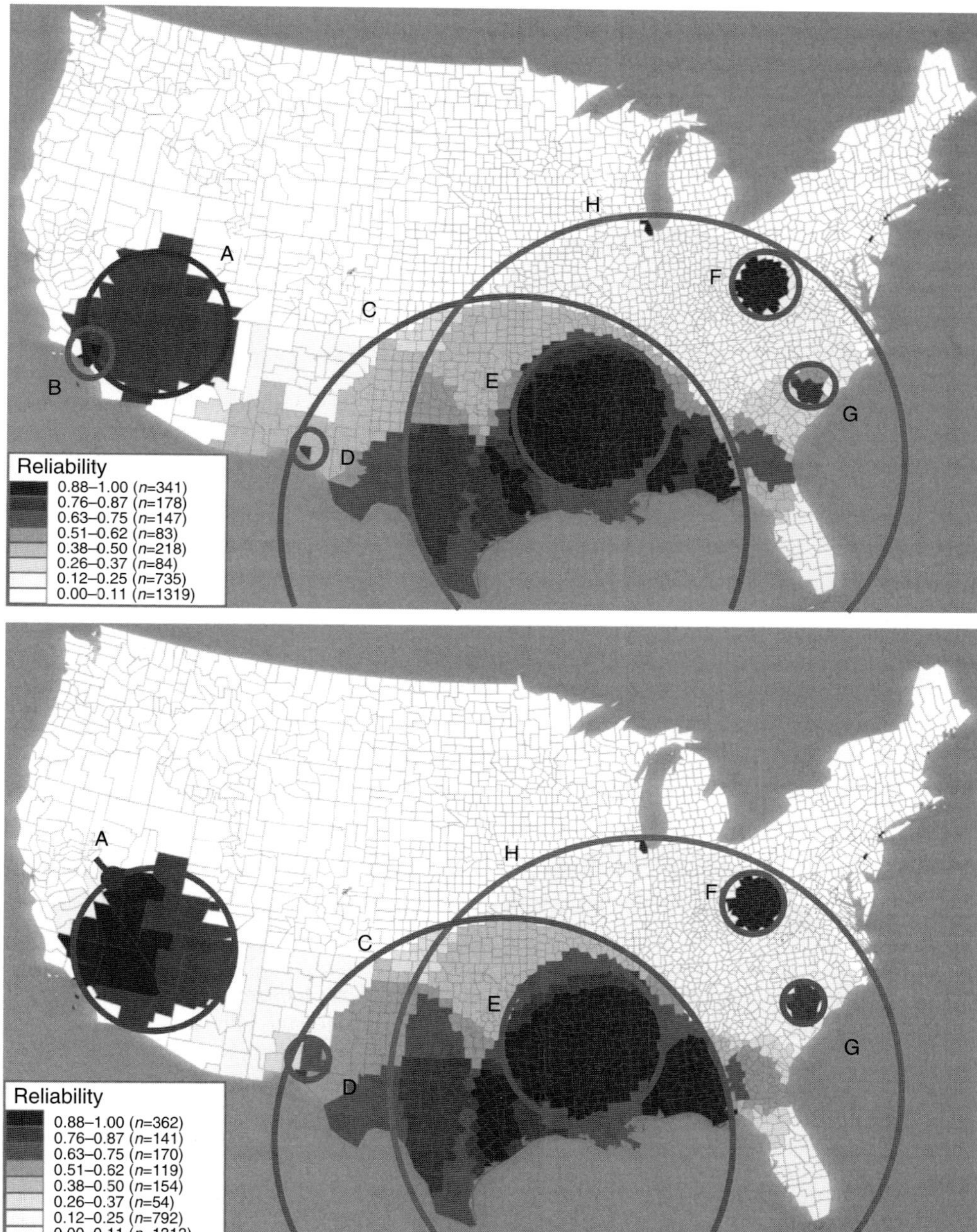

Fig. 7.9. Reliability visualization of clusters of standardized mortality ratio (SMR) data for cervical cancer in the USA using the Visual Inquiry Toolkit (VIT). Top map shows results from the eight runs with the maximum size parameter values of 4%, 6%, 8%, 10%, 20%, 30%, 40% and 50%. Bottom map shows results with maximum size parameter values of 5%, 7%, 9%, 11%, 19%, 29%, 39% and 49%.

map is less accurate in displaying small core clusters than is the map shown in Fig. 7.9, which uses more balanced sizes that treat small and large clusters equally.

In summary, the comparisons described above suggest that the VIT reliability visualization, when applied to multiple SaTScan results produced by systematically chosen maximum

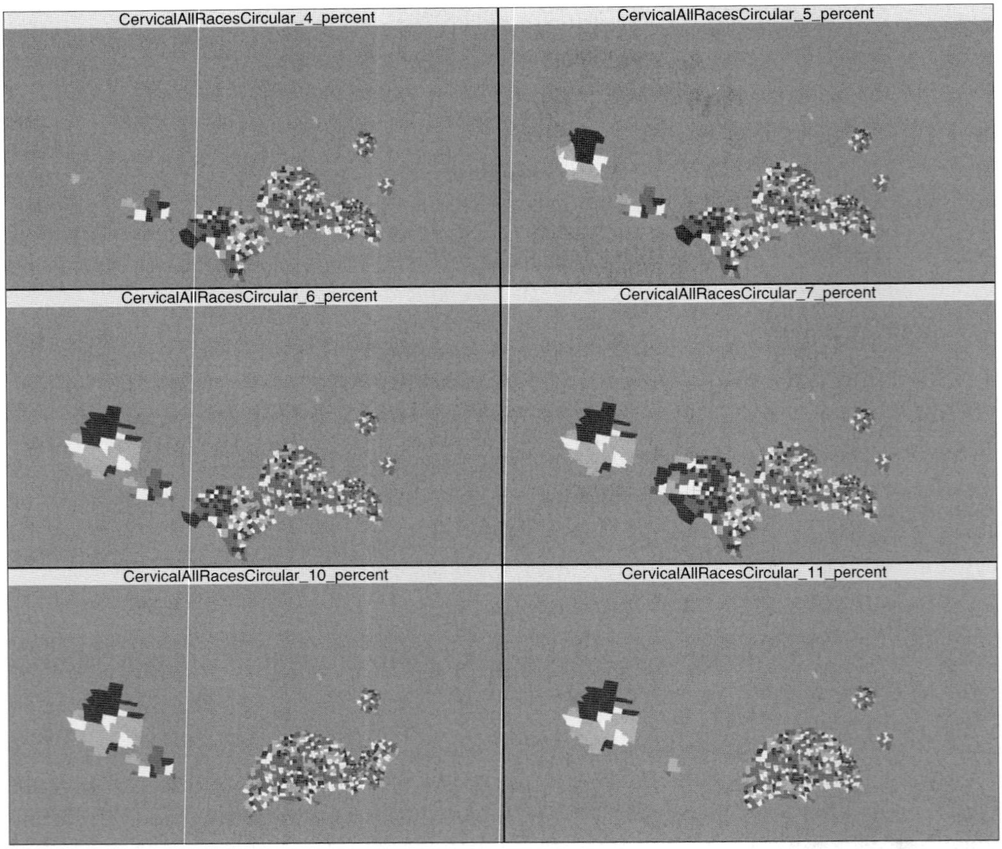

Fig. 7.10. SaTScan (density based) clusters of standardized mortality ratio (SMR) data for cervical cancer in the USA vary considerably when using individual small maximum size parameter values, even with tiny changes.

sizes, can effectively reduce the influence of parameter choices on the interpretation of SaTScan results. In addition, reliability visualization can provide one summary view of multiple SaTScan runs completed with varying maximum size parameter values, and effectively discriminate core clusters from heterogeneous clusters. The discrimination is important both for: (i) identifying spatially small, yet important and stable high-risk core clusters that can otherwise be easily hidden in the reported SaTScan clusters; and (ii) improving the understanding of heterogeneous clusters and their formation. Such discrimination is difficult when interpreting a single scan result using traditional visualization methods. The reliability visualization method can be used in any situation where a method's parameter sensitivity is a concern and when the analysis of multiple outcomes is needed, thus allowing application beyond the maximum size parameter of the Kulldorff spatial scan statistic.

The reliability visualization has also been further developed to show concurrently both disease risk and the reliability of detected clusters, as shown in Fig. 7.12. In this map, the bright regions are reliable, high-risk clusters; less reliable clusters and low-risk regions have been dissolved into the background.

7.6 Conclusion

Cluster analysis of geographic health data requires users to carefully choose clustering

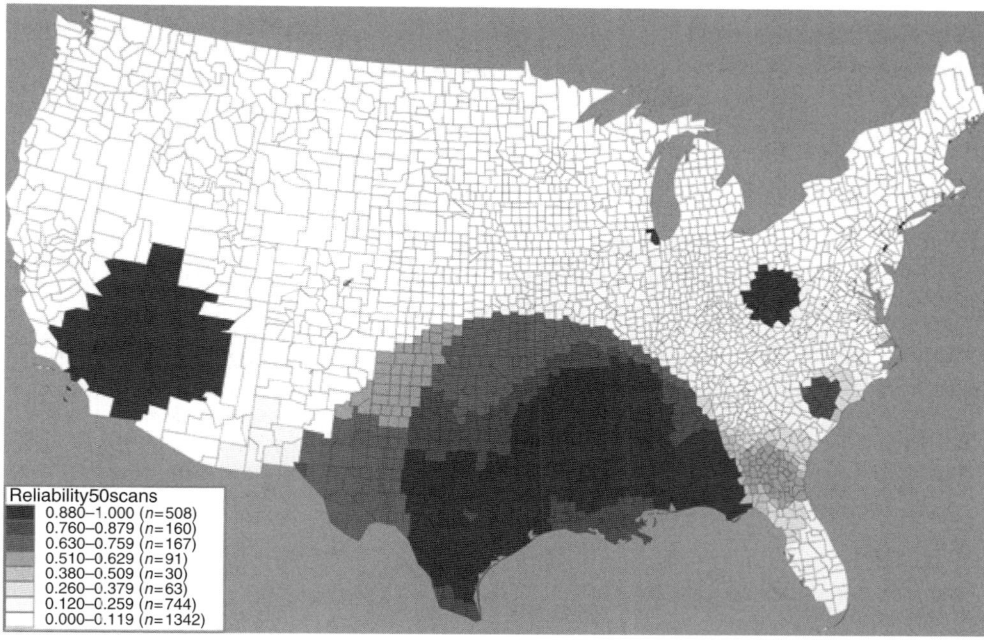

Fig. 7.11. Reliability map of clusters of standardized mortality ratio (SMR) data for cervical cancer in the USA produced by the Visual Inquiry Toolkit (VIT) using all 50 maximum size parameter values (from 1% to 50%).

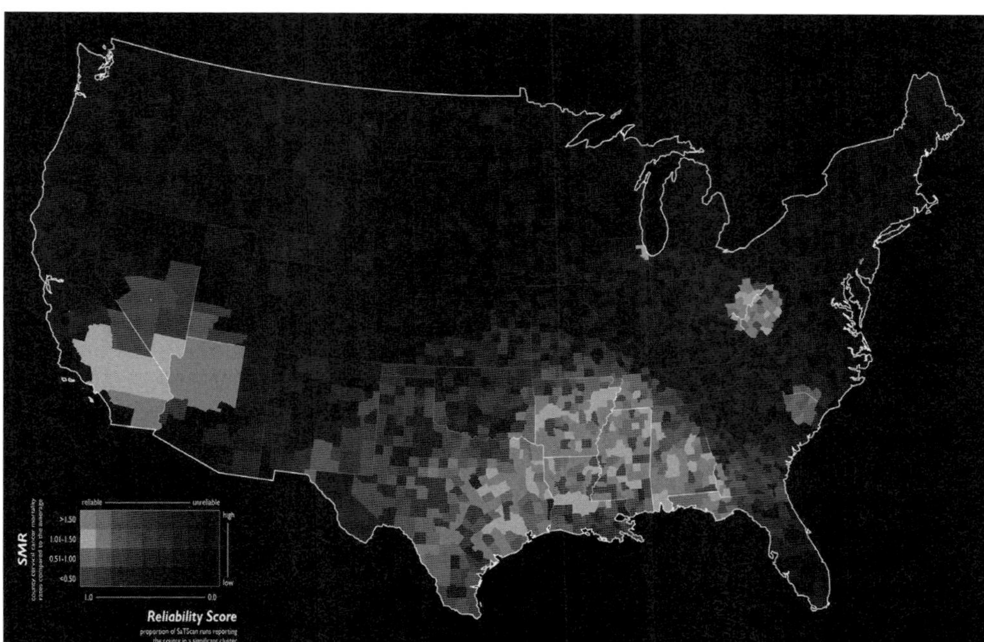

Fig. 7.12. Bivariate map concurrently displaying standardized mortality ratio (SMR) for cervical cancer in the USA and reliability scores for the clusters detected. The map shows the reliable high-risk clusters brightly highlighted, and the less reliable clusters and low-risk regions faded.

algorithms that produce clusters that appropriately represent the geographic processes on the ground. This research emphasizes the concepts of similarity-based clusters and density-based clusters, and suggests the use of density-based clustering for the identification of high (or low) risk regions of disease clusters.

The Kulldorff spatial scan statistic, and its free software implementation, SaTScan, is a density-based clustering method that has been widely adopted for the identification of disease clusters. There are, nevertheless, two issues which make the use of the method and interpretation of its results problematic: (i) SaTScan lacks cartographic support for understanding the clusters in geographic context; and (ii) results from the method are sensitive to the selection of the scaling parameters. SaTScan provides neither direct support for making these choices, nor methods for evaluating the results by the selection of various parameters.

This chapter addresses the first issue by describing a geovisual analytics approach that uses an interactive interface (the Visual Inquiry Toolkit, VIT) for visualizing identified clusters on a geographic map. For the second issue, the example used (cervical cancer mortality in the USA) in the chapter suggests that there is unlikely to be a single optimal maximum size parameter value when scanning a relatively large spatial data set (e.g. US data aggregated by county). Rather, it is probable that the core disease clusters exist at different geographic scales, each requiring a unique maximum size parameter value for detection. Therefore, we recommend completing multiple SaTScan runs while adjusting the maximum size parameter values systematically. The map matrix, reliability visualization and interactive tabular interface of VIT can then be used for the interactive investigation and interpretation of the multiple scans. In summary, the proposed geovisual analytics approach complements statistical approaches in cluster identification, thereby enhancing the interpretation of identified clusters.

References

Aldstadt, J. and Getis, A. (2006) Using AMOEBA to create a spatial weights matrix and identify spatial clusters. *Geographical Analysis* 38, 327–343.

Andrienko, G., Andrienko, N., Jankowski, P., Keim, D., Kraak, M.J., MacEachren, A. and Wrobel, S. (2007) Geovisual analytics for spatial decision support: setting the research agenda. *International Journal of Geographical Information Science* 21, 839–857.

Anselin, L. (1994) Exploratory spatial data analysis and geographic information systems. In: Painho, M. (ed.) *New Tools for Spatial Analysis*. Eurostat, Luxembourg, pp. 45–54.

Anselin, L. (1995) Local indicators of spatial association – LISA. *Geographical Analysis* 27, 93–115.

Anselin, L. (1996) The Moran scatterplot as an ESDA tool to assess local instability in spatial association. In: Fischer, M., Scholten, H.J. and Unwin, D. (eds) *Spatial Analytical Perspectives on GIS*. Taylor and Francis, London, pp. 111–125.

Anselin, L. (2005) *Exploring Spatial Data with GeoDa™: A Workbook*, rev. 6 March 2005. Center for Spatially Integrated Social Science (CISS), Santa Barbara, California. Available at: https://geodacenter.asu.edu/system/files/geodaworkbook.pdf (accessed 20 March 2013).

Bhowmick, T., Griffin, A.L., MacEachren, A.M., Kluhsman, B.C. and Lengerich, E.J. (2008) Informing geospatial toolset design: understanding the process of cancer data exploration and analysis. *Health and Place* 14, 576–607.

Boscoe, F.P., Mclaughlin, C., Schymura, M.J. and Kielb, C.L. (2003) Visualization of the spatial scan statistic using nested circles. *Health and Place* 9, 273–277.

Chen, J. and MacEachren, A.M. (2008) Resolution control for balancing overview and detail in multivariate spatial analysis. *The Cartographic Journal* 45, 261–273.

Chen, J., MacEachren, A.M. and Guo, D. (2008a) Supporting the process of exploring and interpreting space-time, multivariate patterns: the Visual Inquiry Toolkit. *Cartography and Geographic Information Science* 35, 33–50.

Chen, J., Roth, R.E., Naito, A.T., Lengerich, E.J. and MacEachren, A.M. (2008b) Geovisual analytics to enhance spatial scan statistic interpretation: an analysis of U.S. cervical cancer mortality. *International Journal of Health Geographics* 7:57. Available at: http://www.ij-healthgeographics.com/content/7/1/57 (accessed 20 March 2013).

Conley, J., Gahegan, M. and MacGill, J. (2005) A genetic approach to detecting clusters in point data sets. *Geographical Analysis* 37, 286–314.

Cromley, E.K. and McLafferty, S. (2002) *GIS and Public Health*. Guilford Press, New York.

Duczmal, L., Cancado, A.L.F., Takahashi, R.H.C. and Bessegato, L.F. (2007) A genetic algorithm for irregularly shaped spatial scan statistics. *Computational Statistics and Data Analysis* 52, 43–52.

Elliott, P. and Wartenberg, D. (2004) Spatial epidemiology: current approaches and future challenges. *Environmental Health Perspectives* 112, 998–1006.

Fukuda, Y., Umezaki, M., Nakamura, K. and Takano, T. (2005) Variations in societal characteristics of spatial disease clusters: examples of colon, lung and breast cancer in Japan. *International Journal of Health Geographics* 4:16. Available at: http://www.ij-healthgeographics.com/content/4/1/16 (accessed 20 March 2013).

GeoVISTA Center (2010) The Visual Inquiry Toolkit (VIT). GeoVISTA Center, Department of Geography, Pennsylvania State University, University Park, Pennsylvania. Available at: http://www.geovista.psu.edu/VIT/ (accessed 29 March 2013).

Getis, A. (1999) Spatial statistics. In: Longley, P.A., Goodchild, M.F., Maguire, D.J. and Rhind, D.W. (eds) *Geographical Information Systems: Principles, Techniques, Management and Applications*, 2nd edn. John Wiley, New York, pp. 239–251.

Getis, A. and Ord, J.K. (1992) The analysis of spatial association by use of distance statistics. *Geographical Analysis* 24, 189–206.

Glaz, J. and Balakrishnan, N. (1999) *Scan Statistics and Applications*. Birkhauser, Boston, Massachusetts.

Haining, R.R.P. (2003) *Spatial Data Analysis: Theory and Practice*. Cambridge University Press, Cambridge, UK.

Han, J. and Kamber, M. (2006) *Data Mining: Concepts and Techniques*. Elsevier, Amsterdam and Boston, Massachusetts/Morgan Kaufmann, San Francisco, California.

Han, J., Kamber, M. and Tung, A.K.H. (2001) Spatial clustering methods in data mining: a survey. In: Miller, H.J. and Han, J. (eds) *Geographic Data Mining and Knowledge Discovery*. Taylor and Francis, London and New York, pp. 188–217.

Han, J., Lee, J.-G. and Kamber, M. (2009) An overview of clustering methods in geographic data analysis. In: Miller, H.J. and Han, J. (eds) *Geographic Data Mining and Knowledge Discovery*, 2nd edn. Taylor and Francis, London and New York, pp. 149–110.

Hastie, T., Tibshirani, R. and Friedman, J. (2001) *The Elements of Statistical Learning: Data Mining, Inference, and Prediction*. Springer, New York.

Hsu, C.E., Jacobson, H. and Soto Mas, F. (2004) Evaluating the disparity of female breast cancer mortality among racial groups – a spatiotemporal analysis. *International Journal of Health Geographics* 3:4. Available at: http://www.ij-healthgeographics.com/content/3/1/4 (accessed 20 March 2013).

Huang, L., Pickle, L.W. and Das, B. (2008) Evaluating spatial methods for investigating global clustering and cluster detection of cancer cases. *Statistics in Medicine* 27, 5111–5142.

Jemal, A., Kulldorff, M., Devesa, S.S., Hayes, R.B. and Fraumeni, J.F. Jr (2002) A geographic analysis of prostate cancer mortality in the United States, 1970–89. *International Journal of Cancer* 101, 168–174.

Johnson, C.R., Moorehead, R., Munzner, T., Pfister, H., Rheingans, P. and Yoo, T.S. (2006) *NIH/NSF Visualization Research Challenges Report*. IEEE Press, Los Alamitos, California.

Keim, D.A., Mansmann, F., Schneidewind, J. and Ziegler, H.A.Z.H. (2006) Challenges in visual data analysis. In: Mansmann, F. (ed.) *Tenth International Conference on Information Visualization, IV 2006*, 5–7 July 2006, London. IEEE Conference Publications, IEEE Press, Los Alamitos, California, pp. 9–16.

Knox, E.G. (1989) Detection of clusters. In: Elliott, P. (ed.) *Methodology of Enquiries into Disease Clustering*. Small Area Health Statistics Unit, London, pp. 17–20.

Kulldorff, M. (1997) A spatial scan statistic. *Communications in Statistics – Theory and Methods* 26, 1481–1496.

Kulldorff, M. (2001) Prospective time periodic geographical disease surveillance using a scan statistic. *Journal of the Royal Statistical Society* 164, 61–72.

Kulldorff, M. (2006) SaTScan™ User Guide for version 7.0. SaTScan, Boston, Massachusetts. Available at: http://www.plansky.net/bbs/forum.php?mod=attachment&aid=MzA0OXwxMDQ3OWY1OHwxMzYxNjcyMDA3fDB8ODA5Ng%3D%3D (accessed 20 March 2013).

Kulldorff, M. and Information Management Services, Inc. (2006) SaTScan v7.0: software for the spatial and space-time scan statistics. SaTScan, Boston, Massachusetts.

Kulldorff, M. and Nagarwalla, N. (1995) Spatial disease clusters: detection and inference. *Statistics in Medicine* 14, 799–810.

Kulldorff, M., Song, C., Gregorio, D., Samociuk, H. and DeChello, L. (2006) Cancer map patterns: are they random or not? *American Journal of Preventive Medicine* 30(2, Supplement), S37–S49.

Lawson, A.B. (2006) *Statistical Methods in Spatial Epidemiology*. John Wiley, Chichester, UK.

MacEachren, A., Dai, X., Hardisty, F., Guo, D. and Lengerich, G. (2003) Exploring high-D spaces with multiform matrices and small multiples. In: *IEEE Symposium on Information Visualization, 2003 (INFOVIS 2003), 21–21 October, 2003, Seattle, Washington*. IEEE Conference Publications, IEEE Press, Los Alamitos, California, pp. 31–38. Available at: http://www.ncbi.nlm.nih.gov/pmc/articles/PMC3176663/ (accessed 20 March 2013).

Mostashari, F. (2003) Dead bird clusters as an early warning system for West Nile virus activity. *Emerging Infectious Diseases* 9, 641–646.

Openshaw, S., Charlton, M., Wymer, C. and Craft, A. (1987) A Mark 1 Geographical Analysis Machine for the automated analysis of point data sets. *International Journal of Geographical Information Science* 1, 335–358.

O'Sullivan, D.D. and Unwin, D.J. (2003) *Geographic Information Analysis*. John Wiley, Hoboken, New Jersey.

Ord, J.K. and Getis, A. (1995) Local spatial autocorrelation statistics: distributional issues and an application. *Geographical Analysis* 27, 286–306.

Rothman, K.J. and Greenland, S. (1998) *Modern Epidemiology*. Lippincott-Raven, Philadelphia, Pennsylvania.

Sheehan, J.T., DeChello, L.M., Kulldorff, M., Gregorio, D.I., Gershman, S. and Mroszczyk, M. (2004) The geographic distribution of breast cancer incidence in Massachusetts 1988 to 1997, adjusted for covariates. *International Journal of Health Geographics* 3:17. Available at: http://www.ij-healthgeographics.com/content/3/1/17 (accessed 20 March 2013).

Smith, M.J. de., Goodchild, M.F. and Longley, P.A. (2008) *Geospatial Analysis: A Comprehensive Guide to Principles, Techniques and Software Tools*. Troubador, Leicester, UK.

Thomas, J.J. and Cook, K.A. (eds) (2005) *Illuminating the Path: The Research and Development Agenda for Visual Analytics*. IEEE, Los Alamitos, California.

Waller, L.A. and Gotway, C.A. (2004) *Applied Spatial Statistics for Public Health Data*. John Wiley, Hoboken, New Jersey.

8 Methods for Creating Smoothed Maps of Disease Burdens

Chetan Tiwari*
University of North Texas, Denton, Texas, USA

8.1 Introduction

Disease mapping is an important component of the public health planning and intervention process as disease maps provide valuable insights into the geographical spread of a particular disease, information about people and places affected by it and its relationship to risk factors in the environment, as well as information for control and intervention efforts.

In 2010, the New York State Department of Health unveiled a comprehensive statewide cancer mapping web site that provides information on cancer counts at the US Census Block Group level along with information on the locations of potentially hazardous facilities, including chemical storage sites and hazardous waste generators (New York State Department of Health, 2010a). The mapping web site was created as a result of law passed by the New York State Legislature (*2010 New York Code, PBH – Public Health, Article 24 – Control of Malignant Diseases, Title 1 – (2400–2404-B) General Provisions 2401-B: Cancer incidence and environmental facility maps*) and is among the first in the USA to provide comprehensive spatial data on cancer outcomes and risk factors in the environment. While the web site is an important milestone in the use of mapping methods and geographic information system (GIS) technology for disease surveillance and information dissemination, there are also concerns about the possibility of misinterpretation of the data –in terms of both cancer risks and burdens (New York State Department of Health, 2010b).

It is important to note that any map is an abstraction of reality that is constructed by collecting, manipulating and visualizing data using a variety of processes and assumptions. The disease mapping literature has received considerable attention from researchers on issues relating to methodology, representation and visualization, and community participation (Rushton, 2003; Beyer *et al.*, 2010, 2012). In this chapter, a brief overview is provided of disease mapping methods and a method for producing statistically reliable, spatially continuous maps of disease burdens is showcased.

8.2 Sample Data and Software

The data sets used in this chapter were downloaded from the GeoDa Center for Geospatial Analysis and Computation (https://geodacenter.asu.edu/) at Arizona State University, and contained information on malaria incidence and population data in Colombia for the year 1998.

* E-mail: chetan.tiwari@unt.edu

The data are available as a polygon shapefile containing aggregated counts of malaria cases for 1068 municipalities and 33 departments in that country. Spatial analysis tasks, including data manipulation, processing and visualization were done using Quantum GIS (QGIS) software (available from http://www.qgis.org/). QGIS is free, open-source GIS software that is suitable for a variety of platforms, including Microsoft Windows, Mac OS and Linux. Disease maps were created using a combination of the Web-based Disease Mapping and Analysis Program (WebDMAP) (http://www.webdmap.com) and GIS software. WebDMAP is free, open-source, web-based GIS server software for creating and visualizing a variety of disease maps constructed using the spatially adaptive filters method. More details on the software and processing steps are provided in relevant sections in this chapter.

8.3 Types of Disease Maps

8.3.1 Dot density and proportional symbols map

The simplest and also the most unreliable representation of disease data is through the construction of a dot density map where locations representing disease cases or aggregations of disease cases are mapped as point symbols on a map. The point symbols (usually dots) may represent a certain number of disease cases, e.g. the map-maker may decide that one dot represents five disease cases. The dots are then placed randomly on the map, constrained by the administrative unit that contained those observations. This ensures that the dots are spatially distributed in a manner that represents the intensity of the observations. While these maps are useful for providing a broad overview of disease patterns, they do not take population density or population structures (such as age–sex distributions) into account and are therefore inadequate for measuring the spread and impact of diseases in human populations. For example, a cluster of cancer cases may coincide with the location of a centre for seniors where the population characteristics of that location make it more vulnerable to the disease.

Variants of the dot density map include proportional symbol maps, which use different sized symbols (such as circles) to represent different magnitudes of disease counts (Brewer, 2006). The symbols may be used to present data for two variables by using a combination of size and colour. A challenge with using such maps lies in the choice of map density or symbol size. The spatial arrangement of the administrative units, particularly in densely populated urban areas, is likely to result in maps that are cluttered with too much information to discern differences in disease burdens across geographic space.

The map in Fig. 8.1 shows the number of reported malaria cases in Colombia using graduated symbol sizes, with larger symbols indicating larger observed counts. The map was created in QGIS by first converting the polygon shapefile into a point shapefile using the 'Polygon Centroids' option in the software. Point symbols were then classified by population data and scaled by malaria incidence count data using the 'Layer Properties' option. The resulting map uses colour gradients to represent 1998 population and size gradients to represent malaria incidence. It is important to note here that the map represents counts, not rates, of malaria. In general, it is preferable to map rates in a population rather than raw disease counts, as the latter can often be misleading. For example, in Fig. 8.1, the largest symbol has a population that is lower (indicated by the lighter shade) than the smaller symbol with the darkest shade, possibly implying differences in the rates of the disease between the two municipalities.

8.3.2 Choropleth maps

Choropleth maps are an alternative and commonly used method for visualizing disease rates. They are constructed by shading areas (typically representing administrative units) with colours or intensities of colours that are derived by grouping the observed data into classes. This method is particularly useful for mapping diseases as privacy and confidentiality concerns often dictate that such data are released as counts aggregated to some administrative unit. Additionally, census data such as

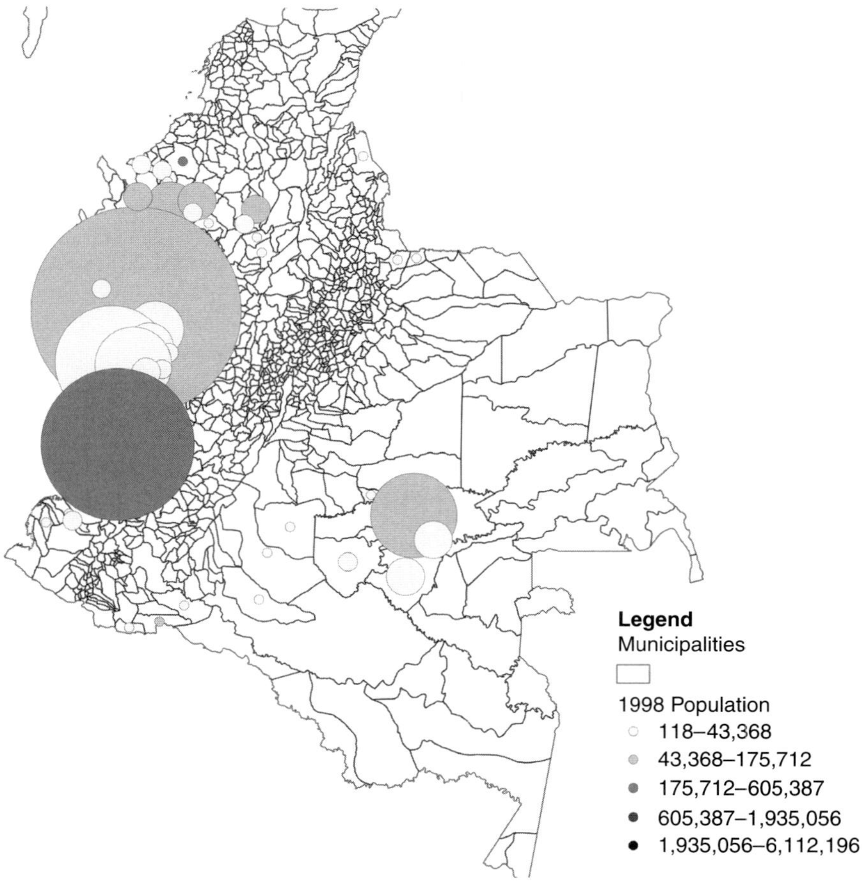

Fig. 8.1. Malaria incidence in municipalities in Colombia in 1998. Disease incidence is represented by graduated colours (different shades of grey and white) and symbols (different sized circles).

population counts and age–sex structures are also collected at the same spatial scales, thereby enabling easy calculation of crude or population age–sex adjusted disease rates. Previous research on mapping disease burdens using choropleth maps has addressed a number of issues relating to classification and colour schemes (Brewer *et al.*, 1997; Brewer and Pickle, 2002; Brewer, 2006), choice of areal units (Boscoe and Pickle, 2003), areal bias (Cressie, 1992) and map unreliability due to the Modifiable Areal Unit Problem (MAUP) (Openshaw, 1977, 1983) and to small numbers (Tiwari and Rushton, 2005).

The MAUP is a well-researched problem that is known to exist with studies that utilize aggregated data. It states that any change in the level of aggregation or shape of areal units will result in changing map patterns. In other words, maps that are produced using disease data that are aggregated to different levels of administrative units (e.g. census units versus postal units) will result in different map patterns. More generally, any change in the shape of the unit being mapped will result in different spatial patterns. The effect of changing scale is shown in Fig. 8.2. The two maps shown were produced using the same malaria incidence data in Colombia. The map on the left uses a coarser administrative unit (departments); that on the right uses a finer administrative unit (municipalities). These maps were produced in QGIS by changing the 'Symbol Style' to a 'Graduated' colour scheme. The 'Natural Breaks' classification

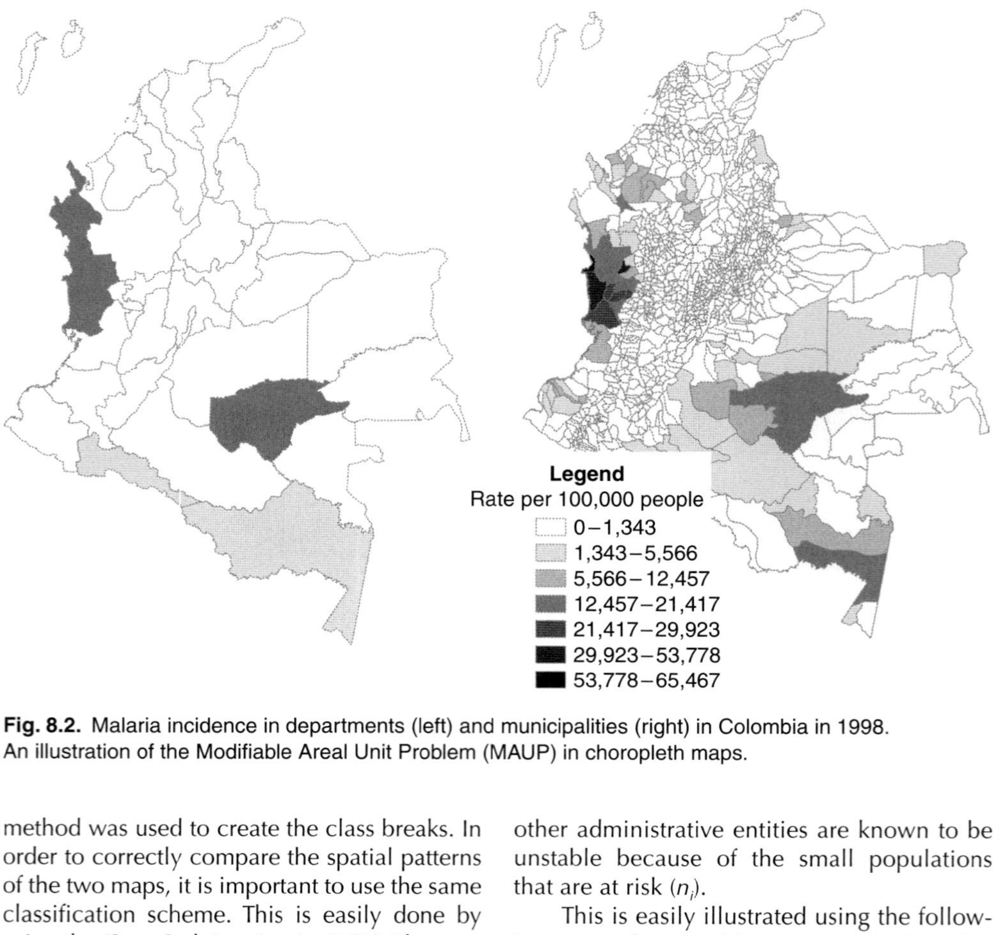

Fig. 8.2. Malaria incidence in departments (left) and municipalities (right) in Colombia in 1998. An illustration of the Modifiable Areal Unit Problem (MAUP) in choropleth maps.

method was used to create the class breaks. In order to correctly compare the spatial patterns of the two maps, it is important to use the same classification scheme. This is easily done by using the 'Save Style' option in QGIS. The geographical patterns of malaria incidence are clearly different between the two maps despite being produced from the same data. This is the result of the MAUP. Further, the discrete nature of the administrative boundaries is not reflective of the spatially continuous nature of the disease risk being mapped.

As noted earlier, it is generally preferable to map rates of disease in a population rather than raw counts of the number of cases. Crude disease rates are calculated as:

$$R_i = \frac{d_i}{n_i} \tag{8.1}$$

where R_i is the rate in area i, d_i represents the number of observed disease cases and n_i represents the at-risk population count in the area. Choropleth maps of disease rates (R_i) produced for small areas such as zip codes or other administrative entities are known to be unstable because of the small populations that are at risk (n_i).

This is easily illustrated using the following example: consider a municipality that contains an at-risk population count of ten persons (n_i). Let us assume that one person ($d_i = 1$) out of these ten dies from cancer. The resulting mortality rate for this municipality is 10%. Let us now assume that two people have died from cancer ($d_i = 2$). The cancer mortality rate now jumps to 20%. When small numbers are used in the denominator, any small change in the numerator will result in a drastic increase or decrease in the estimated disease rate for that area. When several areas of small population sizes (or small numbers) are present in a map, it causes the map to be highly unstable as any increase or decrease in the disease (numerator) counts will likely result in substantially different spatial patterns of disease risk. In other words, the variance in disease rates across the map becomes larger as smaller population sizes (possibly resulting from smaller administrative units) are used.

Figure 8.3 provides an example of this. It shows histograms representing calculations of malaria rates in departments and municipalities that have been overlaid on top of each other. The darker bars represent the larger spatial units (departments) and the lighter bars represent finer spatial units (municipalities). Note that the variance in estimated rates, as indicated by the spread of the histogram, is greater for the finer scale data, indicating possible uncertainty in the map.

While comparing Figs 8.2 and 8.3, it is critical to note that there is always a trade-off between geographic detail and stability of disease rate. In other words, finer spatial units result in high geographic detail and a high rate of instability, whereas coarser spatial units result in low geographic detail and a low rate of instability. Ideally, a map should have high detail and a low rate of instability. This trade-off can be achieved by using a variety of smoothing methods.

8.3.3 Continuous or isopleth maps

A third category of disease maps in addition to the dot and choropleth maps so far described represent disease risk as a spatially continuous function over geographical space. Such maps, known as isopleth maps, are commonly used to represent phenomena that are known to vary continuously across geographic space, including rainfall, elevation and certain ratio measures (Jones, 1930). On the issue of mapping ratios, such as estimates of disease rates in a population, Jones (1930) writes: 'ratios cannot be mapped by the dot method, and in many cases the quantitative relation between phenomena is much more significant than are the absolute values of the individual phenomena'. Kernel density estimation methods are commonly used to produce such maps (Kelsall and Diggle, 1995a,b; Rushton and Lolonis, 1996; Talbot *et al.*, 2000; Tiwari and Rushton, 2005). Maps produced using these methods use a kernel or spatial filter characterized by a particular shape, size and density function to compute the intensity of a spatial point process using a weighted moving average at each point of a regular or irregular grid of points constructed over the study region (Gatrell *et al.*, 1996). The weighted moving average, which is computed from aggregations of case and control populations, results in stable rate estimates as

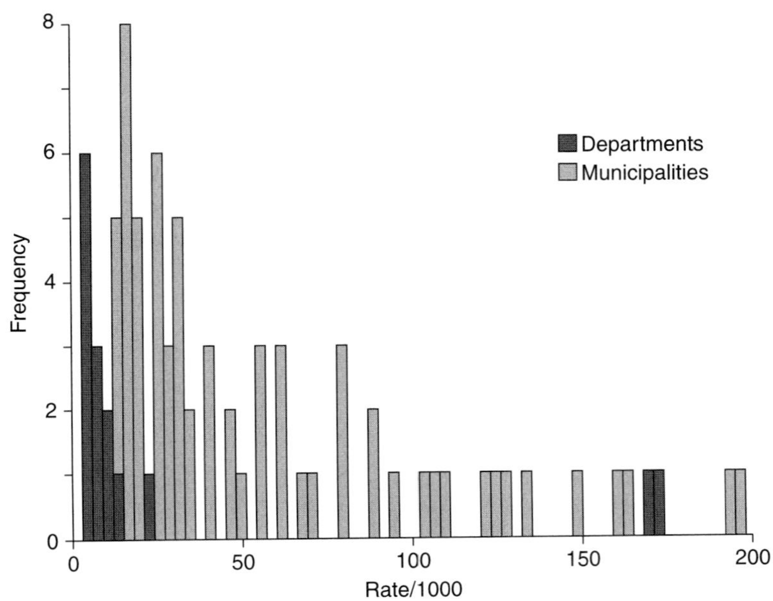

Fig. 8.3. A comparison of rates of malaria in Colombia in 1998 computed using different spatial scales: departments (dark bars) and municipalities (light bars) overlaid on a histogram.

the spatial filter allows the map-maker to control for the denominator population counts. Additionally, the overlapping spatial filters account for spatial autocorrelation. Two kinds of spatial filters are commonly used: fixed width filters and adaptive width filters.

Fixed versus adaptive spatial filters

Rushton and Lolonis (1996) used a kernel density estimation approach for computing rates of infant mortality in Des Moines, Iowa. The method uses a series of overlapping spatial filters that are centred on each point of a regular lattice of grid points that are arbitrarily located at 0.5 mile intervals across the geographic extents of the study area. The spatial filters themselves are of a fixed radius (0.4 mile) and uniform density function. Rates of infant mortality are computed at each grid point by dividing the numerator (case) and denominator (control) populations that fall inside the spatial extents of the filter. Note that the uniform density function implies that all observations within a spatial filter are given equal weights. The density function may take on other shapes – such as a Gaussian function that weights observations closer to the centre of the spatial filter more than observations that are further away.

It is also important to note that the size of the spatial filter is defined using a fixed radius, so it is insensitive to the underlying population density (Fig. 8.4). Consequently, rates estimated

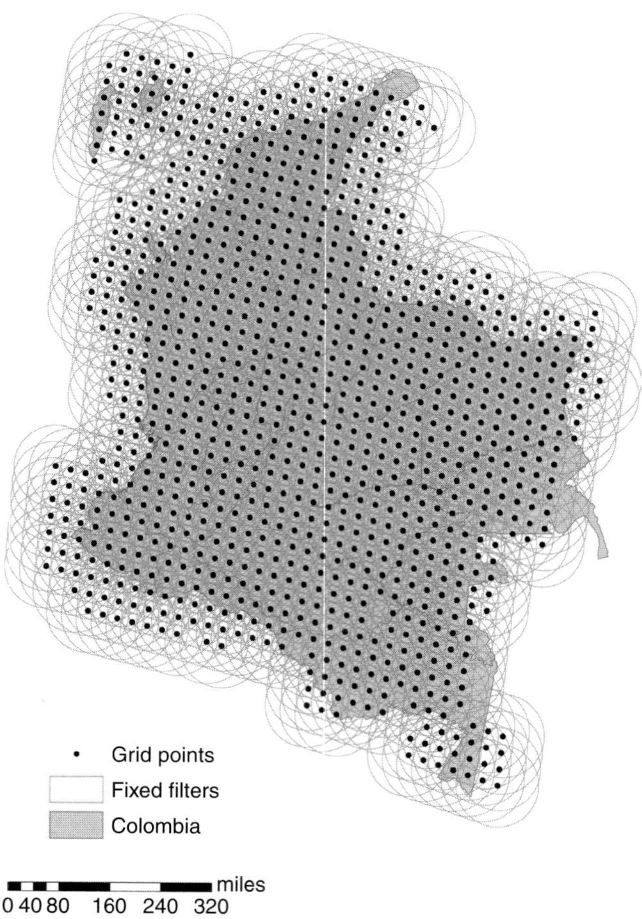

Fig. 8.4. Illustration of the used of fixed size spatial filters and a predefined regular lattice of grid points across Colombia in the production of an isopleth map of, for example, disease incidence.

using fixed-size spatial filters may be undersmoothed or oversmoothed. Undersmoothing refers to a situation where the size of the spatial filter is too small to obtain an adequate control population count and therefore results in unstable estimates. Conversely, oversmoothing refers to a situation where the size of the spatial filter is larger than that needed to calculate a stable disease rate and therefore results in a loss of geographic detail. Undersmoothing is likely to occur in rural areas where population densities are sparse, whereas oversmoothing is likely to occur in densely populated urban areas.

A solution to this problem lies in the use of a modified version of fixed spatial filters so that they dynamically expand or contract depending on the spatial distribution of the control population density (Talbot *et al.*, 2000; Tiwari and Rushton, 2005). This type of filter, known as a spatially adaptive filter, produces maps that have high geographic detail while maintaining low variability in estimated rates. As stated earlier, this is a desirable property to have in a disease map. The method uses kernels (or spatial filters) of varying sizes to estimate rates of disease burdens at each point of a predefined grid of regularly or irregularly spaced points. Rates are computed by dividing the numerator counts by the denominator counts that fall within the area encompassed by each spatial filter. The size of the spatial filter at each grid point is determined based on the underlying density of the control population and a user-defined threshold that defines the minimum number of controls that must be included within the spatial extent of each filter (see Fig 8.5).

When individual level data are used, the spatial filter meets the threshold specification exactly, thereby resulting in perfectly circular

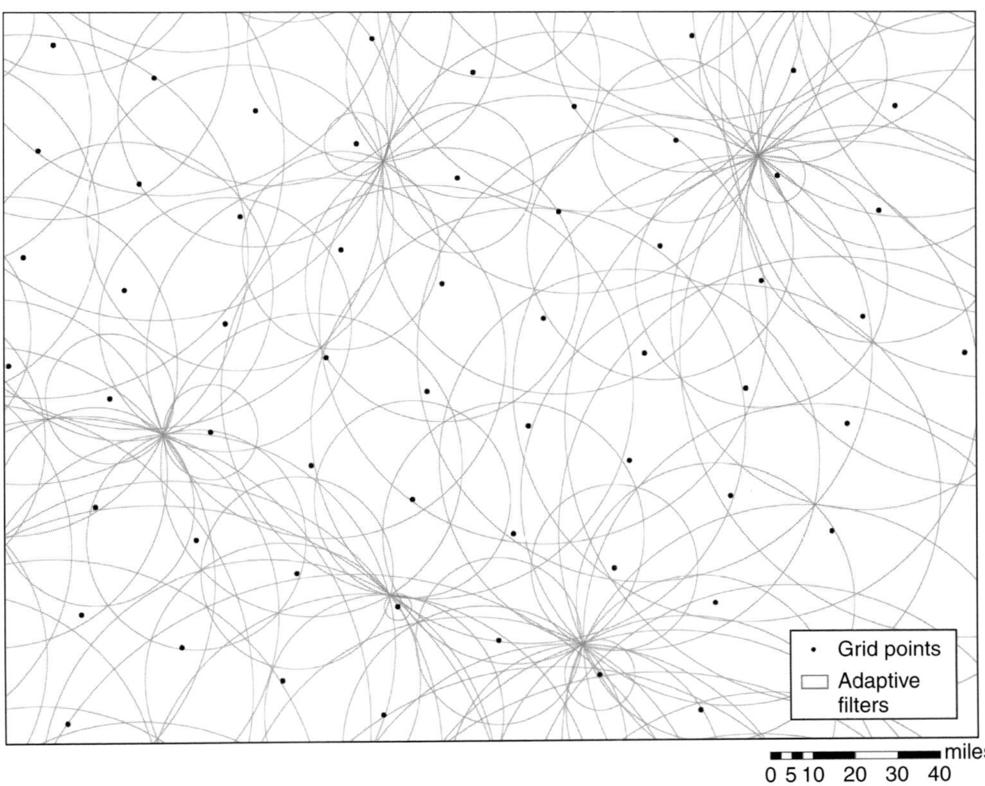

Fig. 8.5. Illustration of the used of spatially adaptive filters and a predefined regular lattice of grid points across an area in the production of an isopleth map of, for example, disease incidence.

filters across the map. However, when data aggregated to different levels of geography are used, the spatial filter is constructed using aggregate counts of individuals that are typically placed at the centroids of the areal units involved in the rate calculations. In such cases, the spatial filter is no longer a circle. Instead, it takes on an irregular shape that is defined by the boundaries of the small areas whose centroids are enclosed within the bounds of the spatial filter. Rates that are estimated at the grid points are then converted into a smooth, continuous surface using the Inverse Distance Weighted (IDW) interpolation method in a GIS. A discussion of the role of the grid and the interpolation is presented in the next section.

The advantage of the spatially adaptive filters method over other forms of disease mapping is that it minimizes the overall variance in estimated rates, while maximizing the amount of geographic detail portrayed on the map. A disadvantage, though, is that the spatial basis of support used to estimate rates across the study region is not constant. This implies that the area of the geography from which disease and population data are drawn is not consistent across disease maps. Consequently, a comparison of such maps becomes difficult. Additionally, because the overlapping filters use shared observations of cases and controls, performing statistical tests on the estimated rates is not recommended as they violate the statistical assumption of independence.

Constructing a grid for the spatially adaptive filters method

As discussed earlier, the spatially adaptive filters method computes disease rates along all points of a regularly or irregularly spaced grid of points. The definition of this grid plays an important role in the disease mapping process as it defines where the spatial filters are placed in the study area. Ideally, disease rates would be estimated using an extremely fine grid that can then be rasterized to create a continuous risk surface. However, this is not practical for two reasons. First, the computational requirements of calculating disease rates for an extremely fine grid become unmanageable as the grid becomes finer and the study area becomes larger. This is explained in the next section on the implementation of the spatially adaptive filters method. Secondly, sparse population densities in many rural areas will result in sparse case and control counts. Constructing a fine grid in such areas, not only results in unnecessary computing time, but also creates spurious detail as a consequence of the IDW interpolation method that is needed to convert the discrete disease rate estimates into a smoothed, continuous surface.

A solution to the problem lies in the use of the underlying density of the control population itself to define the grid. A quadtree based approach that recursively divides the study area based on some user defined threshold value can be used to define polygons that contain approximately the same number of controls (Samet, 1984). The centroids of these polygons can then be used to define the grid. The density of the resulting grid reflects the density of the control population. In other words, areas with sparse population densities are likely to contain fewer grid points and areas with dense population densities are likely to contain a larger number of grid points. As the size of the spatial filter is also driven by population density, a grid that is too sparse may result in certain populations being excluded from the disease rate calculations. In other words, the overall coverage of the spatial filters across the study area may contain gaps, thereby excluding certain populations from rate calculations. Conversely, a grid that is too fine will be computationally inefficient due to repeated calculations of rates that use the same sparsely populated geographic areas within their spatial filters. Additionally, the quadtree approach not only resolves issues of geographic detail, but generally also results in faster compute times especially when working in areas that have a mix of urban and rural populations. Yiannakoulias *et al.* (2007) compared a quadtree based grid with a uniform grid to search for simulated clusters using the spatial scan approach to disease clustering (Kulldorff *et al.*, 2005). They found the quadtree based approach was not only computationally more efficient, but was also more sensitive to high-resolution spatial clusters (Yiannakoulias *et al.*, 2007).

Implementation of the spatially adaptive filters method

The process of creating disease maps using the spatially adaptive filters method relies on the creation of 'distance strings'. Distance strings are data structures that were originally designed for efficiently storing information about travel costs between locations that are encoded as nodes within a GIS (Densham and Rushton, 1992).

This data structure has been used extensively for solving problems in location–allocation modelling. The basic idea behind a distance string is that it stores information about travel costs (i.e. distance) between a base node and all other nodes in an increasing order of distance. In the spatially adaptive filters method, distance strings are adapted to store distance information from each grid point at which a disease rate is computed (which becomes the base node) to all other points representing case and control locations. This information is stored for every grid point location. For a grid of size N1 and a population table (case or control) of size N2, the distance strings are of the order (N1*N2). More simply, it is important to note that distance strings can potentially have large storage requirements and long computing times depending upon the size of the data sets involved. Consequently, optimizing the locations of the grid points as discussed in the previous section is a critical step in this mapping process. Additionally, distance strings can be further optimized by truncating the data values based on some predefined distance criteria. For instance, if spatial filters of sizes greater than 50 miles are unlikely for a particular map, the distance strings can be truncated to only compute distances from case/control locations that are within 50 miles of a base node. Despite this cut-off strategy, there can be situations where these data structures can become unmanageably large. For example, for surveillance purposes, individual level data on disease outcomes is increasingly being collected across large parts of the USA. A nationwide map on infant mortality for a 5 year time period can result in extremely large distance strings despite using the strategies discussed above. These potentially large data requirements are best implemented within a relational database that is equipped to handle large volumes of data efficiently. A description of the implementation of this method, as well as the procedure for creating disease maps is described later in this chapter.

Adjusting for covariates in the spatially adaptive filters method

In addition to creating stable and spatially continuous representations of disease burdens, it is also important to account for differences in population structures (covariates). For age adjustment, there are two commonly used methods – indirect and direct, which are described below.

INDIRECTLY AGE-ADJUSTED MAPS. The indirect method adjusts for differences in population structure by applying age-specific mortality/morbidity rates of a standard population to the age structure of the local study population. The standard population is typically a much larger reference region, such as a state or the country. The indirect age-adjustment procedure gives us the expected number of cases in the local study area if it had the same age–sex specific rates as the standard population. The stability of this expected number is not a problem because it is computed using standardized rates that are generally derived from a large population. Recall that the spatially adaptive filters method requires the user to specify a population threshold value. In the indirect implementation, this value is applied to the expected number of cases. The standardized incidence rate (SIR) or the standardized mortality rate (SMR) is computed at each grid point as the ratio of the sum of the observed number of cases across all population subgroups to the sum of the expected number of cases across all population subgroups. The equation for computing indirectly age-adjusted disease rates is as follows:

$$SIR_k = \frac{O_k}{E_k} \tag{8.2}$$

where: O_k is the observed cases in the local area k; E_k is the expected cases in local area k, equal to

$$\sum_{g=1}^{m} R_g . P_{g,k} \tag{8.3}$$

where m is the number of population subgroups in the *standard* population; R_g is the disease rate in subgroup g of the standard population; and $P_{g,k}$ is the population in subgroup g and local area k of the *study* population.

DIRECTLY AGE-ADJUSTED MAPS. The direct method adjusts for differences in population structure by applying locally observed rates computed from subgroups of the local study population to the age structure of the standard population. Again, the standard population refers to a much larger reference region, such as a state or country. The direct age-adjustment procedure gives us the expected number of cases for each population subgroup as if it had the same composition as that of the standard population. The directly age-adjusted rate (R_k) for the local study area k is defined as:

$$R_k = \sum_{g=1}^{m} \frac{O_{g,k}}{P_{g,k}} . W_g \tag{8.4}$$

where: m is the number of population subgroups; $O_{g,k}$ is the observed cases in population subgroup g and local area k; $P_{g,k}$ is the population in subgroup g and local area k; and W_g is the standard weight for population subgroup g (standard weight is the number of persons in subgroup g of the standard population divided by the total number of persons in subgroup g of the standard population).

In the implementation of the direct age-adjustment method, one has to be careful when computing the disease rate in a subpopulation of the local study area. The primary concern is that locally observed rates that are determined for subgroups of the local study population are likely to be unstable because of small population sizes. Hence, the application of these unstable rates to the standard population can result in unstable age-adjusted rate estimates. A solution to this problem lies in grouping age groups together to ensure that adequate population sizes are available when computing local disease rates.

8.3.4 Other mapping methods

Bithell (2000) categorizes disease mapping methods as falling under two broad classes: non-parametric methods and parametric or model-based methods. Non-parametric methods are useful for describing disease risk surfaces and have the advantage of requiring fewer assumptions and the ability to adjust for covariates (Bithell, 2000). Smoothing methods, including spatial filtering methods, fall into this class. In contrast, parametric methods are useful for constructing risk surfaces based on some pre-specified source of risk. Bayesian and geostatistical methods for smoothing data (Clayton and Kaldor 1987; Wakefield *et al.*, 2000; Berke, 2004; Goovaerts, 2005) fall into this category. Other disease mapping methods include linear smoothers, in which the smoothing function is primarily dependent on the distance and weight of points within a defined neighbourhood, and non-linear methods, which include response-surface analysis. Median polish and head-banging provide local smoothing of the data (Mungiole *et al.*, 1999; Pickle and Su, 2002) while empirical Bayes methods shrink local estimates towards a global mean (Mollie and Richardson, 1991).

Methods under each of these classes may be further classified depending on the type of data being mapped. The data needed to construct a disease map should ideally consist of case data locations and corresponding control or reference population locations. Diggle *et al.* (1999) argues that, at a minimum, the selection of the control population should be spatially neutral. In other words, the control population must represent a random sample of non-case locations. The data can either be at the individual level or at an aggregated scale (typically aggregated to some administrative unit). In the absence of privacy and confidentiality concerns, individual level data is most desirable for disease mapping purposes as it enables the creation of maps that are geographically more detailed than maps that are produced using aggregated data. Bithell (2000) argues that it is inherently wasteful to bin individual data points into geographical regions (such as choropleth maps) that are the equivalent of histograms for non-spatial data. From a geographical point of view, he argues that these geographical regions that usually represent some administrative boundary have little relevance to the disease in question. However, as stated earlier, privacy and confidentiality concerns surrounding health data usually require that the data are made available in an aggregated form. The spatially adaptive filters method described in Section 8.3.3 and its implementation in web-based GIS software called WebDMAP can operate at both the individual level and on aggregated data. Additionally, maps generated using such methods anonymize point- or area-based observations of disease outcomes by converting them to continuous surfaces of risk. The software and procedure for creating such maps is described in the next section.

8.4 WebDMAP: A Software for Creating Maps Using the Spatially Adaptive Filters Method

WebDMAP is a free, open-source, web-based GIS software for constructing crude and age-adjusted maps of disease burdens using the spatially adaptive filters method. The software consists of three main modules – disease mapping, GIS tasks and visualization. The disease mapping module allows users to construct crude maps, indirectly age-adjusted maps and directly age-adjusted maps. It also provides an option for creating maps that permit valid comparison of disease patterns over time. The grid file used for the calculation of disease rates can be created within WebDMAP by using the GIS tasks module. Finally, the visualization module allows users to create maps of disease burdens that can be viewed using either an interactive web browser based interface or Google Earth. The software is designed as a multi-user system that runs on a centralized computer server. Outputs from WebDMAP can also be imported into standard GIS software packages for further analysis.

8.4.1 WebDMAP system architecture, user interface and installation

WebDMAP is a complex collection of web and database server software, spatial databases, open-source GIS programming libraries and custom written code. It was developed as server software for a number of reasons.

First, the capability to manage and manipulate large volumes of data is available through the use of existing relational database server software that is designed specifically for applications like WebDMAP that have large database storage, management and manipulation needs.

Secondly, security and access restriction capabilities that are commonly available in server-based software allow the analysis component of WebDMAP to reside on a database server in a secure environment that is isolated from other users and the public in general. The outputs produced by WebDMAP include spatially continuous maps or shapefiles that contain disease rate estimates computed at all points of an arbitrarily generated grid. Recall that such rates are computed by aggregating case and control data within different sized spatial filters. This process automatically anonymizes the output even though confidential health data might have been used as the input data source. This ability to centrally store, manage and secure confidential data while producing anonymized map outputs is an important capability for public health departments.

Thirdly, the installation and deployment of the software is a centralized process that requires some initial effort by system administrators who manage the information technology infrastructure of a typical public health department. However, as the system is accessed via a web browser based interface, the end user remains unaffected by system updates or changes, thus making the software easier to manage.

Finally, the ability to encapsulate complex algorithms, spatial analysis tasks and database operations in an easy-to-use, web-based graphical user interface is important given that the target audience of this system includes public health researchers and professionals who are well versed in the areas of epidemiology and public health, but may not have the necessary skills to manipulate, process and analyse geospatial data. The system is designed as a series of modules, which are further categorized into tasks that must be performed as a sequence of steps (see Fig. 8.6). These tasks are embedded within web pages that allow a user to easily navigate the system on any machine that has web browser capabilities.

The web server provides access to the user interface via a series of HTML pages. The web server also provides access to analysis outputs. These are stored on password protected web folders that are accessible over the network concerned. Note that the outputs from WebDMAP

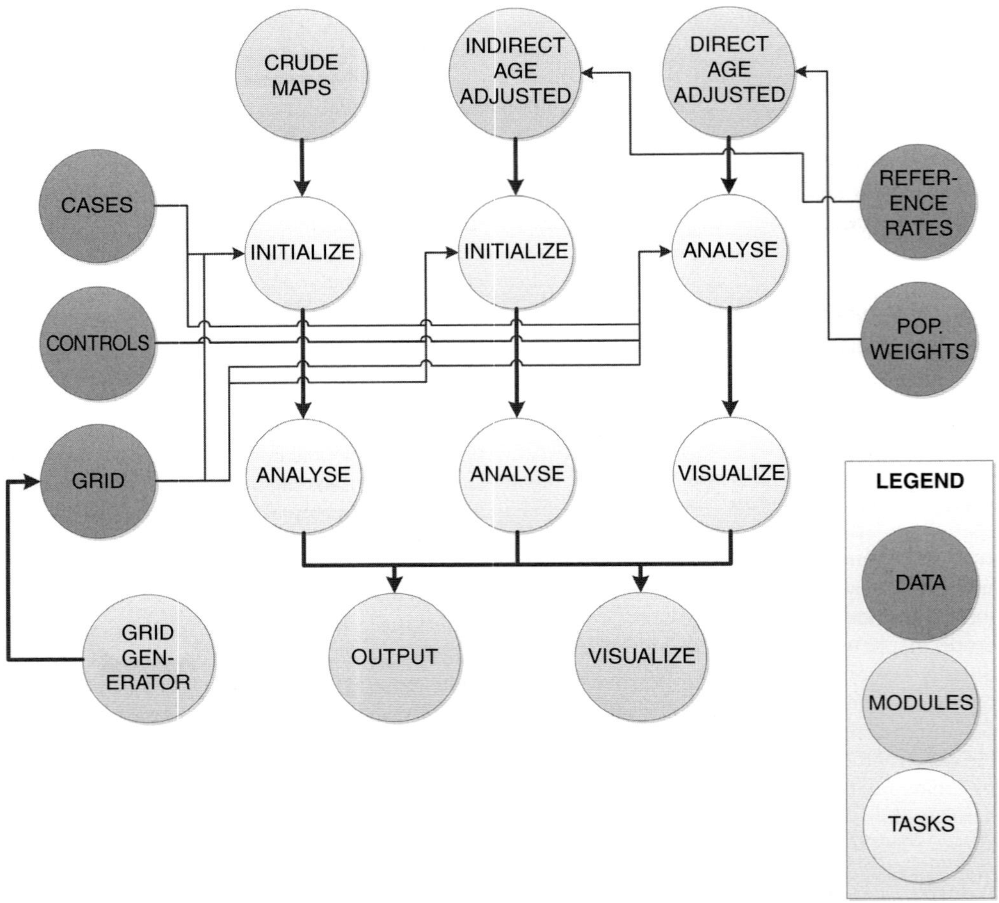

Fig. 8.6. Process for creating disease maps using WebDMAP (Web-based Disease Mapping and Analysis Program) software. POP., population.

do not contain any personally identifiable information. Once the input case/control data are loaded on to the server, they remain isolated from other users as well as from the public.

The software uses a number of PHP (a scripting language) scripts to perform basic tasks, including error checking and data processing. The analysis component of the system is written in a database programming language called Procedural SQL (PL/SQL). PL/SQL scripts have the advantage of executing directly on the database server, and therefore reduce the need to move confidential health data out of the database server for analysis. The database server used is PostgreSQL, which is an object-relational database management system (ORDBMS). PostgreSQL was the selected as the primary choice for hosting the WebDMAP data infrastructure because of its rich spatial data handling capabilities, which are available via an extension called PostGIS. The ability to create customized functions in PostgreSQL using GIS functions provided by PostGIS allows the combination of the capabilities of regular database management systems (DBMS) with the ability to manipulate spatial data, thus resulting in an extremely flexible platform for research and software development.

Although there are other database systems that provide similar functionality, including commercial systems such as Oracle and IBM's DB/2, PostGIS's active development, compliance with

Open GIS standards, use of a robust object-relational DBMS as the back end and an active user community make it a very attractive free alternative. In fact, all of the software components used in WebDMAP are free and open source, like WebDMAP itself. The source code for WebDMAP is publicly available under the Creative Commons Attribution-NonCommercial-Share Alike 3.0 Unported License, and the software, source code and installation instructions can be downloaded from http://www.webdmap.com.

8.4.2 Creating crude and age-adjusted maps of disease burdens using WebDMAP

The process for creating disease maps in WebDMAP is outlined in Fig. 8.6.

Creating crude rate maps of disease burdens

The user starts by preparing the input data, which are in three files – a case file, control file and grid file. The three files must be saved in the Comma-Separated Values (CSV) format. The case file must contain the following data columns: id, longitude, latitude, weight. Each row represents a case location – which may either be at the individual level or at an aggregated scale (in which case each row represents the centroid of the spatial unit). If individual data values are used, then the weight is set to 1. Alternatively, if aggregated data are used, the weight is set to the case count observed within that spatial unit. The control file is similar to the case file, except that it contains the locations and counts of the control population. The grid file must contain the following data columns: id, lon, lat. Each row in the grid file represents the location of a grid point. This file can either be created using external GIS software such as QGIS or ArcMap, or, preferably, by using the 'GIS Tasks' option in WebDMAP. WebDMAP uses information about the spatial extents of the study area and the population density of the control population to define the grid. The user provides the control file as an input in this step and can choose to generate either a regular grid or a densified grid. The regular grid option places grid points that are equally spaced across the study area based on a user-defined distance value. The densified grid option uses the quadtree approach described in Section 8.3.3 to create a grid that reflects the underlying density of the control population.

Once the data files are ready, the user must select the option to 'Initialize a New Project'. At this stage, the data files are processed and uploaded to the server. Distance strings are computed and stored under a database schema object that is created specifically for this project. The schema and all associated data are password protected and only accessible by the user who initialized the project. The user is notified by e-mail when this process is complete. As discussed in Section 8.3.3, the time required for this step depends on the size of the input data.

The final step in the mapping process is the analysis step. There are two options available to the user at this stage. The first option requires the user to specify the population threshold value. This value defines the minimum population size that will be encompassed by each spatial filter before a rate is computed. The threshold value is typically defined in consultation with a public health expert. The second option allows users to specify spatial filter definitions (i.e. spatial filter sizes) from a previously analysed project. This option is useful for constructing maps that compare changes in a particular disease over time. Because maps of disease burdens produced using the spatially adaptive filters method are available as raster surfaces, at each pixel, we can compute a measure of change that is given by the ratio of the estimated rate in time period $t + 1$ to the estimated rate in the time period t. However, one must be careful to ensure that the spatial basis of support that is used to compute the disease rate for the two time periods is exactly the same. The option to use existing filter size definitions guarantees that the spatial basis of support used to compute a rate at each grid point is exactly the same across the different maps being compared. Hence, valid comparisons of change can easily be made.

Creating age-adjusted maps of disease burdens

The process for creating age-adjusted maps is similar to the crude rate mapping process with the exception that it requires additional data. The indirect age-adjustment method requires data on disease rates obtained from some reference population. The direct age-adjustment method requires data on population weights obtained from some standard population. For both the methods, the case, control and supplemental data need to be stratified by age groups. Additional details on creating maps using the two age-adjustment methods can be found in the WebDMAP documentation.

Visualizing the output from WebDMAP

The output from WebDMAP is a shapefile that contains the locations of the grid points and the following attributes: gridid, the size of the spatial filter (ndistance and ddistance), the case count (nsumwt), control population count (dsumwt) and rate. The rate is calculated by dividing the case count by the control population count. The user may choose to multiply the rate by a multiplication factor, e.g. to report rate per 100,000 population, multiply the rate column by 100,000. To construct a continuous raster surface from these data, the IDW interpolation is used. The output from WebDMAP can readily be imported into a variety of different GIS software packages for further analysis or mapping, or it can be visualized directly within the WebDMAP system.

The cartographic capabilities of different GIS software packages vary substantially, with ArcMap providing the most customization options, followed by QGIS and, finally, by the built-in visualization function in WebDMAP. The Geostatistical Analyst extension in Esri's ArcGIS software provides an easy implementation of the IDW method. As the output from WebDMAP has already been smoothed, a small neighbourhood size and high power value for the IDW interpolation parameters is recommended, specifically; a neighbourhood size of 8 and power value of 2. The resulting surface can be classified into a graduated colour map using the 'Layer Properties' option in ArcMap; classification of the data into five or six classes is recommended. The IDW interpolation option in QGIS is not quite as intuitive. The interface in QGIS Version 1.7.4 allows the user to control smoothing by specifying a distance coefficient parameter. Values of 3 or 4 produce results that are comparable to the ArcMap output. Additionally, the symbolization interface for the IDW output in QGIS is rather basic. Choosing the 'Colormap' option under the 'Layer Properties Style' tab and manually specifying the class breaks with 'Discrete' colour interpolation seems to produce the best results.

A continuous surface of disease burdens can directly be created in WebDMAP, which uses the IDW implementation provided by the Geospatial Data Abstraction Library (GDAL). The interpolated surface is then colorized using a quantiles classification method. The colorized raster is converted to a georeferenced image, which is then 'tiled' using the MapTiler software. Tiling refers to the process of breaking an image down into multiple pieces to improve loading times and is particularly useful for web applications that are restricted by network bandwidth availability. The OpenLayers map library is used to overlay these tiles on base data that is obtained from a variety of online map data providers, including Google, Yahoo and Microsoft. This library also provides interactive map functions that include zoom, pan and transparency. Maps produced using the visualization option in WebDMAP can be viewed in any standard web browser. Figure 8.7 compares the three visualization options using malaria incidence data from Colombia. Note that in each case, the implementation of the IDW interpolation method causes the map outputs to be slightly different from one other. To reiterate, it is recommended that the IDW parameters are set in a manner that minimizes any additional smoothing that occurs as a result of the interpolation process.

8.5 Conclusion

Disease mapping methodology and software provide innovative methods for visualizing disease burdens. The spatially adaptive filters method allows control of the spatial basis of support and thereby produces stable estimates of disease rates across a geographical region. The quadtree based approach for defining a grid over which disease rates are estimated using the spatially adaptive filters method provides a mechanism for producing maps that are geographically detailed in areas where they

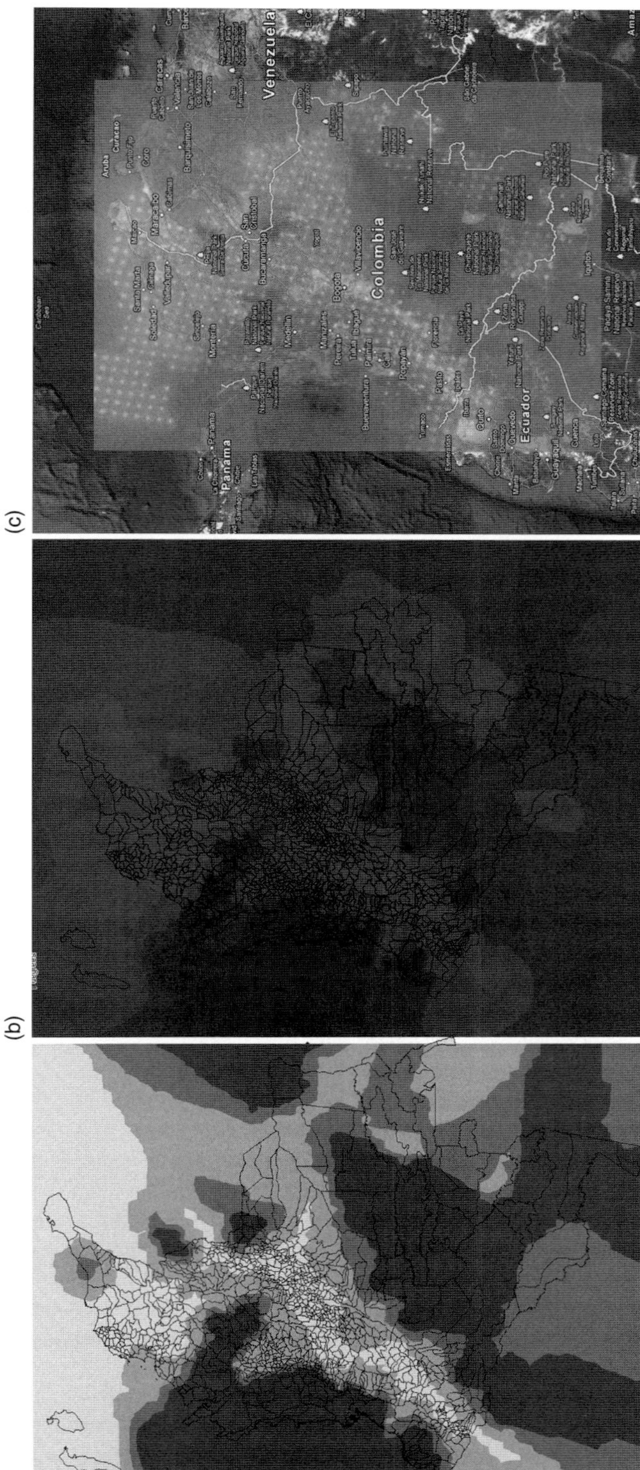

Fig. 8.7. Disease maps visualized using (a) Esri's ArcGIS, (b) QGIS (Quantum GIS) and (c) WebDMAP (Web-based Disease Mapping and Analysis Program). Data are for malaria incidence in Colombia in 1998.

should be (such as urban areas), while making the mapping process computationally efficient. To permit valid comparison of disease burdens across different geographic regions, it is important to account for differences in the population composition of the areas or time periods being compared. Typically, this involves accounting for differences in the age–sex structures of the given populations. WebDMAP combines two commonly used methods of age standardization into the spatially adaptive filters method. The ability to control the spatial basis of support for temporal comparisons is particularly useful for health surveillance applications. The web-based software that implements these methods in an easy to use, web-based interface can improve the capacity of public health departments that do not necessarily have the spatial analysis capabilities for tracking disease burdens over space and time. Further, the software design isolates the data and the analysis components from the end user and therefore provides new directions for analysing and mapping confidential health data.

References

Berke, O. (2004) Exploratory disease mapping: kriging the spatial risk function from regional count data. *International Journal of Health Geographics* 3:1. Available at: http://www.ij-healthgeographics.com/content/3/1/18 (accessed 22 March 2013).

Beyer, K.M.M., Comstock, S. and Seagren, R. (2010) Disease maps as context for community mapping: a methodological approach for linking confidential health information with local geographical knowledge for community health research. *Journal of Community Health* 35, 635–644.

Beyer, K.M.M., Tiwari, C. and Rushton, G. (2012) Five essential properties of disease maps. *Annals of the Association of American Geographers* 102, 1067–1075.

Bithell, J. (2000) A classification of disease mapping methods. *Statistics in Medicine* 19, 2203–2215.

Boscoe, F.P. and Pickle, L.W. (2003) Choosing geographic units for choropleth rate maps, with an emphasis on public health applications. *Cartography and Geographic Information Science* 30, 237–248.

Brewer, C.A. (2006) Basic mapping principles for visualizing cancer data using geographic information systems (GIS). *American Journal of Preventive Medicine* 30, S25–S36.

Brewer, C.A. and Pickle, L. (2002) Evaluation of methods for classifying epidemiological data on choropleth maps in series. *Annals of the Association of American Geographers* 92, 662–681.

Brewer, C.A., MacEachren, A.M., Pickle, L.W. and Herrmann, D. (1997) Mapping mortality: evaluating color schemes for choropleth maps. *Annals of the Association of American Geographers* 87, 411–438.

Clayton, D. and Kaldor, J. (1987) Empirical Bayes estimates of age-standardized relative risks for use in disease mapping. *Biometrics* 43, 671–681.

Cressie, N. (1992) Statistics for spatial data. *Terra Nova* 4, 613–617.

Densham, P.J. and Rushton, G. (1992) Strategies for solving large location–allocation problems by heuristic methods. *Environment and Planning A* 24, 289–304.

Diggle, P.J., Morris, S. and Morton-Jones, A.J. (1999) Case-control isotonic regression for investigation of elevation in risk around a point source. *Statistics in Medicine* 18, 189–197.

Gatrell, A.C., Bailey, T.C., Diggle, P.J. and Rowlingson, B.S. (1996) Spatial point pattern analysis and its application in geographical epidemiology. *Transactions of the Institute of British Geographers* 21, 256–274.

Goovaerts, P. (2005) Geostatistical analysis of disease data: estimation of cancer mortality risk from empirical frequencies using Poisson kriging. *International Journal of Health Geographics* 4:1. Available at: http://www.ij-healthgeographics.com/content/4/1/31 (accessed 22 March 2013).

Jones, W.D. (1930) Ratios and isopleth maps in regional investigation of agricultural land occupance. *Annals of the Association of American Geographers* 20, no. 4, 177–195.

Kelsall, J.E. and Diggle, P.J. (1995a) Kernel estimation of relative risk. *Bernoulli* 1, 3–16.

Kelsall, J.E. and Diggle, P.J. (1995b) Non-parametric estimation of spatial variation in relative risk. *Statistics in Medicine* 14, 2335–2342.

Kulldorff, M., Heffernan, R., Hartman, J., Assunção, R. and Mostashari, F. (2005) A space–time permutation scan statistic for disease outbreak detection. *PLoS Medicine* 2(3): e59. Available at: http://dx.doi.org/10.1371%2Fjournal.pmed.0020059 (accessed 22 March 2013).

Mollie, A. and Richardson, S. (1991) Empirical Bayes estimates of cancer mortality rates using spatial models. *Statistics in Medicine* 10, 95–112.

Mungiole, M., Pickle, L.W., Simonson, K.H. and White, A. (1999) Application of a weighted head-banging algorithm to mortality data maps. *Statistics in Medicine* 18, 3201–3209.

New York State Department of Health (2010a) Environmental Facilities and Cancer Map. Available at: https://apps.nyhealth.gov/statistics/cancer/environmental_facilities/mapping/map/ (accessed 31 May 2012).

New York State Department of Health (2010b) Environmental Facilities and Cancer Maps: Frequently Asked Questions. 1 May 2010 (update). Available at: http://www.health.ny.gov/statistics/cancer/environmental_facilities/mapping/about/frequently_asked_questions.htm (accessed 31 May 2012).

Openshaw, S. (1977) Optimal zoning systems for spatial interaction models. *Environment and Planning A* 9, 169–184.

Openshaw, S. (1983) *The Modifiable Areal Unit Problem*. Geo Books, Norwich, UK.

Pickle, L.W. and Su, Y. (2002) Within-state geographic patterns of health insurance coverage and health risk factors in the United States. *American Journal of Preventive Medicine* 22, 75–83.

Rushton, G. (2003) Public health, GIS, and spatial analytic tools. *Annual Review of Public Health* 24, 43–56.

Rushton, G. and Lolonis, P. (1996) Exploratory spatial analysis of birth defect rates in an urban population. *Statistics in Medicine* 15, 717–726.

Samet, H. (1984) The quadtree and related hierarchical data structures. *ACM Computing Surveys (CSUR)* 16, 187–260.

Talbot, T.O., Kulldorff, M., Forand, S.P. and Haley, V.B. (2000) Evaluation of spatial filters to create smoothed maps of health data. *Statistics in Medicine* 19, 2399–2408.

Tiwari, C. and Rushton, G. (2005) Using spatially adaptive filters to map late stage colorectal cancer incidence in Iowa. In: Fisher, P.F. (ed.) *Developments in Spatial Data Handling: 11th International Symposium on Spatial Data Handling*. Springer, Berlin, pp. 665–676.

Wakefield, J.C., Best, N.G. and Waller, L. (2000) Bayesian approaches to disease mapping. In: Elliott, P., Wakefield, J.C., Best, N.G. and Briggs, D.J. (eds) *Spatial Epidemiology: Methods and Applications*. Oxford University Press, Oxford, UK, pp. 104–127.

Yiannakoulias, N., Karosas, A., Schopflocher, D.P., Svenson, L.W. and Hodgson, M.J. (2007) Using quad trees to generate grid points for application in geographic disease surveillance. *Advances in Disease Surveillance* 3:2. Available at: http://www.isdsjournal.org/articles/32.pdf (accessed 22 March 2013).

9 Geographic Access to Health Services

Kevin A. Henry* **and Kaila McDonald**
University of Utah, Salt Lake City, Utah, USA

9.1 Introduction

Timely access to health care is an important priority among citizens and governments worldwide and is a highly debated political issue owing to the potential social justice and human rights implications of fair access (WHO, 2010). Greater health in a population is most often linked to lower mortality, lower morbidity and fewer disability adjusted life years (DALYs). Policy and research efforts to improve access to health care and eliminate health disparities have mostly focused on access in terms of costs, affordability and health insurance. While these are essential components of access to health care, there are additional components that can influence it too, including the availability of health services in a community (supply), the number of people needing a service (demand) and the travel distance or time between different populations and health service locations. These components are often described in terms of the geographic access to or spatial accessibility of health services.

In this chapter, we review the basic concepts related to geographic accessibility to health services, and describe the most common measures for estimating geographic accessibility. We also explain how various measures of geographic accessibility can be applied in a real world setting and provide several worked examples of how to calculate these measures. While you are reading the chapter, we encourage you to begin thinking about health care in your community and the factors that play into your own decisions in utilizing health care services.

9.2 Geographic Access to Health Services

Health services include services dealing with the diagnosis and treatment of disease as well as the maintenance and rehabilitation of health. They include services such as cancer screening (e.g. mammography), childhood vaccination, home care services, mental health services, cardiac rehabilitation programmes, hospitalization, dental care, physician care, occupational therapy and child medical services. The term *access*, in the context of health services, describes the 'ability to use health services when and where they are needed' (Aday and Andersen, 1981) and the ability to command appropriate health service resources in order to maintain or improve health (Cromley and McLafferty, 2002).

* E-mail: kevin.henry@geog.utah.edu

A population's overall utilization of health services is determined by predisposing factors and enabling factors, along with perceived and actual need (Andersen, 1995). A population's demographic and health composition are important predisposing factors to accessing health services and often drive the demand for services. For example, a population comprising a large number of children and women of reproductive age places substantial demand on paediatric, obstetric and gynaecological services, while a population with mostly older adults places demand on services for preventing and treating chronic disease. Specific predisposing factors include age, sex, religion and psychosocial factors such as attitudes and beliefs about illness and disease prevention.

For health services to be used, personal and community enabling factors must be available as well. Important enabling factors include health insurance, income, free time, family resources and geographic access to health services. Further enabling factors can include resources such as education and the skills necessary to learn a behaviour that might be beneficial to effectively access health services or to interact with health care providers. A lack of enabling factors, or resources, can serve as barriers to accessing care and can lead to a decreased use of services. For example, a man or woman with a family, a busy work schedule and little free time may be less inclined to visit a physician for preventive services than someone with a less demanding daily schedule. What about yourself? Do you visit a doctor annually? When was the last time you visited a dentist? Can you think of enabling factors that either facilitate or impede your use of health services?

Geographic accessibility is an important enabling factor, and it can either facilitate or inhibit the use of health services. Geographic accessibility specifically describes the relationship between the availability of services (supply), the number of people needing a service (demand), the spatial variation of services from one place to another and the spatial interaction between places. In more general terms, geographic accessibility refers to the 'relative ease' (Wang, 2012) by which health services can be reached and utilized by a population when and where the services are needed (Aday and Andersen, 1981; Cromley and McLafferty, 2002).

A deficit or maldistribution of supply and/or populations travelling long distances to health services can result in access barriers to services and possible geographic disparities in health service utilization rates. Such barriers are often related to economic decisions made by physicians who decide not to live or work in certain geographic areas. For example, physicians may decide to locate and live in areas where patients have the ability to pay, or where there are excellent schools for their children, or where there is easy access to recreational and shopping amenities. Sometimes decisions are made not to build a much needed clinic in a poor community because of high crime rates and the inability of local residents to pay for services. Choices such as these can leave some communities without the necessary health services and create barriers to care, possibly forcing people to commute long distances at inconvenient times to receive care. The maldistribution of resources has been demonstrated in several studies. Onega *et al.* (2008), using road network estimates of travel time to cancer care in the population of the continental USA, discovered that Native Americans and non-urban populations had longer travel times to cancer care than other populations (Onega *et al.*, 2008). In another example, Boscoe *et al.* (2011) examined whether women with early stage breast cancer who live far from a radiation therapy facility may be more likely to opt for mastectomy, which does not require follow-up treatment of radiation, versus breast-conserving surgery (BCS), which requires several weeks of radiation after surgery. They found that women travelling over 75 km for treatment were about 1.4 times more likely to receive a mastectomy than those travelling under 15 km.

In addition to spatial factors, non-spatial factors must be considered, as they can both directly and indirectly affect geographic accessibility. Some population groups may have fewer resources with which to overcome geographic constraints (e.g. travelling to care). Demographic and socio-economic determinants of health service utilization are well documented, and provide sufficient evidence that the use of health services is significantly influenced by age, race/ethnicity, household income, education, insurance status, marital status and health status or co-morbidities. Some population groups, for example, may not have access to a car or public transportation, and for older adults or persons with disabilities driving and/or using public transport may not be possible (Peipins *et al.*, 2011; Blanford *et al.*, 2012). If services are located far from an individual's home, it could be cost-prohibitive to get to them. Also, getting time off from work might be too difficult for some, who consequently might delay or even forgo getting treatment and/or preventive services. Moreover, studies have shown that living close to health services is not a guarantee of better utilization of services either as a result of other key factors such as poverty. The individual and contextual effects of poverty can work to counteract any potential benefit gained from the closeness of services (Cromley and McLafferty, 2002; Henry *et al.*, 2011). Geographic barriers can be based on other criteria as well, such as insurance acceptance (particularly for Medicaid enrollees), convenient parking, short waiting times for an appointment (Elkin *et al.*, 2010), physician referral, accessibility by public transportation, costs under different insurance plans and/or providers and the availability of linguistically appropriate services (Wells and Roetzheim, 2007).

An individual's activity space can also affect geographic access to health services. Activity space represents an individual's set of daily activities and the space within which they occur. It usually begins and ends at an individual's home location and might include daily activity locations such as school, work, shopping and recreation. Access to health services can often be constrained or enabled by an individual's activity space, which is related to the daily time demands of work and family responsibilities (Miller, 2004; Vallée *et al.*, 2010, 2011). Activity spaces that encompass larger areas or longer commute times can provide additional opportunities to access health services. For example, someone who regularly commutes to work or school might have the additional opportunity of seeing a doctor near his or her school or workplace.

Thus far, we have summarized some of the key themes in health care access, focusing mostly on geographic accessibility. We hope that after reading this introductory section you have a better understanding of how health care access is multidimensional, and that insurance is only one of many enabling factors. Furthermore, we also hope that you are excited and encouraged to learn more about how geographic access is measured. For the remainder of the chapter, we will discuss why proximity to care is important, while focusing on the methods that are most utilized for measuring geographic accessibility. Additionally, worked problems are provided using both hypothetical data and data from a case study that examined geographic accessibility to colonoscopy providers in northern Utah.

9.3 Measuring Geographic Accessibility

Evaluating geographic accessibility to health services can help to identify areas with poor access and provide information that can be used for service delivery planning and intervention. There are numerous ways of measuring geographic access, and most can be implemented using a geographic information system (GIS) and/or statistical packages such as R and SAS. The next section (Section 9.3.1) discusses the most popular measure of geographic accessibility: provider-to-population ratios.

9.3.1 Provider-to-population ratios

The most popular measure of geographic accessibility is the provider-to-population ratio (or supply-to-demand ratio). It provides a basic way of assessing the geographic distribution of health resources such as hospital beds, nurses, dentists, physicians and pharmacies in relationship to the population. The ratios are often estimated and mapped as summaries over various census enumeration units (e.g. nation, state, county, postal codes) and help to answer such questions as: where are health services located; are there enough resources; and are the distributions fair? Geographic patterns uncovered from estimating and mapping provider-to-population ratios can be used to generate hypotheses about what causes the patterns, as well as to help plan possible interventions.

In the USA, provider-to-population ratios are used by health departments, hospitals and non-profit organizations to assess need, locate medically underserved areas and examine changing patterns of supply and demand of health services.

The provider-to-population ratio (P_i) is calculated as follows:

$$P_i = \frac{\Sigma Prov_i}{\Sigma Pop_i} \quad (9.1)$$

where P_i for location i is computed by summing both the total number of providers ($Prov_i$) and the population (Pop_i) in need of the service within each unique geographic location i, and then dividing the total providers by total population. The number of providers could be any meaningful measure of capacity, such as number of physicians, clinics or screening mammography machines. When preparing population data, you should think carefully about who needs or demands the service that you are interested in measuring before simply calculating ratios. For example, if you were interested in calculating provider-to-population ratios for colorectal cancer screening accessibility, the demand should reflect those who require this service which, based on current screening recommendations in the USA, would be men and women aged 50 years and older (American Cancer Society, 2011). Including people younger than 50 years of age, who are not considered 'at risk', would increase the population estimates (Pop_i) and ultimately overestimate the need for this service.

Data availability for estimating total providers or facilities (e.g. hospitals) varies by country. In the USA, for example, the most common sources of data used for calculating these ratios are the Health Resources and Services Administration Area Resource File (ARF) (US Department of Health and Human Services, 2012) and state medical licensing data from the American Medical Association (AMA) Physician Masterfile (American Medical Association, 2012). Data for populations or demand within an area are most often available from local or national censuses.

In the following example, we review the steps for calculating provider-to-population ratios using data from Utah. We first collected data from several sources to ascertain both the number of providers and the number of physicians in Utah who perform colorectal cancer (CRC) screening. Providers were identified using a comprehensive Internet search and the ARF, and by reviewing lists of gastroenterologists from the AMA and the National Provider Information (NPI) file (Centers for Medicare & Medicaid Services, 2012). We noted discrepancies in the total number of physicians from these sources so health providers in Utah were contacted to confirm the total number of physicians as well as to obtain full-time equivalency (FTE) rates for each provider. Next, we reviewed the colorectal screening guidelines, which recommend screening for colorectal cancer beginning at age 50 using either high-sensitivity fecal occult blood testing, sigmoidoscopy or colonoscopy. County-level population data (denominator data) therefore included men and women of 50 years and older. These data were obtained from the United States Census Bureau. We then used the physician counts and population data to compute provider-to-population ratios for each county in Utah. As an example, the physician-to-population ratio for Davis County is calculated as follows: six physicians who perform CRC screening ÷ 61,008 persons 50 years and older × 10,000= 0.98. So in Davis County there are 0.98 physicians that can perform colonoscopy per 10,000 persons older than 50 years of age. The geographic distributions of provider-to-population ratios for CRC screening (colonoscopy) are illustrated in Fig. 9.1. Overall, the statewide ratio of colonoscopy providers to the population 50 years and older was 4.1 to 10,000 persons. Duchesne and Wasatch counties had the most colonoscopy providers per population 50 years and older and also the highest provider-to-population ratios, while several counties had no providers (Fig. 9.1).

Despite the popularity of provider-to-population ratios, they have some important limitations that should be considered. First, they do not account for border crossings and assume that boundaries are impermeable and that patients do not leave a defined area unit (in our example, county of residence) to access health services. This is a primary reason why provider-to-population ratios are computed for large geographic regions (e.g. counties, nations, provinces) and are not appropriate for small geographic areas (e.g. census tracts).

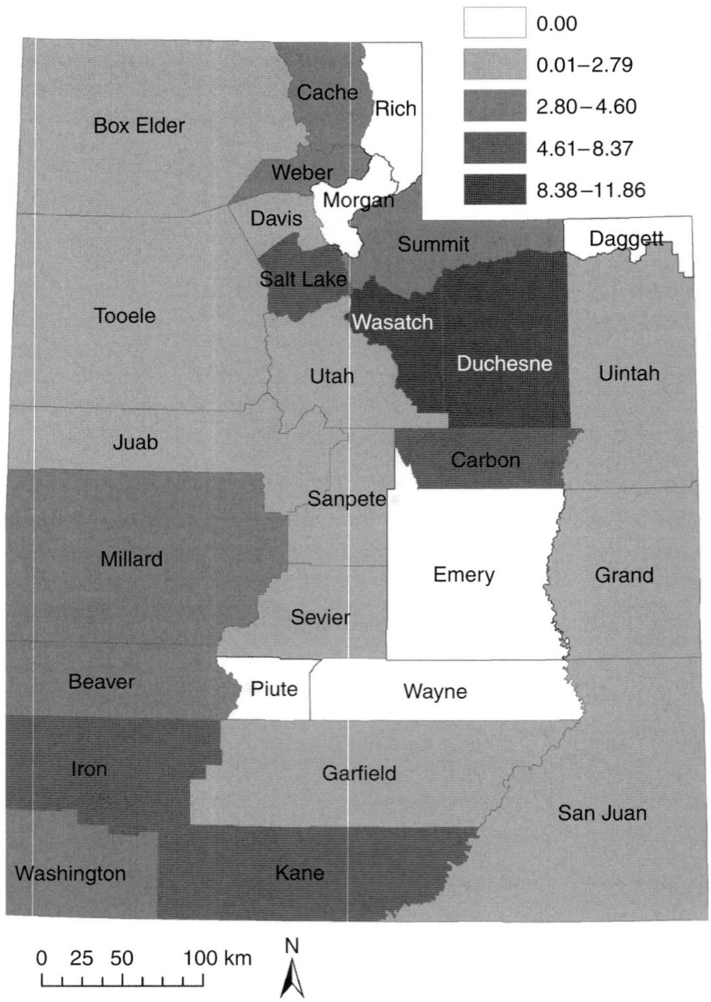

Fig. 9.1. Provider-to-population ratios (providers/10,000 persons of 50+ years) for physicians who perform colorectal cancer (CRC) screening by colonoscopy in Utah.

When considering this problem, think of a place that is part of a large metropolitan area, like northern New Jersey. Would people seeking care here forgo a medical service simply because a county or state boundary must be crossed? It seems very unlikely. While the problem is less pronounced in certain geographic locations, we cannot ignore this limitation when assessing provider-to-population ratios. A second problem with provider-to-population ratios is that nothing is revealed about the detailed spatial variation within a region. In our example, Morgan County had no physicians who perform CRC screening However, a review of the population distribution revealed that the majority of the population lives close to the county border that straddles Weber and Davis counties, which have adequate supplies and are only a short drive for those living in Morgan County. Finally, a third problem with provider-to-population ratios is that the ratios themselves can vary significantly depending on the size, number and configuration of the study zones. This is yet another example of the modifiable areal unit problem (MAUP) that was discussed in Section 8.3.2.

In summary, provider-to-population ratios provide a measure of the availability of health services (i.e. supply, capacity) but they do not provide any information about how far individuals have to travel to get to a specific service. In the next section (Section 9.3.2), we review methods for measuring distance and travel time to health services.

9.3.2 Measuring proximity and travel time to providers

Measuring the proximity or distance between residential locations and features of interest in an effort to identify health risks, gaps, shortages and disparities has become a popular technique in recent years. Proximity measures have been used for many applications. For example, researchers have examined distance and travel time to preventive (e.g. cancer screening, vaccination), primary (e.g. physicians) and emergency (e.g. burn centres) health services (Messina *et al.*, 2006; Patel *et al.*, 2007; Hayanga *et al.*, 2009; Klein *et al.*, 2009; Ludwick *et al.*, 2009; Luo and Qi, 2009; Sasaki *et al.*, 2010; Gabrysch *et al.*, 2011; Gatrell and Wood, 2012). More recently, there has been an interest in measuring proximity and access to healthy amenities in communities, such as bike paths, parks, schools, recreation facilities, supermarkets, farmers' markets and greengrocers (Po'e *et al.*, 2012; Yamashita and Kunkel, 2012). In addition, there have been a number of studies examining proximity to adverse features – such as gambling centres, liquor stores, unhealthy foods, billboards and pollution (Burdette and Whitaker, 2004; Cradock *et al.*, 2005; Gilliland and Ross, 2005; Pearce *et al.*, 2006; Larsen and Gilliland, 2008; Hart *et al.*, 2009; Hay *et al.*, 2009; Hillier *et al.*, 2009; Kearney and Kiros, 2009). The majority of studies have found that proximity or accessibility was a significant explanatory factor in the use of health services, with longer distances (i.e. poor accessibility) corresponding to lower use of services and lower exposure.

So, why is proximity an important consideration when examining geographic access to health services or other features of interest (e.g. parks)? Typically, it is important because of the concept of *distance decay* and its relationship to geographic access to health services. Distance decay refers to the decline of an activity, function or exposure with increasing distance from a point of origin (e.g. residence). The decline in activity is a result of the 'friction' of distance, or the way that distance can impede movement from one location to another. The concept of friction of distance is based on the idea that moving from one location to another requires time and/or money. Therefore, the 'friction', or added time and costs needed to travel long distances to access health services, might result in lower utilization rates.

The actual effect of distance on health care utilization varies with population characteristics such as poverty and demographic structure. Among men and women living in impoverished urban areas, individual and contextual effects of poverty might counteract any potential benefit of the close proximity of health services. For example, men and women from impoverished urban areas with good access to mammography might have to bypass nearby facilities and travel further to care if facilities do not accept their insurance or if they are seeking charity care. Additionally, a study by Probst *et al.* (2007) suggested that the use of public transport, common in impoverished urban areas, adds a substantial amount of travel time. The study found that people who used public transportation or walked to care spent more time in travel than those who drove themselves to care (28.8 versus 20.5 minutes), and that the average trip time to care by public transport was almost the same as average trip time for rural residents. Barriers to transportation in both impoverished and non-impoverished rural areas might compound access problems. In rural areas, public transportation is limited and those without cars must depend on friends and family for transportation, thus possibly limiting their trip timing and route. Furthermore, rural residents who we might expect to have lower utilization rates because of relatively longer travel times to health services may in fact have high utilization rates because they are accustomed to travelling relatively longer distances for services and basic necessities (e.g. groceries). So when examining geographic access to health services for different populations it is important to look beyond measures of proximity and remember that other factors, such as poverty and transportation, can have an impact on the actual effect of proximity to services.

The frictional effect of distance is not the same for all health services and can vary based on the concentration of services in a region, the type of service and the need for that service. For example, an examination of the relationship between distance to hospital on inpatient episodes in Cambridgeshire, Norfolk and Suffolk in the UK found that, after controlling for confounders, distance to hospital was a significant predictor for acute elective, acute emergency, psychiatric and geriatric episodes (Haynes *et al.* 1999). Figure 9.2 shows the effect of distance on these different inpatient episodes. We can see from this graph that for acute episodes, hospital distance had a greater impact on emergency than on elective admissions. Distance to hospital had the greatest impact on acute emergency and psychiatric episodes.

When examining proximity to services, the degree of medical specialization being examined can also affect the frictional effects of distance. Generally, there are fewer specialized health services than general or less specialized services. Consequently, the frictional effect of distance will be more important for more specialized services than for less specialized services because a greater proportion of the population will have to travel further to access these services. As an example, Fig. 9.3 provides a summary of travel times to various cancer care and prevention services among the US population. The graph shows that as the level of service specialization decreases, the proportion of the population that lives within 30 min of that care increases. For instance, approximately 50% of the population lives within 30 min of academic-based care – the most specialized type of cancer care, while 96% of women live within 30 min of mammography screening facilities, the least specialized service. The abundance of mammography facilities in the USA significantly reduces the friction of distance to this particular service as compared with that of the other cancer care services.

9.3.3 Measures of distance and travel time

There are four common types of distance measures used when calculating proximity to services: Euclidean distance (straight line), great

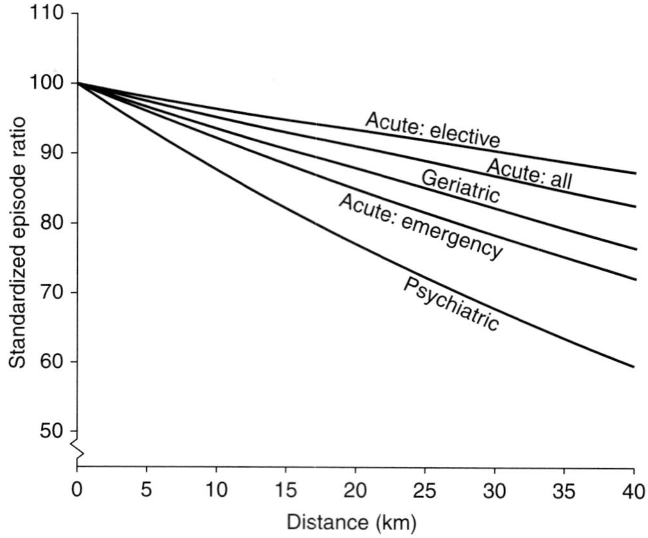

Fig. 9.2. Effects of distance to hospital on inpatient episodes in Cambridgeshire, Norfolk and Suffolk, UK. Source: Haynes *et al.* (1999).

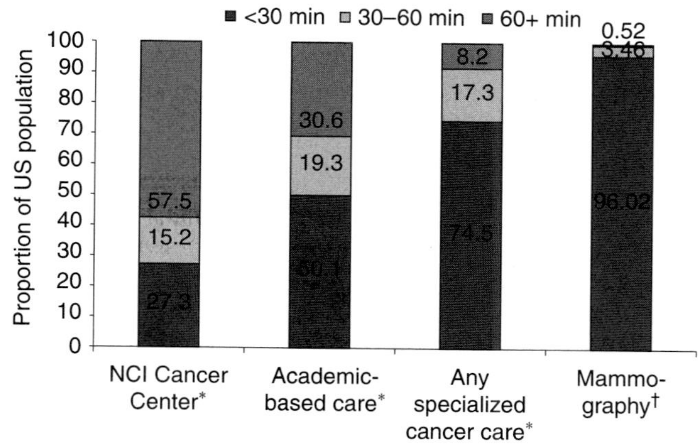

Fig. 9.3. Percentage of the US population by categories of travel time to the nearest type of cancer care. NCI, National Cancer Institute. Source: *Onega *et al.* (2008); †Henry *et al.* (2011).

circle distance, Manhattan distance and shortest network distance. Euclidean and Manhattan distances can easily be computed between two points using only the geographic coordinates of both points. The Euclidean distance, a straight line distance between two points, is appropriate to use when working with projected geographic coordinates such as the Universal Transverse Mercator (UTM), state plane, Australian Map Grid (AMG) or equidistant conic systems. It is important to remember, however, that Euclidean distances do not take into account the curvature of the earth, meaning that the data should be projected before calculating distances, especially when calculating over larger geographic areas. Euclidean distance is calculated using the Pythagorean formula:

$$e_{ij} = \sqrt{(X_i - X_j)^2 + (Y_i - Y_j)^2} \quad (9.2)$$

where location i has the coordinates (X_i, Y_i) and location j has the coordinates (X_j, Y_j), the Euclidean distance (e_{ij}) is computed by taking the squared difference of the two X coordinates and the two Y coordinates, adding them together and then taking the square root.

As an example, Fig. 9.4 shows the distance between a patient's home and a hospital. The UTM coordinates at location (residence) A are 12N/N 4,632,991/E 406,380; at destination B (health care facility) they are 12N/N 4,619,331/E 401,200. The Euclidean distance between these two locations is computed as 14.61 km (see equation bottom of page):

A limitation of Euclidean distance is that it does not take into account geographic barriers (e.g. mountains, lakes) or road networks. As illustrated in Fig. 9.4, Euclidean distance does not follow the path of the road network and so underestimates the true travel distance. In densely populated or urban areas, an alternative measure of distance is the Manhattan distance, also known as the taxicab distance. This measures the distance between two points based on a Cartesian grid. Manhattan distances are the sum of the distances of the horizontal and vertical components connecting the start and end points. The Manhattan distance can be calculated as:

$$m_{ij} = |X_i - X_j| + |Y_i - Y_j| \quad (9.3)$$

$$\begin{aligned} e_{ij} &= \sqrt{(401{,}200 - 406{,}380)^2 + (4{,}619{,}331 - 4{,}632{,}991)^2} = \sqrt{(26{,}832{,}400 + 186{,}595{,}600)} \\ &= \sqrt{213{,}428{,}000} = 14{,}609\ \text{m} = 14.61\ \text{km} \end{aligned}$$

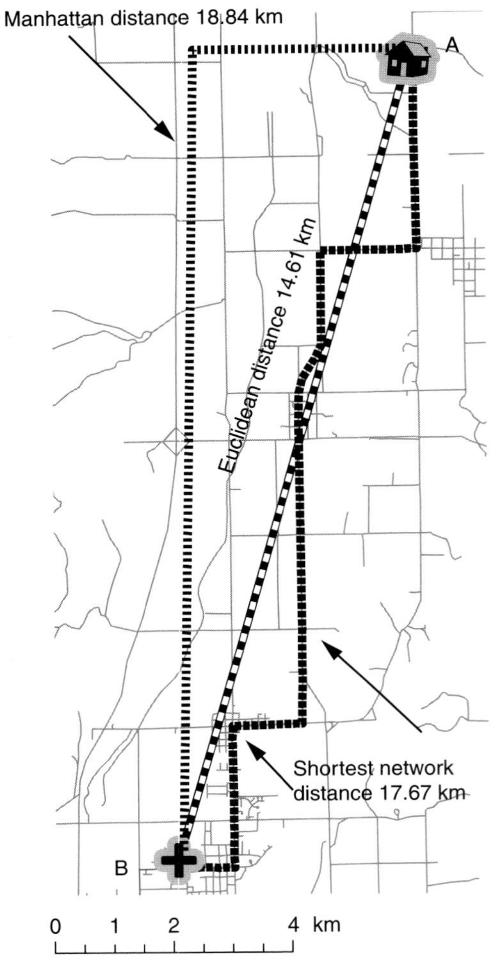

Fig. 9.4. Euclidean, Manhattan and road network distances from client (residence) A to health care facility B.

where location i has the coordinates (X_i, Y_i) and location j has the coordinates (X_j, Y_j).

Using the same location data as for the previous example and Eqn 9.3, the Manhattan distance (m_{ij}) between these two locations is computed as:

$$m_{ij} = |401{,}200 - 406{,}380| + |4{,}619{,}332 - 4{,}632{,}991| = 5180 + 13{,}659 = 18{,}839 \text{ m} = 18.84 \text{ km}$$

So the Manhattan distance between residence A and facility B is 18.84 km. This is larger than the Euclidean measure of 14.61 km, and is much closer to the actual road network distance of 17.67 km (see Fig. 9.4). Manhattan distances may not be as accurate as road network calculations, but in a study area where roads networks follow a grid pattern, this measure is a very good surrogate for street network distances.

When calculating distances over large regions (e.g. state, continent), or when using unprojected geographic coordinates (e.g. latitude and longitude), distance measurements should be calculated along the curved surface of the earth or the measurements will not be correct. This measurement is referred to as great circle distance, or a spherical distance. It is the shortest distance between two points on the surface of a sphere, a curved line whose visualization is familiar from representations of airplane flight paths. The calculations for great circle distances are different from Euclidean geometry because there are no straight lines; instead, there are geodesics (great circles) on the sphere. There are several ways of calculating great circle distances, including the spherical law of cosines, Haversine or Vincenty formulas. The last two methods are better for calculating small distances.

The great circle distance in kilometres between two points i (X_i, Y_i) and j (X_j, Y_j) can be calculated using the spherical law of cosines as:

$$C_{ij} = (\arccos[\sin(Y_i)\sin(Y_j) + \cos(Y_i)\cos(Y_j)\cos(X_i - X_j)]) \times 6371.01 \quad (9.4)$$

where: c_{ij} = great circle distance (in km); Y = latitude (in radians) at locations i and j; X = longitude (in radians) at locations i and j; and 6371.01 represents the mean radius of the earth in kilometres.

Using the location data from Table 9.1, the projected coordinates of latitude and longitude must first be converted from degrees into radians. This is done by multiplying degrees by $\pi/180$, the results of which are displayed in the Table 9.1 and are now added into our equation (see equation bottom of page):

$$c_{ij} = (\text{arcos}([\sin(0.7303) \times \sin(0.7282)) + (\cos(0.7303) \times \cos(0.7282)) \times \cos(1.9570) - (1.9578)]) \times 6371.01 = 13.91\text{km}$$

Table 9.1. Converting from latitude/longitude to radians.

		Degrees	× Radian conversion factor (π/180)	= Radians
Y_i	Latitude 1	41.8433	(3.1416/180)	0.7303
Y_j	Latitude 2	41.7199	(3.1416/180)	0.7282
X_i	Longitude 1	−112.1277	(3.1416/180)	1.9570
X_j	Longitude 2	−112.1731	(3.1416/180)	1.9578

While these three distance measures (Euclidean, Manhattan and great circle) are still routinely used in GIS, recent technological advances have essentially eliminated the cost of calculating street network distances, allowing most personal computers to now easily and quickly perform these more accurate distance calculations. Network distances are quickly becoming the most popular method for calculating geographic distances in health services research. Network distance is the shortest path (or least cost) distance through a road network. A road network is made up of a set of nodes (junctions) that connect a set of arcs (edges), which form the basis of network connectivity. In addition to connectivity, attribute features can be added to control navigation through the networks. Popular features that are often added to networks include driving direction, speed limits and turning restrictions. There are several algorithms currently proposed for obtaining the shortest path between two places on a network. A widely used approach, discussed in Section 1.8, is the algorithm developed by Dijkstra (1959).

Travel times to health services can also be calculated using network data sets and Dijkstra's algorithm if average travel speeds and/or speed limits are available as attributes for the network data set. The effects of traffic on travel time at certain times of the day can be integrated as well by incorporating additional traffic data into the network data set. When considering access to care, travel times may be a more relevant alternative measure of geographic access than travel distance because it is more reflective of the overall effort and costs to get to and from a location. Street network data can be purchased from commercial vendors (e.g. NavTeq) and integrated into GIS software programs. Traffic data can be purchased from local or state transportation departments or third party vendors. United States Census TIGER files can be converted into street networks, although they lack attribute data such as speed limits and turn restrictions, and hence are limited in their ability to depict flow through networks. Additionally, there are commercial web sites (e.g. Google, Yahoo!, Mapquest and Bing, and in North America, Rand McNally) available that offer precise driving directions between nearly all locations in the developed world. Programs written in SAS or in open source programming languages, such as Python or Perl, can be used to make repeated calls to these sites, thus automating data acquisition (Zdeb, 2009). While these sites do not require additional GIS software for processing data, many of them have restrictions on how many records can be processed daily. At the time of writing, Google's limit was 2500 records a day.

9.4 Travel Impedance and Geographic Accessibility

Travel impedance is a measure or the amount of resistance or cost required to move from one location to another along a path in a network. Resistance can be measured as travel time, distance or cost. An impedance value of 0 indicates no resistance, while higher impedance values (e.g. longer travel times) imply more resistance to movement.

The application and potential usefulness of travel impedance measures, specifically distance and time, rely on the concept of distance decay. Therefore, it is often assumed that those living closer to a needed service have better accessibility and perhaps better utilization rates than those living further away from the service. Travel impedance (or travel cost) from a client's residence to the closest health service location is one of the simplest and most intuitive methods of measuring potential geographic access to health services (Guagliardo, 2004). Distance or travel time to the closest health service facility has been utilized in countless studies and provides a simple way to assess the availability of services and the relative ease by which those resources can be reached (Aday and Andersen, 1981; Cromley and McLafferty, 2002; Ray and Ebener, 2008; Wang, 2012). Of course, when distance or travel time to the closest facility is used as a travel impedance measure, it is assumed that clients and patients will use the closest facility. In some health care systems, for certain procedures or visits, there may be efficiencies built into the system whereby clients and patients do in fact go to the closest screening facility or primary care centre.

However, this scenario is likely to be the exception, not the rule. In a private market health care system, the provider assigned to a patient may not be the closest provider to their residence. In some situations, patients may elect to bypass the facility closest and instead seek care at a facility with what they perceive as better services, even though it is located further away from their home (Adams and Wright, 1991; Tai *et al.*, 2004; Baldwin *et al.*, 2008; Boscoe *et al.*, 2011; Gauthier and Wane, 2011). One study that examined Medicare beneficiaries in a rural market found that 60% of patients living in rural areas used the hospital services at their closest rural hospital and 40% used either hospitals in urban areas or hospitals other than the closest (Adams and Wright, 1991). Another study found that Medicare patients had a strong preference for closer hospitals and those with greater service capacity. The study noted that patients with complex acute medical conditions and those with more resources were more likely to bypass their closest rural hospitals. Other factors noted for bypassing the closest facility included not having a regular physician, preferences for certain hospital attributes, longer travel time to a physician's office and dissatisfaction with the availability of health care (Tai *et al.*, 2004). Because clients do not always receive care at the closest facility, several researchers have suggested that a single measure of distance or time to nearest facility is not appropriate when measuring geographic access to care; instead, they favour measures that combine the availability of services (supply) and travel impedance (distance or time) (Fryer *et al.*, 1999; Guagliardo, 2004).

One such measure, which combines travel impedance and availability of services, is average travel impedance from a client location to all service providers within a service or catchment area. Average travel impedance can be calculated for individual client locations or for population nodes, such as census blocks or census tracts or postal codes. It is computed by averaging all travel impedance measures (e.g. travel time or distance) from an origin point to all service providers in a defined study area. Average travel impedance is given by:

$$Z_i^c = \frac{\sum_{(b \in i)} \omega_b I_{bs}}{\sum_{(b \in i)} \omega_b} \qquad (9.5)$$

where: Z_i^c = average travel impedance between the population in area i and all services; ω_b = total population of spatial unit b contained within area i; and I_{bs} = impedance (distance or time) between the centroid of spatial unit b and service s. Generally, the higher the average travel impedance Z_i^c, the farther clients must travel, on average, to access facilities in their service area, meaning that they have poorer geographic access.

There are a number of alternatives to average travel impedance, including the average distance or time to n number of services and the average number of services within n distance or time. Let us look at a simple example of travel impedance. Figure 9.5 illustrates the straight line and road network paths for 12 clients to their nearest colorectal cancer screening (colonoscopy) provider in northern Utah. Table 9.2 shows the nearest provider for each client, distance measures, average distance to all facilities and the number of facilities within 45 min. If you examine the map in Fig. 9.5, you will see how physical features, such as mountains and lakes, can sometimes result in Euclidean distances being imprecise, even inappropriate, proxies for network distance. Client 12, for example, has a network distance to the nearest facility that is two times more than the Euclidean distance (63.66 km versus 136.67 km). This discrepancy is because the

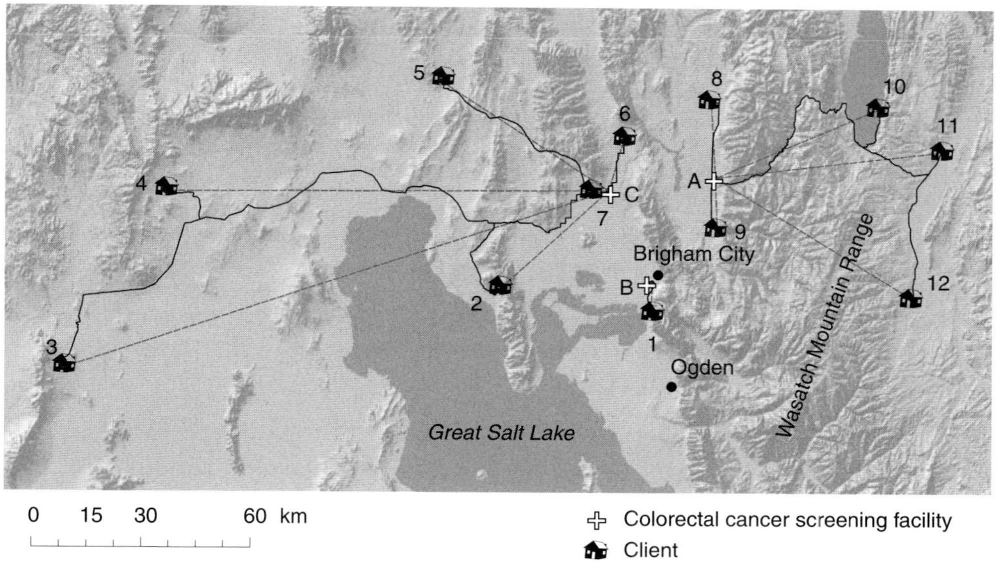

Fig. 9.5. Paths of Euclidean and road network distances to closest colonoscopy providers (A, B, C) from 12 client locations (1–12) in northern Utah.

straight line distance calculation runs straight through a mountain range, a path that has no roads. If you examine the average distance calculation (Table 9.2), you will see that clients 1, 6, 7 and 9 have the best accessibility on average, as calculated by average network distance to all facilities.

Based on this example, you might be inclined to believe that that actual travel distances over road networks are superior measurement alternatives, which would be a correct assumption. Distances calculated utilizing networks are currently the preferred method (whenever possible), and more researchers routinely use network distances in geographic access studies, a trend that is likely to continue to increase, especially as it is less expensive and no longer the labour intensive or GIS lab-dependent undertaking that it once was.

While network distance is a superior measurement, numerous studies have noted that the correlation between straight line distance and network distance is very high, especially for urban areas (Martin *et al.*, 2002; Wood and Gatrell, 2002; Jordan *et al.*, 2004). In one study, Boscoe *et al.* (2011) used travel distances obtained from Google Maps to compare straight line and travel (road network) distances to community hospitals from a representative sample of more than 66,000 locations in the 50 states of the USA, the District of Columbia and Puerto Rico. The authors found that in nearly all locations within the USA, straight line distance is an adequate proxy for road network distance. Important deviations between the two measures were mostly limited to areas located either near uncrossable physical features, such as lakes, rivers and mountains, or in wilderness areas of the western USA and Alaska. The authors also noted that the correlation between straight line and road network distance was strongest after applying a detour index of 1.42. A detour index is a measure of network efficiency, or of how directly travel can be made on a network. It is calculated as the ratio of driving distance to straight line distance. The minimum possible resulting value for a detour index is 1, which represents a direct route, whereas high ratios suggests an inefficient network or indirect routes.

Let us look at a simple example of the detour index. If you examine the network routes for clients 5, 7, 8 and 9, illustrated in Fig. 9.5, you will notice the network driving routes do not deviate substantially from the straight line routes and that the distances of the two are similar (Table 9.2). These routes therefore have the lowest detour index compared

Table 9.2. Summary of proximity measures from 12 client locations (1–12) in northern Utah to closest colonoscopy provider (A, B, C).

Client residence	Closest colorectal cancer screening provider	Euclidean (straight line distance) (km)	Network distance (km)	Detour index	Distance based on the average detour index of 1.43	Average distance to all facilities	No. of facilities within 45 min
1	B	8.93	12.3	1.38	12.77	37.2	2
2	C	41.19	69.76	1.69	58.9	89.1	0
3	C	157.79	204.5	1.3	225.64	223.9	0
4	C	121.47	154.35	1.27	173.7	173.9	0
5	C	54.81	61.94	1.13	78.38	97.59	1
6	C	14.22	17.67	1.24	20.33	33.6	2
7	C	5.78	6.48	1.12	8.27	31.05	2
8	A	21.33	24.73	1.16	30.5	52.3	1
9	A	14.1	17.1	1.21	20.16	36.08	2
10	A	48.94	91.69	1.87	69.98	118.8	0
11	A	62.97	106.42	1.69	90.05	133.19	0
12	A	63.66	136.67	2.15	91.03	142.86	0

with the other routes. In contrast, if you examine the network routes for clients 10, 11 and 12, you will notice that the network distance to the nearest facility deviates substantially from the straight line distance to the nearest facility. These routes have the highest detour index compared with the other routes. This large deviation is a result of clients having to drive all the way around a mountain, a much longer route than the straight line distance, which runs directly through the mountain. Finally, a detour index can be used to estimate network distances from straight line distances. This exercise is completed by multiplying the straight line distances by a detour index. In our example, we multiplied the straight line distances for each client by the average detour index for all 12 clients, which is 1.43. The results are shown in Table 9.2. While this estimation is straightforward, the difficulty arises in knowing the appropriate detour index to use for a specific geographic area or region.

9.5 Supply and Demand Models

9.5.1 Gravity models

Geographic accessibility measures based on travel impedance measures, such as distance or time, offer information about access and availability, but fail to capture information about both supply (e.g. number of physicians, number of mammography screening machines) and demand. When supply and demand relationships are of interest, researchers often turn to the gravity model. The gravity model, which is based on Isaac Newton's theory of gravity, measures the interaction or attraction between a given population (or individual) and all service locations within a study area. It specifies that the attraction between any two locations is proportional to their mass (e.g. population) and inversely proportional to the distance or travel time separating them. Consequently, as travel distance or time increases between an origin and a potential destination, clients are increasingly less likely to make trips to that location. The overall strength of attractiveness of potential destinations can depend on economic activities or services at the destination. For example, health facilities with more specialized and/or lifesaving health services will tend to have a lower distance decay function, as people are likely to travel longer distances for essential services. Cancer patients, for instance, might bypass a local hospital, and travel much further to obtain care at a larger cancer centre with more specialized treatment services or clinical trials. Conversely, clients are less likely to travel long distances to receive basic and elective services.

A simple model that uses gravity model concepts in describing geographic accessibility is the potential model. The potential model provides a measure of an area's overall potential geographic accessibility to services. The model is given by Eqn 9.6:

$$A_i = \sum_{i=1} \frac{S_j}{\left(d_{ij}^b\right)} \qquad (9.6)$$

where A_i is the potential geographic accessibility measure calculated for an individual or area i, S_j is the service capacity at provider j, and d is the measure of travel impedance (e.g. distance or time) between points i and j. The exponent b is the distance decay function. When b is set to equal 0, it has no frictional effect and does not affect access. Therefore, access, in the case of $b = 0$, would only depend on the attractiveness (e.g. capacity) of the providers, but when b is >0, the frictional effect does have an impact on measures of access to services. Higher values of A_i indicate higher levels of (i.e. better) potential geographic accessibility.

Let us now look at how to calculate geographic accessibility using the potential model. Table 9.3 summarizes the northern Utah colonoscopy provider data used for this example and Fig. 9.6 shows the study area. The grid cells shown in Fig. 9.6 (bottom) represent populated locations in the study area. The three crosses represent the locations of colonoscopy providers. The population is not distributed evenly through the study area, because mountains and deserts cover large parts of the region. To keep it simple, we will estimate A_i for only one grid cell (Fig. 9.6 (top) and cell 1, Table 9.3). The travel distances from grid cell 1 to facilities A, B, and C are 6.28 km, 44.31 km, and 35.98 km, respectively. The corresponding network routes are displayed in Fig. 9.6 (top), and details of the numbers of physicians per facility are provided in Table 9.3.

A_i is the sum of $(s_j)/(d_{ij}^d)$, where $b = 2$. For facility A, this is calculated as: six physicians/ $(6.28\ \text{km})^2 = 0.15214$. This calculation is repeated for grid cell 1 to separately account for facilities B and C. The total potential accessibility measure A_i for grid cell 1 is then the sum of the estimates for each of the facilities 1A + 1B + 1C, or 0.15214 + 0.00153 + 0.00023, which is 0.15390. Typically, A_i is not computed for just one location, but instead will be computed for an entire study region, which allows for meaningful relative comparisons of magnitude between locations. We have already estimated A_i for all of the grid cells in the entire study area and these results are shown in Fig. 9.6 (bottom). Not surprisingly, the results indicate that the best potential accessibility (highest values) surrounds the providers, while areas of lower accessibility are further away from the providers. The worst potential accessibility (lowest) values are northeast of the three providers, on the east side of a large mountain range.

While the potential model is a useful tool for assessing potential deficiencies in access, the measure of A_i is not as intuitive as provider-to-population ratios, or travel time and distance measures. The potential model only examines supply and does not adjust for demand. As a result, A_i would be the same for facilities located at similar distances and with similar capacity (e.g. number of physicians, number of hospital beds), regardless of the differences in

Table 9.3. Potential geographic accessibility to physicians performing colorectal cancer (CRC) screening (colonoscopy) in northern Utah based on travel distance and supply and calculated using the potential model.

Grid cell	Facility	Travel distance (d_{ij} in km)	Physicians per facility (S_j, FTE)[a]	Potential geographic accessibility (A_i) measure for each facility ($S_j/d_{ij}^{b=2}$), where b = distance decay function
1	A	6.28	6	0.15214
1	B	44.31	3	0.00153
1	C	35.98	0.3	0.00023
Potential geographic accessibility including facilities A,B,C:				**A_i = 0.15390**

[a]full-time equivalent.

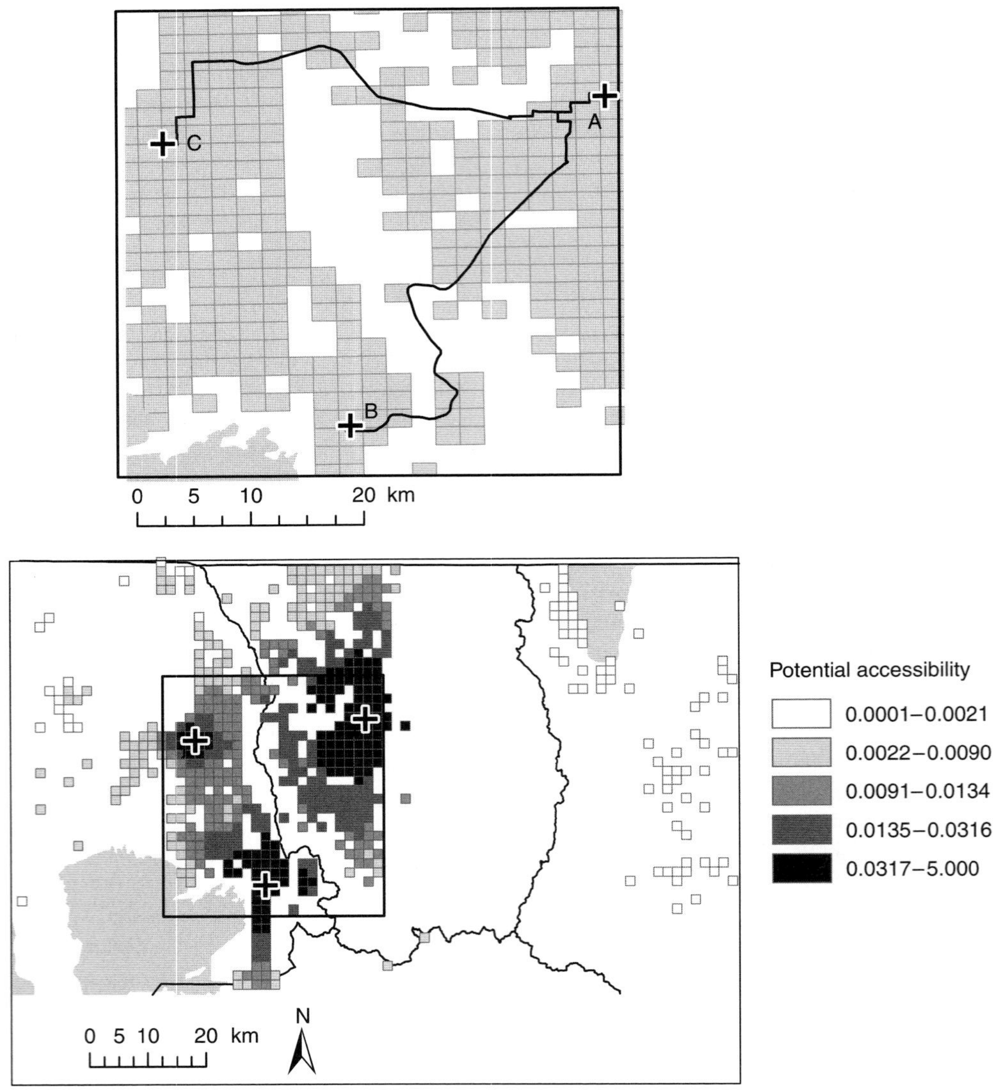

Fig. 9.6. Potential accessibility to physicians performing colorectal cancer screening (by colonoscopy) in northern Utah. Top, grid cell 1 for estimating the potential accessibility model for facilities A, B and C (see Table 9.3); and bottom, map of final values of potential accessibility for study area.

population sizes or demand. Because of this limitation, the potential model probably does not fully capture a population's experience in accessing a health service. If a researcher is interested in measurements that incorporate both supply and demand, a gravity model can be utilized, as demonstrated in our next example.

Below we present a hypothetical worked example of a gravity model, as originally proposed by Wang (2006), and using three colonoscopy providers and the locations of two populations in need of services. The gravity model is given by:

$$A_i^G = \sum_{j=1}^{n} \frac{\left(S_j t_{ij}^{-b}\right)}{(V_i)} \tag{9.7}$$

where: A_i^G = gravity-based accessibility index; n = total number of supply locations; t_{ij} = travel time between population i and facility j; $-b$ = decay function (time); S_j = supply at facility j; and V_j = population demand potential.

The population demand potential, V_j, represents service availability, and is given by Eqn (9.8):

$$V_j = \sum_{k=1}^{m} D_k t_{kj}^{-b} \quad (9.8)$$

where: V_j = population demand potential; m = total number of demand locations; D_k = population demand at location k; t_{kj} = travel distance or time between population demand location and supply location; and $-b$ = decay function (time).

Figure 9.7 shows the locations of three colonoscopy facilities (A, B, C), the number of FTE physicians at each facility, the population total at demand locations k_1 and k_2, and the network travel times between each facility and each population and/or demand location. In this example, the population cell i and demand location k are in the same location. The data and subsequent calculations are given in Table 9.4. Following the gravity model equation above, we first calculate the population potential (demand) V_i for each facility. This is calculated by first estimating the population demand potential for each facility, and then summing these values by each facility. For example, the calculation for facility A and demand location k_1 is 10,000 × (5 min)$^{-1}$ = 2000; for facility A and demand location k_2, it is 20,000 × (15 min)$^{-1}$ = 1333. The estimate of V_i is completed by summing the population potential values for each unique facility. In our example for A, the sum would be 2000 + 1333, which equals 3333.

Next, for each demand or population location we estimate geographic accessibility to each facility based on supply. For example, to describe population i_1 from location k_1 accessing facility A, we calculate the following: (6 physicians × (5 min)$^{-1}$)/3333 = 0.00036.

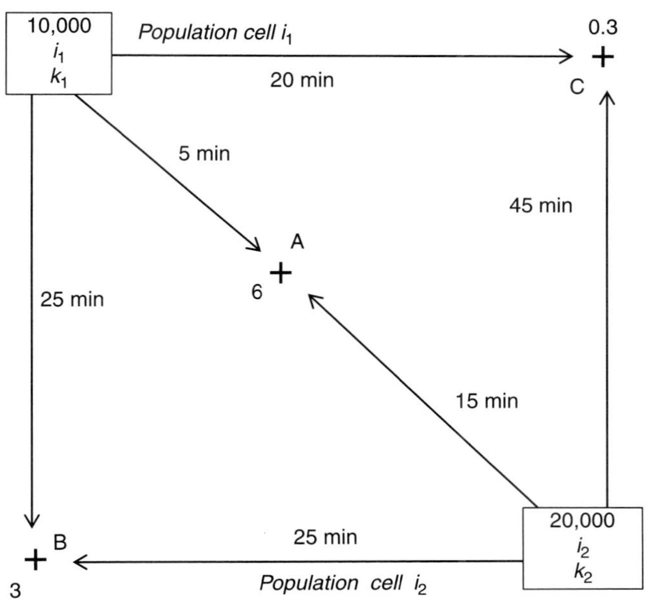

Fig. 9.7. Illustration of accessibility to physicians performing colorectal cancer (CRC) screening (by colonoscopy) in northern Utah based on supply and demand: the use of the gravity model method. A, B, C, colonoscopy facilities; 6, 3, 0.3, CRC physician supply at each facility; 10,000, 20,000, demand populations at cells i_1 and i_2 and demand locations k_1 and k_2. Travel times shown in min.

Table 9.4. Accessibility to physicians performing colorectal cancer (CRC) screening (colonoscopy) in northern Utah based on both supply and demand, and calculated using the gravity model.

Population cell (i)	Demand location (k)	Facility (j)	Demand population (i)	Time (min)	Population demand potential, V_j ($i \times$ time^{-1})	Sum of population demand potential by facility (ΣV_j)	Supply/ies CRC physicians per facility	Σi: accessibility to each facility based on physician supply (no. $\times$ time^{-1}) $\div \Sigma V_j$	Accessibility measure per 100 persons
i_1	k_1	A	10,000	5	2,000	3,333	6	0.000360	
i_1	k_1	B	10,000	25	400	1,200	3	0.000100	
i_1	k_1	C	10,000	20	500	944	0.30	0.000016	
								Σi_1 = 0.000476	**4.76**
i_2	k_2	A	20,000	15	1,333	3,333	6	0.000120	
i_2	k_2	B	20,000	25	800	1,200	3	0.000100	
i_2	k_2	C	20,000	45	444	944	0.30	0.000007	
								Σi_2 = 0.000227	**2.27**

The values for i_1 accessing facility B and C are 0.000100 and 0.000016, respectively. Lastly, to obtain a final accessibility measure for population location i_1 these values for geographic accessibility of each facility are summed. In this example, A_i^G for population cell i_1 is 0.00036 + 0.000100 + 0.000016 = 0.000476 (see Table 9.4).

The gravity-based geographic accessibility measures for populations i_1 and i_2 are 0.000476 and 0.000227, respectively (Table 9.4). Larger values denote better accessibility, and therefore, location i_1 has better geographic accessibility to colorectal cancer screening than does location i_2. While the gravity model is commonly used in health services, it is difficult to calibrate, because we often do not know the decay function (–*b*) between two locations. Remember that the decay function represents the decline in an activity due to increasing travel time or distance between populations and providers. The type of health service being studied can dictate the most appropriate decay function to use, and the decay function can have many possible forms, such as log–logistic, exponential and power. The only way to truly know the most appropriate decay function to use is to derive it from actual data on travel patterns of clients and/or patients to services. This is often not possible, because these data are often unavailable, restricted for certain analysis or are too costly.

Because of these difficulties, many researchers have opted to use the two-step floating catchment method (2SFCA), developed by Luo and Wang (2003), to estimate geographic accessibility. This method does not rely on a time impedance measurement, and is discussed in the next section (Section 9.5.2). For useful modifications of the gravity model for estimating geographic access to health care see Schuurman *et al.* (2009).

9.5.2 Floating catchment method

Like the gravity model, the two-step floating catchment method (2SFCA) also considers supply and demand of services. This method requires that the geographic locations (i.e. coordinates) of supply locations, their service capacities (e.g. physicians) and demand locations (i.e. populations in need of services locations) be known. These data can be examined at the individual level, or aggregated over regions, such as census units or postal codes. The 2SFCA method (Wang, 2006) is given as:

$$A_i^F = \sum_{j\in(t_{ij}\le t_0)} R_j = \sum_{j\in(t_{ij}\le t_0)} \left(\frac{S_j}{\Sigma_{j\in(t_{ij}\le t_0)} D_i} \right) \quad (9.9)$$

where: A_i^F = geographic accessibility at location i; R_j = supply-to-demand ratio within a catchment area; t_0 = travel time threshold; i = demand location (population); j = supply location (e.g. physician); D_i = demand at location i; and $S_j = S_j$ supply at location j.

The 2SFCA measures geographic accessibility as a ratio of providers to the population in need of services using a two-step process: first, within a given catchment area $j \in (t_{ij} \le t_0)$ (e.g. 30 min drive time), we calculate a supply-to-demand ratio for each supply location j. The catchment area can be derived using distance, travel time or some other impedance measure. Next, for each demand location i, we search for all supply locations j that are within the catchment area, and then sum the supply-to-demand ratios, *Rj*, for each demand location i calculated in the previous step. Summing *Rj* at each location provides A_i^F (the geographic accessibility) at location i. As with the potential and gravity models, a larger 2SFCA access score indicates better geographic accessibility within the study area.

Now we will examine how to calculate geographic accessibility by the 2SFCA method, using a hypothetical set of data that includes the location of three physician practices (A, B, C) and seven populations (1–7). The study area is displayed in Fig. 9.8, and data on the supply (physicians) and demand (populations) are provided in Table 9.5 (a and b). In Fig. 9.8, you will see that there are three physician practices (A, B, C) and seven populations (1–7). Next to the physician practices are the number of physicians per practice (e.g. P = 2). Next to the population locations are the total number of people in need of services (e.g. pop. = 100). Notice the dotted line surrounding each of the physician practices; these are the catchments for each practice. In this example, we set the

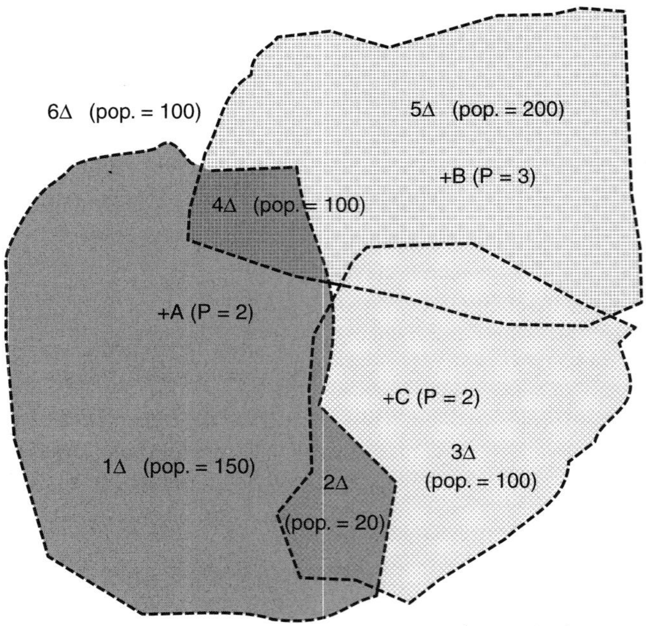

Fig. 9.8. Example of the two-step floating catchment area (2SFCA) method for calculating geographic accessibility to physician practices A, B and C of seven populations (1Δ–7Δ). P, no. of physicians per practice; pop., no. people in need of services; - - - - -, dotted lines enclose physician catchment areas.

catchment area to a 30 min drive time. Using the map and the data provided, we first estimate a supply-to-demand ratio for each physician practice. To do this, we sum the total population in each of the catchment areas and divide the total number of physicians at each practice by the total population for each physician location (Table 9.5a). For example, if you examine physician practice A, you will notice that three populations (1, 2, 4) fall within the catchment area of 30 min drive time.

Next, we add the three populations (150 + 20 + 100 = 270) served by facility A, and then divide the total physicians at facility A by the total population in the catchment (2/270 = 0.00741) to obtain the supply-to-demand ratio (Table 9.5a). After we have estimated the supply-to-demand ratio for each physician practice in each catchment, we then add up the supply-to-demand ratios for physician facilities for each population. In this case, for each of the populations (1–7), we locate all of the physician practices within each catchment that supply each population, and sum the supply-to-demand ratios (Table 9.5b). For example, if you look at the map (Fig. 9.8) you will see that population 2 is located in two catchment areas, denoting that it is served by two facilities (B and C) that are each within a 30 min drive times, so we add the supply-to-demand ratio for each of these practices to calculate the accessibility score for population 2. This makes the accessibility score for population 2 B:0.00741 + C:0.01667 = 0.02408. The calculations and results for this example population and the six others are found in Table 9.5 (a and b).

Overall, the floating catchment method is very flexible, and the use of provider-to-population ratios makes this geographic accessibility measure easy to understand. For further reading on the gravity models and the 2SFCA method, see Wang's *Quantitative Methods and Applications in GIS* (Wang, 2006), which book provides a thorough review of geographic accessibility, as well as a step-by-step guide for calculating the 2SFCA method and gravity

Table 9.5. Hypothetical example of the two-step floating catchment area (2SFCA) method for calculating geographic accessibility to physician practices.

(a) Step 1 of calculation.

		Populations (1–7)								
Practice	No. of physicians (P)	1	2	3	4	5	6	7	Sum of populations	Supply/demand ratio
A	2	150	20	X	100	X	X	X	270	0.00741
B	3	X	X	X	100	200	X	X	300	0.01000
C	2	X	20	100	X	X	X	X	120	0.01667

X, denotes population not within any practice catchment area.

(b) Step 2 of calculation.

Population no.	Geographic accessibility at location i ($A_i^F = \sum_{j \in (t_{ij} \le t_0)} R_j$)	A_i^F	Accessibility measure per 1000 persons
1	0.00741	0.00741	7.41
2	0.00741 + 0.01667	0.02408	24.08
3	0.01667	0.01667	16.67
4	0.00741 + 0.01000	0.01741	17.41
5	0.01	0.01	10.00
6	No access within 30 min	0	0.00
7	No access within 30 min	0	0.00

model in ArcGIS. This method has been recently enhanced by Luo and Qi (2009) to include a distance decay function within defined catchment areas, and this is referred to as the enhanced two-step floating catchment method.

9.6 Conclusion

In this chapter we have reviewed the basic concepts related to geographic accessibility to health services and described the most common measures for estimating geographic accessibility. We have also provided numerous worked examples of how to calculate these measures and various examples of how these measures can be applied in a real world setting. After reading this chapter, we hope that you now have a better understanding of how measuring geographic access to health services can help identify areas with poor access and provide vital information for service delivery planning. As you will have learned, geographic access to health services can depend on the geographic distribution and location of services in relation to those requiring services.

It is important to remember that health delivery systems are dynamic as well. For example, the expansion and contraction of health services can alter how health care is provided, where it is located and for whom it is provided, and therefore geographic access needs constant attention in the form of analysis and reanalysis. The different measures and mapping techniques that have been presented are useful for monitoring geographic access to health services. In addition, they are useful for showing policy makers the impacts that a policy change (e.g. closing a facility) might have on a population's ability to access health services. As the saying goes, 'a map is worth a thousand words,' and maps illustrating geographic access to health services can provide the evidence necessary to inform policy decisions and ultimately help to reduce geographic barriers to health services.

References

Adams, E.K. and Wright, G.E. (1991) Hospital choice of Medicare beneficiaries in a rural market: why not the closest? *The Journal of Rural Health* 7, 134–152.

Aday, L.A. and Andersen, R.M. (1981) Equity of access to medical care: a conceptual and empirical overview. *Medical Care* 19, 4–27.

American Cancer Society (2011) *Cancer Facts & Figures 2011*. American Cancer Society, Atlanta, Georgia. Available at: http://www.cancer.org/acs/groups/content/@epidemiologysurveilance/documents/document/acspc-029771.pdf (accessed 25 March 2013).

American Medical Association (AMA) (2012) AMA Physician Masterfile. Available at: http://www.ama-assn.org/ama/pub/about-ama/physician-data-resources/physician-masterfile.page (accessed 15 September 2012).

Andersen, R.M. (1995) Revisiting the behavioral model and access to medical care: does it matter? *Journal of Health and Social Behavior* 36, 1–10.

Baldwin, L.M., Cai, Y., Larson, E.H., Dobie, S.A., Wright, G.E., Goodman, D.C., Matthews, B. and Hart, L.G. (2008) Access to cancer services for rural colorectal cancer patients. *The Journal of Rural Health* 24, 390–399.

Blanford, J.I., Kumar, S., Luo, W. and MacEachren, A.M. (2012) It's a long, long walk: accessibility to hospitals, maternity and integrated health centers in Niger. *International Journal of Health Geographics* 11:24. Available at: http://www.ij-healthgeographics.com/content/11/1/24 (accessed 25 March 2013).

Boscoe, F.P., Johnson, C.J., Henry, K.A., Goldberg, D.W., Shahabi, K., Elkin, E.B., Ballas, L.K. and Cockburn, M. (2011) Geographic proximity to treatment for early stage breast cancer and likelihood of mastectomy. *Breast* 20, 324–328.

Burdette, H.L. and Whitaker, R.C. (2004) Neighborhood playgrounds, fast food restaurants, and crime: relationships to overweight in low-income preschool children. *Preventive Medicine* 38, 57–63.

Centers for Medicare & Medicaid Services (2012) National Provider Identifier Standard (NPI). Available at: CMS, Baltimore, Maryland. Available at: http://www.cms.gov/Regulations-and-Guidance/HIPAA-Administrative-Simplification/NationalProvIdentStand/index.html?redirect=/nationalprovidentstand/ (accessed 25 March 2013).

Cradock, A.L., Kawachi, I., Colditz, G.A., Hannon, C., Melly, S.J., Wiecha, J.L. and Gortmaker, S.L. (2005) Playground safety and access in Boston neighborhoods. *American Journal of Preventive Medicine* 28, 357–363.

Cromley, E.K. and McLafferty, S. (2002) *GIS and Public Health*. Guilford Press, New York.

Dijkstra, E.W. (1959) A note on two problems in connexion with graphs. *Numerische Mathematik* 1, 269–271.

Elkin, E.B., Ishill, N.M., Snow, J.G., Panageas, K.S., Bach, P.B., Liberman, L., Wang, F. and Schrag, D. (2010) Geographic access and the use of screening mammography. *Medical Care* 48, 349–356.

Fryer, G.E. Jr, Drisko, J., Krugman, R.D., Vojir, C.P., Prochazka, A., Miyoshi, T.J. and Miller, M.E. (1999) Multimethod assessment of access to primary medical care in rural Colorado. *The Journal of Rural Health* 15, 113–121.

Gabrysch, S., Simushi, V. and Campbell, O.M.R. (2011) Availability and distribution of, and geographic access to emergency obstetric care in Zambia. *International Journal of Gynecology and Obstetrics* 114, 174–179.

Gatrell, A.C. and Wood, D.J. (2012) Variation in geographic access to specialist inpatient hospices in England and Wales. *Health and Place* 18, 832–840.

Gauthier, B. and Wane, W. (2011) Bypassing health providers: the quest for better price and quality of health care in Chad. *Social Science and Medicine* 73, 540–549.

Gilliland, J.A. and Ross, N.A. (2005) Opportunities for video lottery terminal gambling in Montreal: an environmental analysis. *Canadian Journal of Public Health* 96, 55–59.

Guagliardo, M.F. (2004) Spatial accessibility of primary care: concepts, methods and challenges. *International Journal of Health Geographics* 3:3. Available at: http://www.ij-healthgeographics.com/content/3/1/3 (accessed 25 March 2013).

Hart, J.E., Laden, F., Puett, R.C., Costenbader, K.H. and Karlson, E.W. (2009) Exposure to traffic pollution and increased risk of rheumatoid arthritis. *Environmental Health Perspectives* 117, 1065–1069.

Hay, G.C., Whigham, P.A., Kypri, K. and Langley, J.D. (2009) Neighbourhood deprivation and access to alcohol outlets: a national study. *Health and Place* 15, 1086–1093.

Hayanga, A.J., Waljee, A.K., Kaiser, H.E., Chang, D.C. and Morris, A.M. (2009) Racial clustering and access to colorectal surgeons, gastroenterologists, and radiation oncologists by African Americans and Asian Americans in the United States: a county-level data analysis. *Journal of the American Medical Association Surgery* 144, 532–535.

Haynes, R., Bentham, G., Lovett, A. and Gale, S. (1999) Effects of distances to hospital and GP surgery on hospital inpatient episodes, controlling for needs and provision. *Social Science and Medicine* 49, 425–433.

Henry, K.A., Boscoe, F.P., Johnson, C. J., Goldberg, D.W., Sherman, R. and Cockburn, M. (2011) Breast cancer stage at diagnosis: is travel time important? *Journal of Community Health* 36, 933–942.

Hillier, A., Cole, B.L., Smith, T.E., Yancey, A.K., Williams, J.D., Grier, S.A. and McCarthy, W.J. (2009) Clustering of unhealthy outdoor advertisements around child-serving institutions: a comparison of three cities. *Health and Place* 15, 935–945.

Jordan, H., Roderick, P., Martin, D. and Barnett, S. (2004) Distance, rurality and the need for care: access to health services in South West England. *International Journal of Health Geographics* 3:21. Available at: http://www.ij-healthgeographics.com/content/3/1/21 (accessed 25 March 2013).

Kearney, G. and Kiros, G.E. (2009) A spatial evaluation of socio demographics surrounding National Priorities List sites in Florida using a distance-based approach. *International Journal of Health Geographics* 8:33. Available at: http://www.ij-healthgeographics.com/content/8/1/33 (accessed 25 March 2013).

Klein, M.B., Kramer, C.B., Nelson, J., Rivara, F.P., Gibran, N.S. and Concannon, T. (2009) Geographic access to burn center hospitals. *JAMA: The Journal of the American Medical Association* 302, 1774–1781.

Larsen, K. and Gilliland, J. (2008) Mapping the evolution of 'food deserts' in a Canadian city: supermarket accessibility in London, Ontario, 1961–2005. *International Journal of Health Geographics* 7:16. Available at: http://www.ij-healthgeographics.com/content/7/1/16 (accessed 25 March 2013).

Ludwick, A., Fu, R., Warden, C. and Lowe, R.A. (2009) Distances to emergency department and to primary care provider's office affect emergency department use in children. *Academic Emergency Medicine* 16, 411–417.

Luo, W. and Qi, Y. (2009) An enhanced two-step floating catchment area (E2SFCA) method for measuring spatial accessibility to primary care physicians. *Health and Place* 15, 1100–1107.

Luo, W. and Wang, F. (2003) Measures of spatial accessibility to health care in a GIS environment: synthesis and a case study in the Chicago region. *Environment and Planning B: Planning and Design* 30, 865–884.

Martin, D., Wrigley, H., Barnett, S. and Roderick, P. (2002) Increasing the sophistication of access measurement in a rural healthcare study. *Health and Place* 8, 3–13.

Messina, J.P., Shortridge, A.M., Groop, R.E., Varnakovida, P. and Finn, M.J. (2006) Evaluating Michigan's community hospital access: spatial methods for decision support. *International Journal of Health Geographics* 5:42. Available at: http://www.ij-healthgeographics.com/content/5/1/42 (accessed 25 March 2013).

Miller, H.J. (2004) Tobler's First Law and spatial analysis. *Annals of the Association of American Geographers* 94, 284–289.

Onega, T., Duell, E.J., Shi, X., Wang, D., Demidenko, E. and Goodman, D. (2008) Geographic access to cancer care in the U.S. *Cancer* 112, 909–918.

Patel, A.B., Waters, N.M. and Ghali, W.A. (2007) Determining geographic areas and populations with timely access to cardiac catheterization facilities for acute myocardial infarction care in Alberta, Canada. *International Journal of Health Geographics* 6:47. Available at: http://www.ij-healthgeographics.com/content/6/1/47 (accessed 25 March 2013).

Pearce, J., Witten, K. and Bartie, P. (2006) Neighbourhoods and health: a GIS approach to measuring community resource accessibility. *Journal of Epidemiology and Community Health* 60, 389–395.

Peipins, L.A., Graham, S., Young, R., Lewis, B., Foster, S., Flanagan, B. and Dent, A. (2011) Time and distance barriers to mammography facilities in the Atlanta metropolitan area. *Journal of Community Health* 36, 675–683.

Po'e, E.K., Neureiter, C., Escarfuller, J., Gesell, S.B., Tempesti, T., Widman, P. and Barkin, S.L. (2012) Systematic exposure to recreation centers increases use by Latino families with young children. *Childhood Obesity (formerly Obesity and Weight Management)* 8, 116–123.

Probst, J.C., Laditka, S.B., Wang, J.Y. and Johnson, A.O. (2007) Effects of residence and race on burden of travel for care: cross sectional analysis of the 2001 US National Household Travel Survey. *BMC Health Services Research* 7:40. Available at: http://www.biomedcentral.com/1472-6963/7/40 (accessed 25 March 2013).

Ray, N. and Ebener, S. (2008) AccessMod 3.0: computing geographic coverage and accessibility to health care services using anisotropic movement of patients. *International Journal of Health Geographics* 7:63. Available at: http://www.ij-healthgeographics.com/content/7/1/63 (accessed 25 March 2013).

Sasaki, S., Comber, A.J., Suzuki, H. and Brunsdon, C. (2010) Using genetic algorithms to optimise current and future health planning – the example of ambulance locations. *International Journal of Health Geographics* 9:4. Available at: http://www.ij-healthgeographics.com/content/9/1/4 (accessed 25 March 2013).

Schuurman, N., Berube, M. and Crooks, V. (2009) Measuring potential spatial access to primary health care physicians using a modified gravity model. *The Canadian Geographer* 54, 29–45.

Tai, W.T.C., Porell, F.W. and Adams, E.K. (2004) Hospital choice of rural Medicare beneficiaries: patient, hospital attributes, and the patient–physician relationship. *Health Services Research* 39, 1903–1922.

US Department of Health and Human Services (2012) Area Resource File (ARF). Maintained under contract to National Center for Health Workforce Analysis, Rockville, Maryland by Quality Resource Systems, Inc. (QRS), Fairfax, Virginia. Available at: http://arf.hrsa.gov/ (accessed 15 September 2012).

Vallée, J., Cadot, E., Grillo, F., Parizot, I. and Chauvin, P. (2010) The combined effects of activity space and neighbourhood of residence on participation in preventive health-care activities: the case of cervical screening in the Paris metropolitan area (France). *Health and Place* 16, 838–852.

Vallée, J., Cadot, E., Roustit, C., Parizot, I. and Chauvin, P. (2011) The role of daily mobility in mental health inequalities: the interactive influence of activity space and neighbourhood of residence on depression. *Social Science and Medicine* 73, 1133–1144.

Wang, F. (2006) *Quantitative Methods and Applications in GIS*. CRC Press/Taylor and Francis, Boca Raton, Florida.

Wang, F. (2012) Measurement, optimization, and impact of health care accessibility: a methodological review. *Annals of the Association of American Geographers* 102, 1104–1112.

Wells, K.J. and Roetzheim, R.G. (2007) Health disparities in receipt of screening mammography in Latinas: a critical review of recent literature. *Cancer Control* 14, 369–379.

WHO (2010) *The World Health Report 2010: Health Systems Financing, the Path to Universal Coverage*. World Health Organization, Geneva, Switzerland.

Wood, D.J. and Gatrell, A.C. (2002) *Equity of Geographical Access to Inpatient Hospice Care within North West England: A Geographical Information Systems (GIS) Approach*. Institute for Health Research, Lancaster University, Lancaster, UK.

Yamashita, T. and Kunkel, S.R. (2012) Geographic access to healthy and unhealthy foods for the older population in a U.S. metropolitan area. *Journal of Applied Gerontology* 31, 287–313.

Zdeb, M. (2009) Driving Distances and Drive Times using SAS and Google Maps. Available from sasCommunity.org at: http://www.sascommunity.org/wiki/Driving_Distances_and_Drive_Times_using_SAS_and_Google_Maps (15 September 2012).

10 Location–allocation Modelling for Health Services Research in Low Resource Settings

Nathaniel Bell*
University of South Corolina, College of Nursing, Columbia, South Carolina

10.1 Introduction

Where to locate health care services and how best to rationalize the allocation of these services are routine challenges for many health services providers. As health care goods and services are often provided at fixed locations, inherent inequity in access to services arises from the need to provide them from a small number of widely dispersed sites that satisfy the needs of a spatially dispersed demand. As cost precludes the provision of every demand site, population or region with its own hospital, services must be provided from a few centralized locations. In some modelling scenarios, the number of locations may be known in advance, while in other instances it may be desirable to identify the optimum number of sites from a list of candidate sites. The location–allocation problem is made up of two elements: (i) where to build or *locate* the facilities; and (ii) how to assign or *allocate* demand points to receive services from each facility. The objective of each of these elements is to derive an optimal solution that either maximizes or minimizes a mathematical function. The solutions could include minimizing the total distance that clients must travel to obtain health care services, identifying a select number of sites from a list of candidate sites that is optimal for servicing local populations, or simultaneously optimizing the location and allocation of health care services to populations.

This chapter reviews and provides examples of building location–allocation models for estimating accessibility to health care services. Study examples and process steps are provided using spatial data that are typically available for low- and middle- income countries, thereby providing content examples that reflect the data availability and contexts of health services research specific to many of the world's geographic regions. This is an important emphasis as traditional location–allocation models assume access to robust spatial data, which may not be available or representative of how the majority of the global population accesses health care goods or services.

The first part of the chapter discusses sources of the key data that are required for building location–allocation models using a geographic information system (GIS). All the data examples are derived using the Esri ArcGIS 10.0 GIS software, as currently there is no free GIS software capable of providing extensive support for location–allocation modelling. Examples are presented from a number of sources and provide a number of recommendations for health

* E-mail: natejbell@gmail.com

services research using publically available data sources. The second section of the chapter defines core location–allocation models and their application in health services research. The relevant formulas and conceptual frameworks are also explained. Examples of the use of these models, and details of the strengths and weaknesses of each approach, are also given, thereby providing a rich context for both the potential usage of these tools and of the issues that should be considered in their application.

10.2 Data Sources for Location–allocation Modelling of Health Care Services Using GIS

Location–allocation models require two types of descriptors to model health services coverage: a description of the population and resources that are present, and spatial representations of where resources are located and how they are accessed. Typically, this will include the following data:

- Health care delivery points, such as ambulatory clinics, physician offices, or palliative care facilities.
- Population points representing the area or regional population that will access these service points.
- Street or equivalent transportation network data that can connect the reference population to the service points.
- When possible, information on the type or quantity of health care goods and resources provided at each delivery point to enrich the model parameters.

Estimation of the levels of health service utilization or of limitations in service distribution therefore requires an understanding of the physical location of health care facilities, the geographic origin of the surrounding populations, the type of services offered at the facilities and the mode of travel used to acquire these services. Though not mandatory for access modelling, core attribute information that describes these data, including hospital bed size, services offered (e.g. neurosurgery) and population size, as well as road speed limits, surface grades and transportation barriers, will strengthen the model's representation of geographic or service limitations that populations might experience in attempting to access these services.

Prospective surveillance of population access to health care services typically requires small area population data from a census or from hospital registries for estimating utilization frequency or deficiency patterns. When these data are not available or insufficient, epidemiologists often rely on high-resolution global gridded population data sets for analyses and evaluation of population health outcomes (Linard *et al.*, 2010). Gridded population data sets attribute population counts to sub-national geographic locations by merging administrative data derived from national censuses with finer resolution ancillary (secondary) data sources. Secondary data sources can include paper maps, high-resolution aerial photography, night-time lights and street road networks, as well as satellite imagery (Salvatore *et al.*, 2005).

The resolution of gridded population data sets is typically about 1 km^2, which provides detail fine enough to map the spatial distribution of urban and rural populations globally – and with a precision that was until very recently unobtainable. Some data sets, including the Global Demography Project global population data sets, which were originally developed at the National Center for Geographic Information and Analysis (NCGIA, at the University of California at Santa Barbara), and are currently available from the NASA Socioeconomic Data and Applications Center (SEDAC; http://sedac.ciesin.columbia.edu/data/collection/gpw-v3) allocate populations using pycnophylactic interpolation (Tobler *et al.*, 1995), while others, including the LandScan™ data set developed by the Oak Ridge National Laboratories in Tennessee, use an interpolation method that assesses the relative likelihood of population occurrence on the basis of road proximity, slope, land cover and night-time lights (Dobson *et al.*, 2000). Additional data sources for country or region-specific population data sets are also available (Gakidou and King, 2006; Linard *et al.*, 2010).

Table 10.1 outlines popular gridded population data sets currently used in epidemiological studies and key features of each. A significant value of each is that the data are publically

Table 10.1. Popular gridded population data sets currently used in epidemiological studies. Adapted from Galway *et al.* (2012).

Data set	Gridded Population of the World (GPW), v3 (GPWv3)	Global Rural–Urban Mapping Project (GRUMP), v1 (GRUMPv1)	LandScan™
Source (URL)	http://sedac.ciesin.columbia.edu/gpw/global.jsp	http://sedac.ciesin.columbia.edu/data/collection/grump-v1	http://www.ornl.gov/sci/landscan/landscan_data_avail.shtml
Resolution	2.5′ (~5 km²)	0.5′ (~1 km²)	0.5′ (~1 km²)
Population source	United Nations Development Program (UNDP) census data	UNDP census data	Population Division of the United States Census Bureau
Interpolation method	Areal weighting	Dasymetric mapping	Smart interpolation
Ancillary data	None	Night-time lights Satellite imagery Populated places	Land cover Road networks Digital elevation models Night-time lights Satellite imagery
Year/s available	1990, 1995, 2000	2000	2008

available for research and public health purposes and are accessible online. Each data set is easily integrated into most GIS platforms, allowing for a wide number of data analysis operations using population data at a high-resolution sub-national spatial scale. Alternatively, country- and region-specific population data sets, including the Afripop Project 2011 and the United Nations Environment Programme (UNDP) Gridded Population Databases also provide gridded population data sets that have shown to be a more accurate and precise option when they are available. Figure 10.1 illustrates key attribute information and spatial coverage of the GPW 3.0, GRUMPv1 and LandScan gridded population data sets, which are three of the global population data sets that are most widely used in epidemiological studies to estimate population distributions. All three data sets can be used to approximate service demand points when used for location–allocation modelling.

Following the requirement for population data just discussed, the second requirement in building location–allocation models is obtaining information on the geographic location of health care services. In many instances, access to spatial population and infrastructure data for modelling case scenarios is relatively straightforward. For example, in Canada, higher education institutions participate in a Data Liberation Initiative (DLI) in which academic institutions pay a fixed fee that allows students, faculty and staff of Canadian universities to access georeferenced data depicting population counts, transportation networks and health services administrative units. Topological structures built from these data can then be used in the development of health indicators that represent either current access statistics or areas requiring further surveillance or intervention (Schuurman *et al.*, 2008). However, the quantity and quality of digital data varies across the globe and, in many areas, suitable spatial population or infrastructure data are difficult to obtain or may not be representative of service patterns for small area projects.

In the absence of these data sources, one alternative illustrated in Fig. 10.2 is to identify facility locations by extrapolating data points identified in Google Earth™. Healthcare facility location names referenced on the Web, as well as spatial representation of these features stored in Google Earth, can be obtained to represent individual health care facilities. Hospital lists can be obtained from government and non-government sources. In the event that there is no spatial reference for hospital facilities available through Google Earth, geographic place names can be created manually using address information for each facility. Data points for each of these facilities can then be exported as

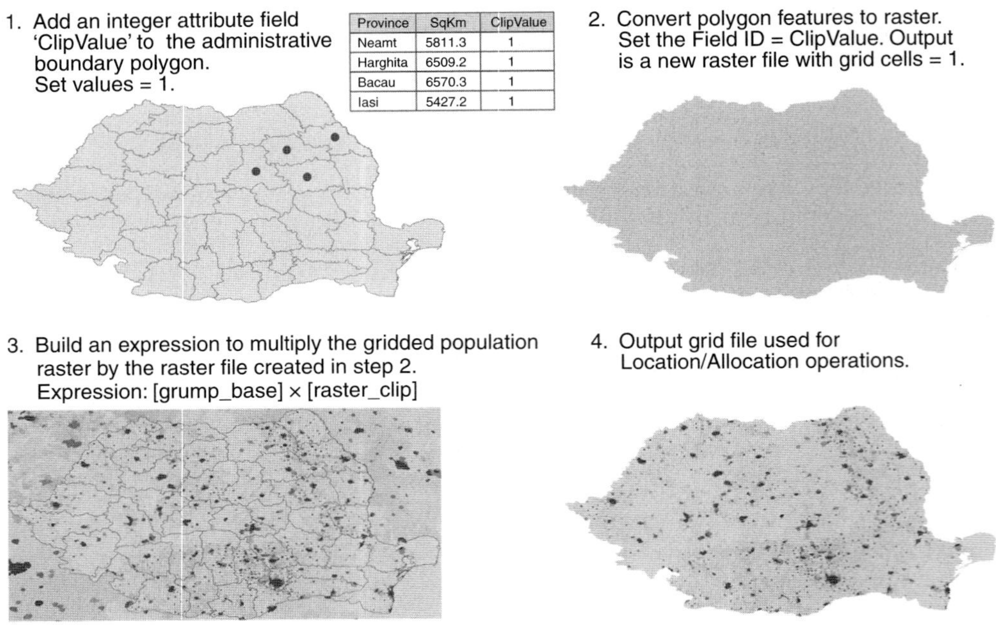

Fig. 10.1. The steps involved in the use of high resolution georeferenced population data for mapping sub-national rural and urban areas in Romania using the 2000 GRUMPv1 (Global Rural–Urban Mapping Project, v1) population grid. Similar data can be modelled using global population data files from GPW (Gridded Population of the World, v1) and LandScan, as well as from GRUMP.

Keyhole Markup Language (KML) data files and subsequently converted into any number of GIS-supported data files using freely available conversion software and scripts. In this example, the KML data file of service location points was imported into ArcGIS and converted into shapefile (SHP) format.

The purpose of a street network file is to connect demand points with service points. In Canada, as in other high-income countries, transportation network data can be obtained from national vendors as well as being available for purchase through private companies. Minimal data sets, such as Statistics Canada's Road Network File (RNF) have been digitized from small-scale topographic maps (1:25,000) and provide digital representation of provincial road networks, including street names and street types. Depending on the level of detail contained in the RNFs, attribute data to measure the cost to travel from one node to the next can be modelled as distance or time. Other descriptors, including road types or speed limits, are used in conjunction with cost features to create cost attributes (e.g. drive time) to model road impedance (the amount of resistance or cost required to move from one location to another along a road path in a network). Restriction attributes, such as one-way or divided highway classes, are common components that can be placed on road networks to control how populations move from one node to the next.

As is often the case, more robust description of the road segments, such as speed limits, road types (e.g. highway, divided highway, logging road) are only available by purchasing spatial street network data from commercial vendors. Many of these data sets have been constructed from the global positioning system (GPS) with centre line accuracy to within 5 m, although in the absence of these attribute points the cumulative travel time between origins and destinations along a street network can be estimated from categorical data associated with each road segment (e.g. road type or road grade).

Figure 10.3 illustrates how to estimate the cumulative cost of travelling between origins

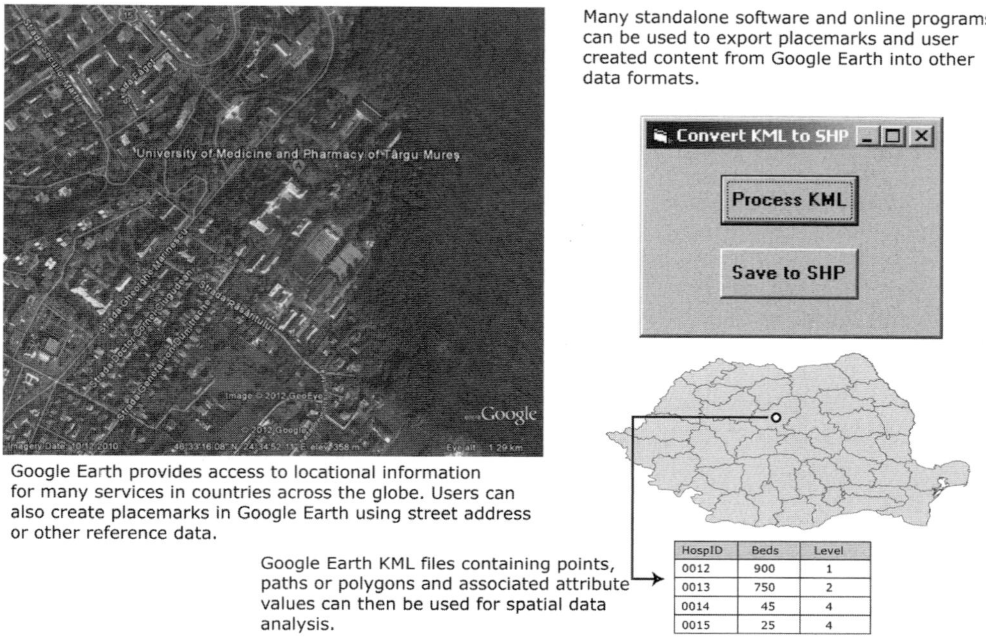

Fig. 10.2. Spatial data for health care facilities can be obtained from numerous electronic data holdings, but Google Earth™ based maps can be used to build these features when such data are not available, as illustrated here for Romania. Numerous software packages and scripts can be used to convert the Google Earth data into other GIS-based data files for further analysis. Here, the Keyhole Markup Language (KML) data file of service location points was imported into ArcGIS software and converted into shapefile (SHP) format.

and destinations along a road network. Each RNF line segment contains at least two vertices, or start and end points, that define its length, as well as where one segment connects to another. Each vertex, or node, can contain attribute information describing features about the road segment (e.g. road type). The total travel time required to traverse the distance between each vertex can be calculated by multiplying each attribute type by a constant representing the estimated speed limit for the road type. In the hypothetical example in Fig. 10.3, the estimated travel time of traversing all five road segments, starting at top left, would be calculated as: $(((\[4550]/100)/1000) \times 60) + (((\[175]/60)/1000) \times 60) + (((\[1247]/60)/1000) \times 60) + (((\[2130]/45)/1000) \times 60) + (((\[995]/45)/1000) \times 60) = 8.32$ min. In contrast, assuming a constant travel speed of 85 km/h in the absence of information on road class type would yield a travel time estimate of 6.42 min for the same spatial distance. The cumulative effect of these differences over large areas is great, emphasizing the value of access to even a relatively small amount of information about the road features.

In many instances, it may also be useful to geocode or address match spatial reference information for each demand point on to an RNF, though it should be pointed out that gridded population data do not contain the same spatial characteristics as many health or population registry records, such as address location, street intersection, postal codes or zip codes. The defining spatial characteristic of gridded population data is raster cells that represent population estimates. One alternative is to convert the gridded population data set from a raster data file into a point layer file. This allows for the creation of topological relationships between point and polyline vector data sources. Once all demand points, facility locations and street network files are built and topological relationships are constructed, flow characteristics

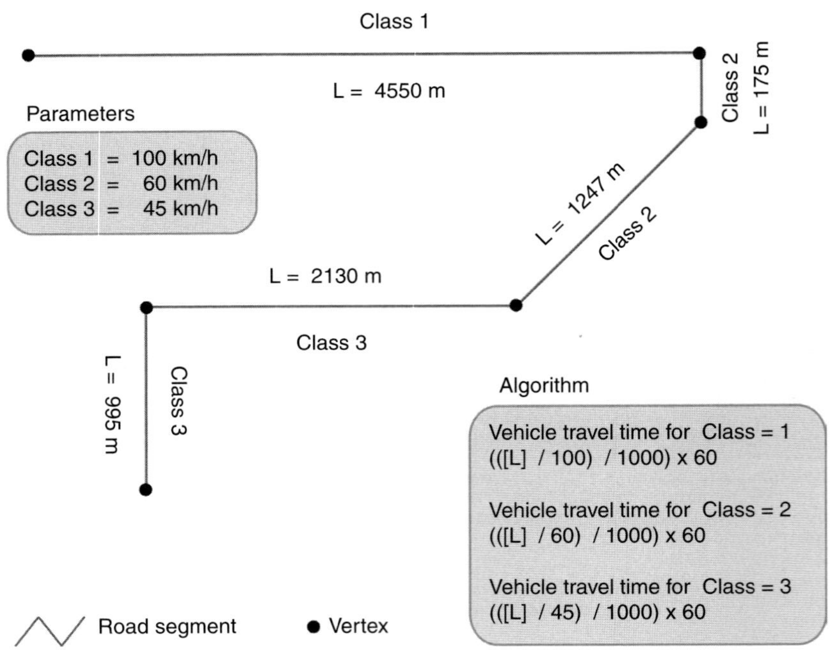

Fig. 10.3. Illustration of building cost impedances for road network files for instances where access to high-resolution spatial data are unavailable. L is the field attribute name that holds the value for the road segment length. From top left, the road segments are class 1 (4550 m), class 2 (175 m, then 1247 m), class 3 (2130 m, then 995 m).

between population points and health care services can be calculated for generating new hypotheses of where to locate health care services, as well as for deciding how best to rationalize how these services are allocated.

10.3 Location–allocation Models for Health Services Research

In developing countries, geographic proximity to health care services has been shown to influence the use of those services (Baume *et al.*, 2000; Tanser *et al.*, 2001; Buor, 2003; Tsoka and le Sueur, 2004). However, specialized and primary care facilities tend to be located in a limited number of locations and to have limited capacity. Location–allocation models provide a prospective measure to evaluate and improve deficiencies in the coverage of health services by identifying specific geographic areas where the placement of additional facilities can in some way be 'optimized' for certain subsets of demand, such as a cost or distance. GIS-based location–allocation methods provide health care researchers with an array of tools for better understanding of how the spatial organization between health care services and populations influences outcomes.

This section reviews the core data and mathematical models that can be used to construct location–allocation models in low resource settings using GIS-based methods. The core functions illustrated in this chapter – including spatial accessibility functions, transportation problems, *p*-median location placement problems, maximal coverage problems and gravity models – represent fundamental techniques used to explore the distribution of health services and offer practical solutions for health care policy and planning in many settings. The primary examples that are presented throughout the chapter use population and health services data for Romania. All the data were freely obtained from GIS data clearing houses, Google Earth and government- and non-government based sources. The data and examples are thus from a varied context and can be used for location–allocation modelling at sub-national geographic scales.

10.3.1 Spatial accessibility methods and functions

A number of spatial accessibility measures of the distances between facility locations and demand points can be generated in a GIS to better understand the relationship between the distribution of resources and the surrounding population (Cromley and McLafferty, 2002). The simplest approach is to calculate straight line distances between facilities and demand points. Straight line calculations are measurement operations that assign attribute information from one map feature to another based on a defining characteristic, such as geographic distance or proximity. Straight line measurements, though, do not take account of topography and have no specified constraints such as slope, elevation or street geometry.

Network accessibility measures that take into account the descriptors (e.g. road type) and restrictions involved in traversing road networks use mathematical models to calculate all plausible routes from a resource location to all demand points for purposes of highlighting the most direct route. Accessibility measures that use network analysis are now common tools in health services research. From a pragmatic point of view, the context of *how* populations access health care services in developing countries must be considered, as populations may use walking rather than motor vehicles as their primary mode of transport to and from health care facilities. Although research has shown that the relationship between geographic distance and health service utilization is not always best depicted using straight line (e.g. 'crow fly') distance calculations (Martin, 2002), in some rural settings this method may be more appropriate than cost-based or network-based travel models as populations may use walking as their primary means for accessing services (Tanser *et al.*, 2006). Consideration of which accessibility model is the most appropriate for the analysis to be undertaken is an important component of early exploratory data analysis and is also important in choosing the methodology that is most suitable for modelling population coverage in relation to health care.

An illustration of this problem is shown in Fig. 10.4. The map depicts two proposed service catchments around a single (hypothetical) health care facility. In one model, a 10 km 'crow fly' buffer was constructed to approximate a geographic constraint between demand points and service centres. A second model used transportation network analysis to identify all demand points within 10 km of the health care facility; for this, all demand points were identified based on unimpeded travel distance along the street network. The differences between the two models in both the number of demand points captured and the total population that would probably be affected by the proposed hospital catchment are clearly shown, and illustrate the effect of using two different approaches for measuring spatial accessibility to health care services. In some instances, the differences in geographic distance between simple and more complex spatial accessibility measures can be insignificant over small distances, but the variation can grow substantially when taking into consideration demand points that are hundreds of kilometres away.

However, many geographic analyses are in fact based on straight line distances, owing in part to the ease of calculating relationships between population points and facility locations; such data can be obtained without requiring either a GIS or road network data files (in Canada, RNFs). In an analysis of more than 66,000 locations in the USA, Boscoe *et al.* (2011) found that straight line calculations were highly correlated with travel time statistics generated using specialized GIS software and road network data ($r^2 > 0.9$) after applying a 'detour index' to all road segments. The detour index value is a constant that represents the ratio (typically about 1.2–1.6) of travel time distance to straight line distance. This was an important finding, as it supports the utility of many freely available Web-based GIS tools as opposed reliance on specialized and often expensive GIS systems for fundamental location–allocation research questions.

In some instances, socio-economic vulnerabilities may be amplified by geographic

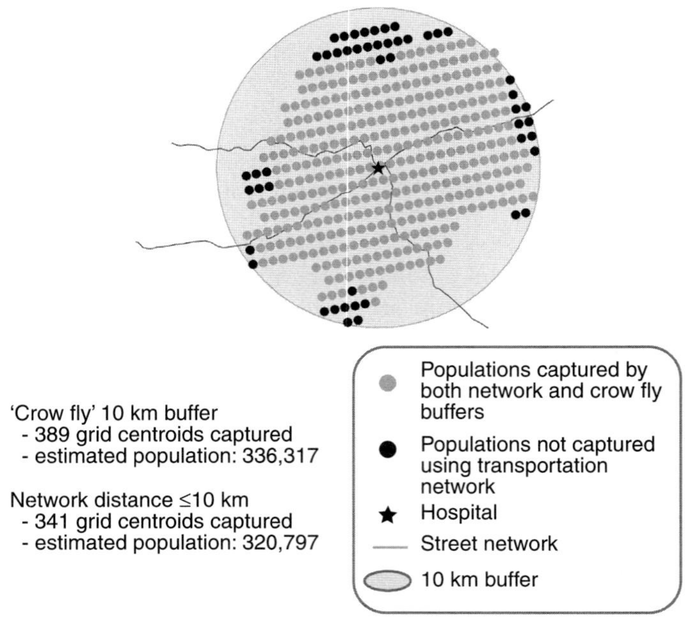

Fig. 10.4. A comparison of two spatial accessibility measures for calculating access to a single health care facility. The service catchment was set to 10 km travel distance from the facility. The use of (i) transportation (street) network and (ii) 'crow fly' representations of accessibility for modelling population access to the facility (in this case a hospital) results in quite different representations of access.

conditions, especially when access to definitive care is delayed. In these instances, better characterization of socio-economic and geographic vulnerabilities may be useful for identifying populations with both high risk of poor health outcomes and poor access to trauma services. Previous studies have combined census data on population distribution and socio-economic deprivation within the network accessibility measures in GIS to characterize isolation from health care facilities in rural communities (Schuurman *et al.*, 2008). The parameters used for this approach are shown in Fig. 10.5. The model described here – the Population Vulnerability Amplifier (PIVA) – is based on the premise that larger populations with *in situ* hospitals located further than an hour from a trauma hospital are more likely candidates for increased services than smaller communities. However, the socio-economic vulnerability component coalesces both population and geographic distance factors to either raise or lower the need for trauma services. This type of strategy accounts for geographic isolation from health care facilities as well as social vulnerability. When combined, exploratory spatial accessibility models drawn from population health theory can inform policy decisions on the delivery of health care services and identify regions where public health prevention strategies may be most effective. These approaches highlight the utility of spatial accessibility models for investigating spatial patterns in accessing health services. Importantly, the value of these methods varies according to the geographic region and the population, the geographic unit of analysis, the measures used to calculate distance and data limitations due to incompleteness, inaccuracy or availability.

10.3.2 Transportation problems

Although spatial accessibility models are useful tools for initially exploring the relationship between resource locations and population areas, they do not allow researchers to model how changing the number of locations or the geographic placement of locations can create

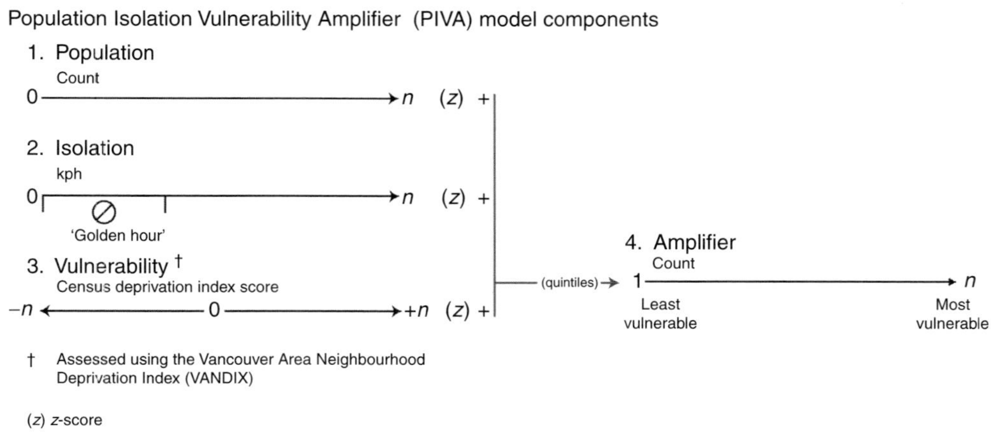

Fig. 10.5. Spatial accessibility to trauma centres in Canada analysed using a multivariate strategy that combines geographic distance (isolation) with combined census data on social vulnerability and population demographics. These three variables are standardized and combined to produce a single index score (PIVA – the Population, Isolation and Vulnerability Amplifier) that ranks the need for trauma services in rural and remote areas. 'Golden hour', time period (*h*) after traumatic injury when prompt medical treatment is most likely to prevent death. After Schuurman *et al.*, 2008.

more efficient relationships. Transportation problems refer to a class of problems that arise as a result of spatially varying demand points having to access health care services from fixed locations. The goal is to minimize the geographical distance required to supply health care services to the largest number of demand points. Constraints, such as including a minimum or maximum number of facilities that can be introduced to meet demand, allow users to create different scenarios that resemble the limitations of real world resources.

Figure 10.6 illustrates this problem using demographic and health services data from Romania. In this illustration, an attempt is made to assign all grid cells with populations ≥500 to one of 12 health care facilities across the country. The spider diagrams indicate which facility each population (or demand point) is nearest to as measured using geographic distance along the street network, with the inclusion criteria that the demand point must lie within 5 km of a road segment. Impedance constraints of 60 min and 120 min are illustrated. Demand points are mapped using the centroids from the GRUMPv1 gridded population of the world raster imagery and weighted by the population within each grid cell. GRUMPv1 population estimates are constructed from dasymetric mapping, using ancillary data from night-time lights, satellite imagery and populated places, thus providing a high-resolution description of settlement patterns in the absence of small area population data (see Table 10.1). Though this is a common analysis step in many GIS modelling exercises, users should be mindful that these processes are dependent on the quality of the spatial data used in the analysis. Line or section breaks, missing roads or misplaced population points within many publically available spatial data sources can detract from the quality of the analysis and lead to errors in location–allocation models.

Allocation models that seek to address the transportation problem have well-known usages in health research. For example, in their analysis of health care facility siting in rural Ghana, research scientists compared changes that occurred in accessibility to health care services when adding one to four new facilities using two transportation models (Møller-Jensen and Kofie, 2001). The first model attempted to minimize the total weighted distance from the demand points to the health care facilities; here, the weighted distance was the network distance multiplied by the number of people living in each demand point. The second approach

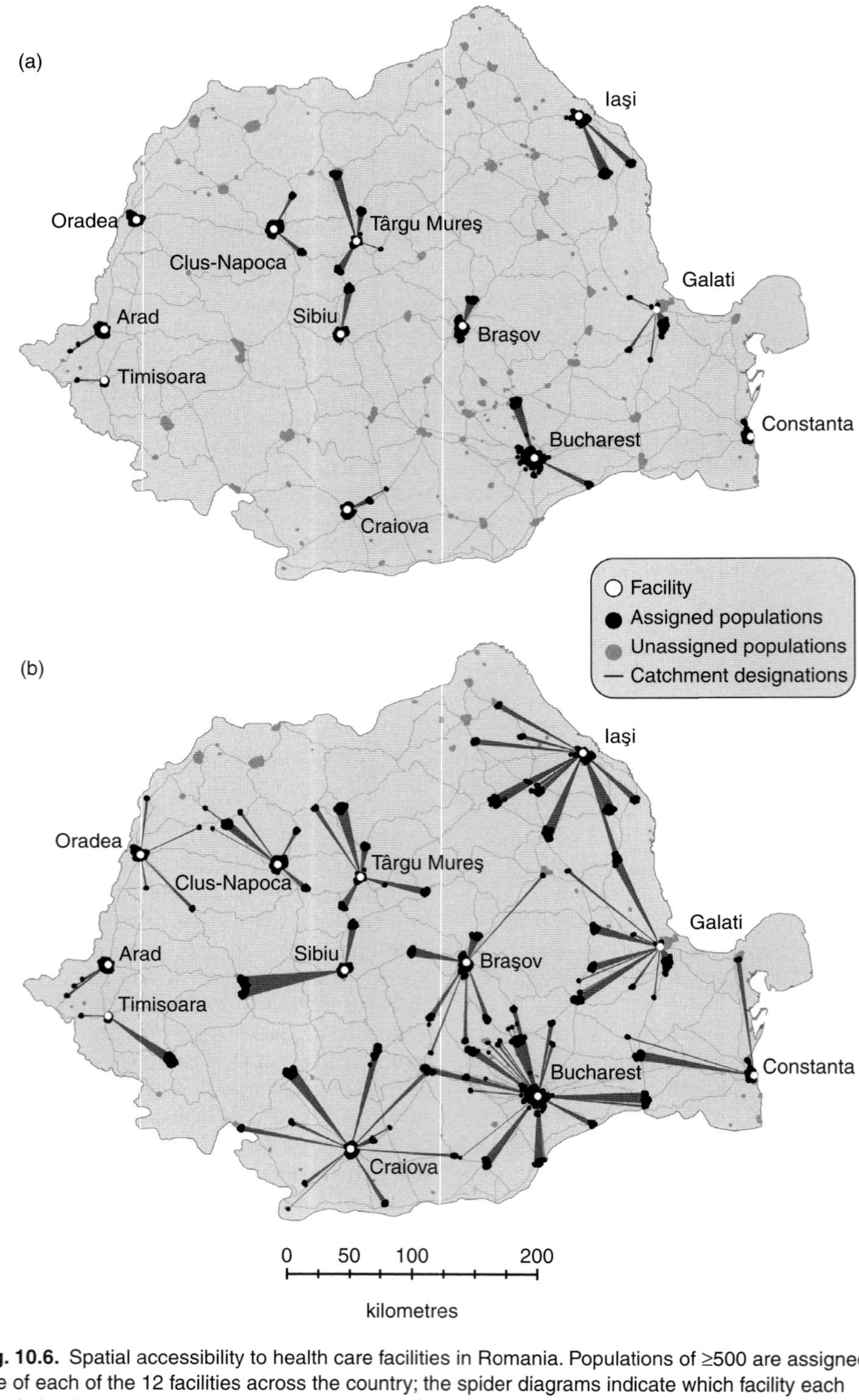

Fig. 10.6. Spatial accessibility to health care facilities in Romania. Populations of ≥500 are assigned to one of each of the 12 facilities across the country; the spider diagrams indicate which facility each population is nearest to along the street network. Travel time variations in population coverage are shown using impedance constraints of (a) 60 min and (b) 120 min.

attempted to maximize health care coverage based on a threshold (or buffer) distance; in this case, all demand within the critical distance was thought to have acceptable coverage and all persons outside the buffer were presumed to have poor provision (Møller-Jensen and Kofie, 2001). In the first model, one additional, optimally located centre reduced the average person distance from 5.35 km to 4.60 km, while four new centres reduced the average (or global) person distance between demand points and resource locations to 3.28 km. The second model demonstrated that distance-based optimization models (the first model) and person-based optimization models (the second model) are often mutually exclusive, as the addition of four optimally located centres allocated by population increased the average person distance to care from 3.28 km to 3.70 km. However, the second model also ensured that almost 95% of all persons were within 8 km of a centre, compared with a lower total of 88% when the minimum distance (first) model was used. It should be noted that while minimizing total person distance between care facilities and demand points is useful for scenarios when centralized facilities are responsible for delivering services to surrounding populations, as the number of facility locations increases, service utilization at each site decreases. This may produce economically unfeasible solutions if the addition of new facilities results in underutilization.

10.3.3 The *p*-median problem

The *p*-median problem is a specific type of transportation problem. Unlike transportation problems, in which the number and locations of resource locations is known a priori, the *p*-median problem specifies only the number of facilities, *p*, to be located from a larger set of possible resource sites (Cromley and McLafferty, 2002). The objective of *p*-median solutions is to optimize the supply of services to demand points, such that each demand point is allocated to a single service supply point and the average costs (median distance or travel time) between demand points and resource locations are minimized. Thus, the *p*-median location model locates facilities such that the average distance from demand points to the resource centres is minimized. Although there are many variables to consider when assigning resources (e.g. cost, planning, staffing, etc.), *p*-median problems can help researchers to identify how to reduce the overall costs (measured either by distance or travel time) of delivering health care goods and services to surrounding populations. The solution to the *p*-median problem is the identification of the optimal relationship between a set of resource centres and population demand points, whereby all persons are allocated to the closest facility. In the *p*-median model, all population points are allocated to a single facility under the assumption that there are no capacity constraints placed on the facilities.

Health services modelling has used *p*-median problems for over three decades. Both Harvey *et al.* (1974) and Narula *et al.* (1975) used a *p*-median model to identify the optimal location of health care facilities within a hierarchical service model. The objective was to locate the optimal number of services within each level of a service network (e.g. tertiary, intermediate, ambulatory) and minimize patients' total travel to services. The model constructed by Narula *et al.* (1975) incorporated referral networks, and allowed certain proportions of patients to be treated at some facilities, while other demand points were assigned to neighbouring facilities. Berlin *et al.* (1976) used a *p*-median model to study hospital location problems in an effort to identify the minimum distance between hospitals and demand points based on response times. Within low and middle income countries, *p*-median problems take on new challenges in that seasonal weather patterns (e.g. floods, monsoons) result in significant coverage problems that have an impact on road surface conditions. Oppong (1996), examined *p*-median problems using Primary Health Care centres in Ghana. Multiple modelling environments were constructed to take into account climate differences during the year, thereby providing more realistic decision support estimates that might reflect real world conditions.

The solution to a *p*-median problem is subject to a set of constraints, including the establishment of: many-to-one relationships between each demand point and facility locations; a maximum capacity to be serviced from each demand point; a cut-off that controls the total number of facilities that can be created; and the number of facilities to be chosen. The ArcGIS interface allows users to set a maximum capacity to be serviced from each demand point, or to choose not to set an optimal capacity constraint on the model (e.g. to use all available facilities). Impedance values or weights are used to define the cost of moving along a transport network between demand points and resource centres. One of the limitations of the *p*-median problem is that it attempts to reduce the global cost of travel, which does not necessarily reduce geographic distances between individual demand points and service locations. This type of problem is typically of value for locating goods and services, as the objective is to reduce the overall costs of supplying health services. Consequently, it may have limitations for allocating many health care services, such as emergency medical services, which typically must be able to reach population areas within critical time limits. A similar caveat is that a *p*-median scenario that is accepted by health care planners as resulting in an adequate configuration of resources may not in fact be representative of real world conditions. Additionally, allocating resources for rural populations that may frequently reside outside critical response times to care must also be considered.

Despite these limitations, *p*-median models offer health services researchers many opportunities to model access to care. For example, obtaining information about access to care in the presence of real world scenarios such as floods, road closures or avalanches is an important aspect of community planning and the provision of health care services. Location–allocation models derived from *p*-median formulae provide a number of techniques for comparing how populations may access health care services in the event of changing conditions.

An example of a *p*-median health services problem is shown in Fig. 10.7, and the associated values are shown in Table 10.2. In this scenario, a *p*-median formulation was constructed for access to the tertiary health care systems across Romania such that each population centre was allocated to the facility that was within the minimum travel distance. An impedance of 120 min was established so that all populations who could not access a facility within this time were identified, with an additional constraint that all population points must be within 5 km of a road segment to be included in the model. In this example, an optimal number of eight facilities was chosen from the existing 12, under the rationale that the remaining four facilities would serve as transitional or overflow care centres in the event of a mass casualty incident (Fig. 10.7A). A polyline 'barrier' was then digitized over the road network north of Bucharest to simulate an environmental constraint to care, such as road closures, flooding, earthquake or other environmental effects (Fig. 10.7B).

Constraints represent an additional time component that populations have to negotiate when attempting to access care. In this event, crossing each barrier requires an additional 15 min of travel time. Table 10.2 illustrates the change in the provider catchments as a result of this barrier. It is apparent from this illustration that the barrier has a considerable impact on where populations would be routed in the event of severe weather or other environmental impact and where new deficiencies would exist. This information can be readily extended to link with data on hospital capacity, staffing levels or surgical services to improve decision support planning and surveillance.

10.3.4 Maximal coverage models

Although distance constraints can be placed on *p*-median problems to ensure that solutions are derived within a specified cut-off value (e.g. 60 min, 10 km, etc.), the minimum number of facilities required to meet all demand points may not be known a priori (Cromley and McLafferty, 2002). While it is possible to identify the minimal number of facilities to provide coverage to a demand area, such a solution is rarely practical given the cost required to provide health services coverage to all populations, as well as the excessive number of services that may be created to provide total coverage. In these cases, demand may best be conceptualized as a maximal coverage problem, through which prospective facilities are located so that as many demand points as possible are allocated within a specified

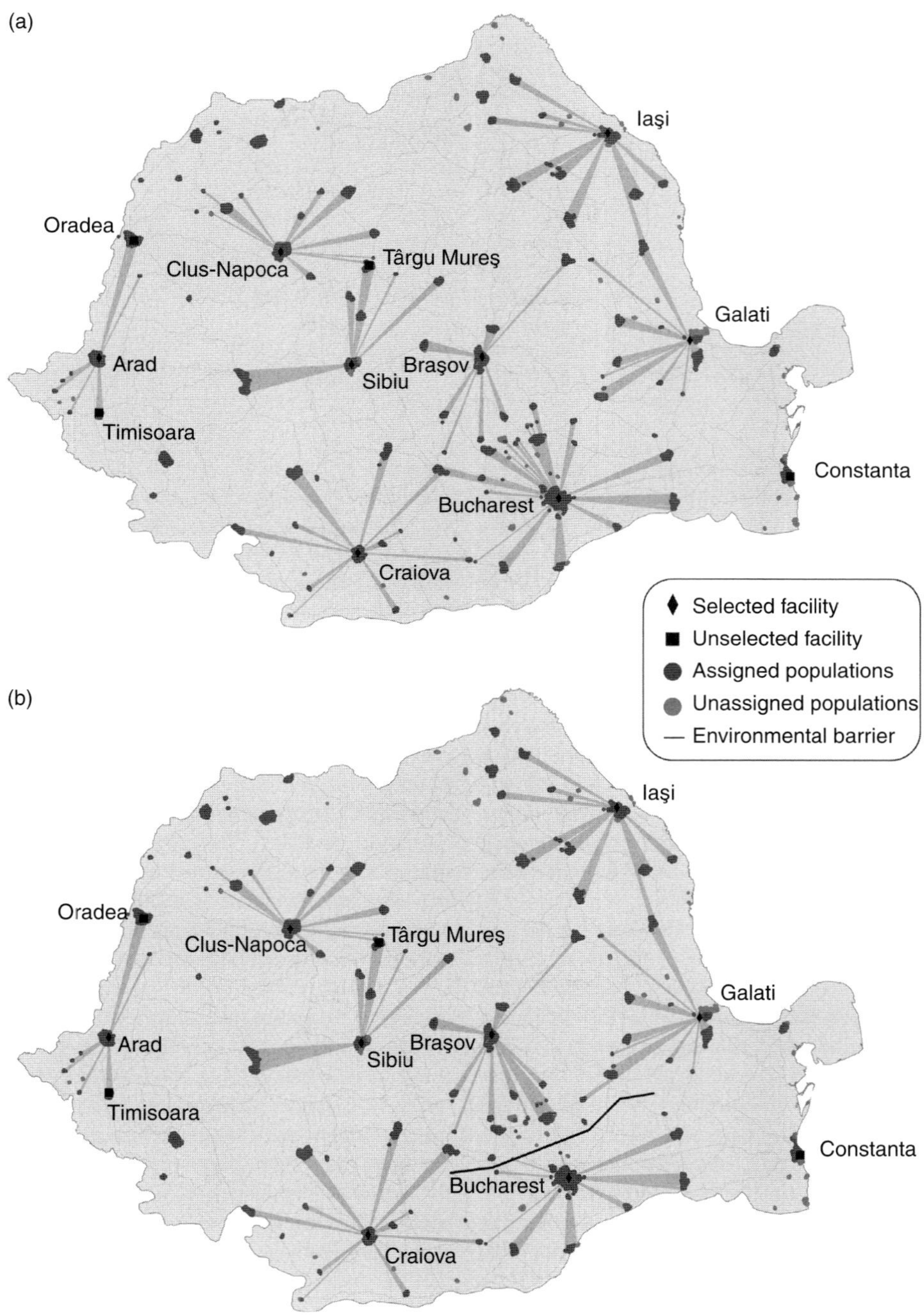

Fig. 10.7. The application of the *p*-median location–allocation problem to optimize the supply of health care services (tertiary facilities) to populations in Romania. (a). Each population centre was allocated to a facility within a minimum travel time of 120 min (and also had to be within 5 km of a road), resulting in the selection of the optimal number of eight facilities out of the 12 available (the remaining four facilities to serve as transitional/overflow centres in the event of a mass incident. (b). A polyline barrier (crooked black line) was digitized over the road network north of Bucharest to simulate real time environmental barriers and show where populations would be routed in an emergency.

Table 10.2. Population assignments to each of the optimal number of eight health care facilities in Romania selected for application of the *p*-median problem. Increased travel time (in this case 15 min) as a result of environmental barriers can be used to identify potential strains on health care systems.

Facility	No barrier	With barrier	Change (%)
Arad	584,632	584,632	0.0
Cluj-Napoca	509,990	584,632	14.6
Craiova	602,129	579,360	–3.8
Bucharest	2,726,140	2,216,939	–18.7
Braşov	436,068	688,012	57.8
Iaşi	878,292	878,292	0.0
Sibiu	480,714	480,714	0.0
Galati	480,714	480,714	0.0
Unassigned (facilities (4)	1,632,045	1,904,027	16.7

distance of the closest facility. Maximal coverage models have been utilized in many health care studies, including the allocation of emergency medical services, as the objective is to locate service points where they can cover the most people within a certain drive time (Daskin and Stern, 1981; Messina *et al.*, 2006). Maximal coverage models are subject to a number of constraints, including a defined number of service points and potential supply points, the distance or time that all demand points should be from a service point, a distance or time impedance cut-off whereby demand can no longer be allocated, and the demand weight specifying the volume required at each demand point that can allocated to a facility.

Maximal coverage models can be formulated to analyse a variety of health planning scenarios, including changing the number of facilities that will provide services, changing the minimum and maximum response times to provide services, as well as placing constraints on the type of geographic locations where potential facilities can be placed. Previous researchers have used maximal response models as a compromising tool among competing objectives that have included minimizing response times, minimizing the number of vehicles to deploy and maximizing services coverage (Eaton *et al.*, 1985).

10.3.5 Gravity models

Another way to conceptualize the geographic relationship between service locations and demand points is by spatial interaction. For example, it is often valuable to know where patients would go in the event of hospital closures and how much additional time or distance would be required for them to obtain services elsewhere (Taket and Mayhew, 1981; Taket, 1989). In addition, situations may also arise in which populations must make a compromise between two or more factors when choosing care. Understanding how compromises between efficiency, equity or market forces affect where populations go to access health care services is important for developing services to meet demand. Spatial interaction models allow researchers to estimate accessibility, or flow, between locations and to evaluate how supply side and demand side forces affect movement between locations (Fotheringham, 1984).

Gravity models are one of the most common type of spatial interaction models used to measure interactions between locations, and these were introduced in the previous chapter. In physics, gravity is defined as the force attraction between two bodies and is proportional to their mass and inversely proportional to the squared distance between them. Gravity models are derived from Newton's analogy of gravity, whereby:

$$T_{ij} = k\frac{W_i^{\lambda} W_j^{\alpha}}{d_{ij}^{\beta}} \quad (10.1)$$

where T_{ij} is the interaction between origins, *i*, and destinations, *j*. Both W_i and W_j are measures of the sizes of the origin and destination, and d_{ij} is the distance between them. The distance friction between origins and locations is measured by a positive parameter, α, and a proportional constant k, which is a calibration parameter. The exponent values (α, λ and β) are parameters used to ensure that the estimated results are similar to observations of flow. Geographers and GIS developers have integrated these concepts into the study of interactions between locations and other measurable attributes, such as population, hospital capacity or commercial space, thus allowing the calculation of spatial interaction, or flow, between two or more points based on their characteristics and proximity (Isard, 1975).

A study of the interaction between emergency hospitalizations and both demand and supply effects by Congdon (2001) used a gravity model to measure relative accessibility to services in the event that hospitals were closed so that flows to emergency rooms could be predicted under 'new' access patterns. Other, similar, studies have employed gravity models to estimate travel to hospitals before and after closures (McLafferty, 1988). Unlike the allocation models previously described, spatial interaction models are designed specifically to predict flow between locations. A significant challenge to the use of gravity models in health services research is related to the calibration parameter, k. In the study by McLafferty (1988), despite the significant inverse relationship found between geographic distance and service utilization, this relationship did not remain constant when changing the set of hospitals used to simulate facility closures. Further, simple assumptions about alternatives proposed in the model require empirical evidence to support the value of using spatial interaction models in health services research.

These challenges to the use of gravity models are illustrated in Table 10.3. In this example, a gravity model was constructed using the Romanian population data set to simulate how a subset of tertiary health care facilities across the country might 'compete' in the provision of elective surgical services. Prior to the analysis, an impendance criterion was established such that only populations within 120 km of each facility were eligible for inclusion. The results illustrate that reducing the number of facilities that offer surgical services from 12 to 11 would result in no loss of total service capacity among populations within the designated catchment area. However, the closure of this one facility – at Arad – would result in a mean increase in travel time of nearly 10% and, as a result, the facilities at both Timisoara and Oradea would be required to increase their service capacities so that the services previously offered at Arad were covered. Table 10.3 shows that as more facilities are removed, the overall mean travel time between facilities and demand points increases. Furthermore, the overall service capacity starts to decrease. This is a consequence of a loss of access among populations who now fall outside the catchment area of the neighbouring facility which, otherwise, would compensate for the loss of services. The resulting figures suggest that, over the whole population, reducing the number of facilities by three would eliminate access for approximately 182,000 people, or just over 2.5% of the original population.

The example just discussed suggests that there may be redundancy in the geographic placement of the current services as evidenced by the lack of movement between demand points and facilities when only one facility is removed. The analysis also illustrates which facilities would experience no disruption in service capacity or require populations to travel further to continue to access care as a result of the closures. This exploratory study allows researchers and planners the opportunity to model potential service disruptions under different delivery scenarios. As the cost of running national health care services runs into many billions of dollars (or other currencies) each year, questions of redundancy are an important component in evaluations of health care. Gravity models provide an opportunity to explore whether services can be reduced while also remaining accessible.

10.4 Conclusion

In this chapter, a review of key data sources and components required for location–allocation modelling in a GIS environment have been discussed. A summary of core methods used for location–allocation models were described and examples provided that illustrated how similar projects could be replicated. In addition,

Table 10.3. Location–allocation of demand points to health care facilities using a gravity model. Incremental reductions in the number of facilities within a 'care network' can be used to identify whether closures increase the distances that populations must travel (i.e. the travel times) to access care or result in lower service capacity.

	No. of facilities: 12		No. of facilities: 11		No. of facilities: 10		No. of facilities: 9	
Facility	Population	Time (mean)	Population	Time (mean)	Population	Time (mean)	Population	Time (mean)
Timisoara	398,893	17.7	527,993	26.9	527,993	26.9	–	–
Arad	142,090	8.3	–	–	–	–	584,632	56.3
Oradea	222,330	10.2	235,320	15.9	235,320	15.9	–	–
Cluj-Napoca	414,693	26.3	414,693	26.3	575,929	43.6	575,929	43.6
Târgu Mureş	290,179	28.5	290,179	28.5	–	–	–	–
Sibiu	349,524	60.8	349,524	60.8	475,508	66.1	475,508	66.1
Craiova	566,938	50.2	566,938	50.2	566,938	50.2	566,938	50.2
Bucharest	2,660,348	26.1	2,660,348	26.1	2,660,348	26.1	2,660,348	26.1
Constanta	283,059	19.2	283,059	19.2	283,059	19.2	283,059	19.2
Braşov	466,846	35.8	466,846	35.8	466,846	35.8	466,846	35.8
Iaşi	882,587	58.1	882,587	58.1	882,587	58.1	882,587	58.1
Galati	504,362	53.9	504,362	53.9	504,362	53.9	504,362	53.9
Total	7,181,848	32.9	7,181,848	36.5	7,178,889	39.6	7,000,208	45.5
Change	–	–	0%	9.8%	–0.04%	16.9%	–2.53%	27.7%

the implications of using these models for location–allocation modelling in resource poor settings were discussed.

These models can be applied to better identifying and addressing geographic differences in access to health care services, and the findings can subsequently be used to analyse associations with adverse health events. Over the past three decades, location–allocation models have been applied in a variety of settings to solve a number of health services-related questions. It is often the case that demand on a primary care facility, clinic or emergency room can exceed its capacity to provide care. When the evidence suggests that delays or constraints to accessing care increase the likelihood of adverse health events, it is not uncommon for health policy makers or planners to propose the development of a new facility to restore a tenable balance between demand and supply. While site location problems are often determined by cost or political motivation, GIS analysis offers a number of applications for proposing equitable facility locations when the consequence of accessibility arises as a result of a spatially dispersed demand.

Health care goods and services tend to be located in particular places and require certain social or financial resources to benefit from their availability. As such, their placement may affect the health of persons simply because they live far away or socio-economic conditions constrain or delay access to services. GISs offer many advantages for location–allocation modelling in health care settings. Data overlay procedures increase the capacity to build and analyse complex representations of real world relationships, and visual representation of these relationships can be used for decision support and planning.

Exploring spatial relationships further aids our understanding of how populations access health care services and where improvements can be made. Health services researchers and medical geographers have long used GISs to study how the social, physical and spatial organizational structures, uses and outcomes of health care delivery affect the health of individuals and populations (Joseph and Phillips, 1984; Gesler, 1986; Gatrell and Löytönen, 1998; Cromley and McLafferty, 2002; Maheswaran and Craglia, 2004). This research has a direct bearing on our understanding of disparities in access to care (Perry and Gesler, 2000; Arcury *et al.*, 2005), whether the placement of new facilities corresponds with populations in need

(Schuurman *et al.*, 2008), or among which populations the take-up of new interventions and therapies is being under-realized (Rosero-Bixby, 2004). Establishing strategies to improve access to health care is important as all populations, not just the poor or those who live in rural areas, realize improvements in health when resources are more equitably distributed across the social and geographic spectrum (Marmot, 2007).

References

Arcury, T., Gesler, W.M., Preisser, J.S., Sherman, J., Spencer, J. and Perin, J. (2005) The effects of geography and spatial behavior on health care utilization among the residents of a rural region. *Health Services Research* 40, 135–155.

Baume, C., Helitzer, D. and Kachur, S.P. (2000) Patterns of care for childhood malaria in Zambia. *Social Science and Medicine* 51, 1491–1503.

Berlin, G., ReVelle, C. and Elzinga, J. (1976) Determining ambulance–hospital locations for on-scene and hospital services. *Environment and Planning A* 8, 553–561.

Boscoe, F.P., Henry, K.A. and Zdeb, M.S. (2011) A nationwide comparison of driving distance versus straight-line distance to hospitals. *The Professional Geographer* 64, 188–196.

Buor, D. (2003) Analysing the primacy of distance in the utilization of health services in the Ahafo-Ano South district, Ghana. *International Journal of Health Planning and Management* 18, 293–311.

Congdon, P. (2001) The development of gravity models for hospital patient flows under system change: a Bayesian modelling approach. *Health Care Management Science* 4, 289–304.

Cromley, E.K. and McLafferty, S. (2002) *GIS and Public Health*. Guilford Press, New York.

Daskin, M. and Stern, E. (1981) A hierarchical objective set covering model for emergency medical service vehicle deployment. *Transportation Science* 15, 137–152.

Dobson, J.E., Bright, E.A., Coleman, P.R., Durfee, R.C. and Worley, B.A. (2000) LandScan: a global population database for estimating populations at risk. *Photogrammetric Engineering and Remote Sensing* 66, 849–857.

Eaton, D., Daskin, M.S., Simmons, D., Bulloch, B. and Jansma, G. (1985) Determining emergency medical service vehicle deployment in Austin, Texas. *Interfaces* 15, 96–108.

Fotheringham, A. (1984) Spatial flows and spatial patterns. *Environment and Planning A* 16, 519–543.

Gakidou, E. and King, G. (2006) Death by survey: estimating adult mortality without selection bias from sibling survival data. *Demography* 43, 569–585.

Galway, L.P., Bell, N., Al Shatari, S.A.E., Hagopian, A., Burnham, G., Flaxman, A., Weiss, W.M., Rajaratnam, J. and Takaro, T.K. (2012) A two-stage cluster sampling method using gridded population data, a GIS, and Google Earth™ imagery in a population-based mortality survey in Iraq. *International Journal of Health Geographics* 11:12. Available at: http://www.ij-healthgeographics.com/content/11/1/12 (accessed 26 March 2013).

Gatrell, A.C. and Löytönen, M. (eds) (1998) *GIS and Health*. Taylor and Francis, London.

Gesler, W. (1986) The uses of spatial analysis in medical geography – a review. *Social Science and Medicine* 23, 963–973.

Harvey, M., Hung, M. and Brown, J. (1974) The application of a *p*-median algorithm to the identification of nodal hierarchies and growth centers. *Economic Geography* 50, 187–202.

Isard, W. (1975) A simple rationale for gravity model type behavior. *Papers of the Regional Science Association* 35, 25–30.

Joseph, A. and Phillips, D. (1984) *Accessibility and Utilization: Geographical Perspectives on Health Care Delivery*. Harper and Row, New York.

Linard, C., Alegana, V.A., Noor, A.M., Snow, R.W. and Tatem, A.J. (2010) A high resolution spatial population database of Somalia for disease risk mapping. *International Journal of Health Geographics* 9:45. Available at: http://www.ij-healthgeographics.com/content/9/1/45 (accessed 26 March 2013).

Maheswaran, R. and Craglia, M. (eds) (2004) *GIS in Public Health Practice*. CRC Press, Boca Raton, Florida.

Marmot, M. (2007) Achieving health equity: from root causes to fair outcomes. *The Lancet* 370, 1153–1163.

Martin, D. (2002) Increasing the sophistication of access measurement in a rural healthcare study. *Health and Place* 8, 3–13.

McLafferty, S. (1988) Predicting the effect of hospital closure on hospital utilization patterns. *Social Science and Medicine* 27, 255–262.

Messina, J.P., Shortridge, A.M., Groop, R.E., Varnakovida, P. and Finn, M.J. (2006) Evaluating Michigan's community hospital access: spatial methods for decision support. *International Journal of Health Geographics* 5:42. Available at: http://www.ij-healthgeographics.com/content/5/1/42 (accessed 26 March 2013).

Møller-Jensen, L. and Kofie, R. (2001) Exploiting available data sources: location/allocation modeling for health service planning in rural Ghana. *Geografisk Tidsskrift* 101, 145–153.

Narula, S.C., Ogbu, U. and Samuelsson, H. (1975) Location of health facilities in developing countries. Paper presented to: ORSA/TIMS Meeting, Chicago, Illinois. Working Paper No. 221, School of Management, State University of New York at Buffalo, New York.

Oppong, J. (1996) Accommodating the rainy-season in third world location-allocation applications. *Socio-Economic Planning Sciences* 30, 121–137.

Perry, B. and Gesler, W. (2000) Physical access to primary health care in Andean Bolivia. *Social Science and Medicine* 50, 1177–1188.

Rosero-Bixby, L. (2004) Spatial access to health care in Costa Rica and its equity: a GIS-based study. *Social Science and Medicine* 58, 1271–1284.

Salvatore, M., Pozzi, F., Ataman, E., Huddleston, B. and Bloise, M. (2005) *Mapping Global Urban and Rural Population Distributions*. Environment and Natural Resources Series, No. 24, Food and Agriculture Organization of the United Nations, Rome.

Schuurman, N., Bell, N., Hameed, S.M. and Simons, R. (2008) A model for identifying and ranking need for trauma service in non-metropolitan regions based on injury risk and access to services. *Journal of Trauma* 65, 54–62.

Taket, A. (1989) Equity and access: exploring the effects of hospital location on the population served – a case study of strategic planning. *Journal of the Operational Research Society* 40, 1001–1010.

Taket, A. and Mayhew, L. (1981) Interactions between the supply of and demand for hospital services in London. *Omega* 9, 519–526.

Tanser, F., Hosegood, V., Benzler, J. and Solarsh, G. (2001) New approaches to spatially analyse primary health care usage patterns in rural South Africa. *Tropical Medicine and International Health* 6, 826–838.

Tanser, F., Gijsbertsen, B. and Herbst, K. (2006) Modelling and understanding primary health care accessibility and utilization in rural South Africa: an exploration using a geographical information system. *Social Science and Medicine* 63, 691–705.

Tobler, W.R., Deichmann, U., Gottsegen, J. and Maloy, K. (1995) *The Global Demography Project*. NCGIA Technical Report 95–6, National Center for Geographic Information and Analysis, University of California at Santa Barbara, Santa Barbara, California.

Tsoka, J.M. and le Sueur, D. (2004) Using GIS to measure geographical accessibility to primary health care in rural South Africa. *South Africa Journal of Science* 100, 329–330.

11 Multilevel and Hierarchical Models for Disease Mapping

Jarvis T. Chen*
Harvard University School of Public Health, Boston, Massachusetts, USA

11.1 Introduction

Georeferenced health data make it possible to locate cases in space and to analyse spatially varying patterns of health, disease and well-being. By linkage to geocoded data on exposures and covariates, it is also possible to enrich health data and the individual level variables contained therein with a variety of information on environmental exposures, socio-economic context and other variables. As these rich and diverse sources of georeferenced data have become more available in recent decades, increasingly sophisticated statistical methods have been developed for modelling them. With these methods at their disposal, epidemiologists, sociologists and environmental scientists can explore such questions as: (i) how do population rates of health, disease and well-being vary over space and across different levels of geographic aggregation; (ii) to what extent are observed spatial variations in health driven by geographically varying exposures; (iii) to what extent are the observed spatial variations driven by the different characteristics of populations living in those areas; and (iv) which geographic areas exhibit unusually high or unusually low rates of disease, taking into account known exposures?

In this chapter, I discuss modelling frameworks that enable the exploration of the spatial variation in health outcomes in relation to observed covariates, and the derivation of estimates of meaningful quantities for data presentation. The modelling approaches that are useful for spatial data are part of a broad family of models known as hierarchical or multilevel models, which have arisen from parallel lines of development in the biostatistical literature on disease mapping, the analysis of longitudinal data and methods for handling clustered data (Gelman *et al.*, 2003; Banerjee *et al.*, 2004; Gelman and Hill, 2007). The broad class of models includes so-called mixed effects, random effects, variance components and generalized linear mixed models (GLMM). Latent variable models can also be viewed as hierarchical models because random effects can also have a latent variable interpretation.

What these approaches have in common is that they are useful in complex data sets where information is available on several different levels of observational units, the distributions of which are controlled by multiple parameters that can be regarded as connected by the structure of the problem. Because they are 'related', the joint probability model for these parameters needs to reflect the dependence

* E-mail: jarvis@hsph.harvard.edu

among them. An appealing approach is to model such data hierarchically, with observable outcomes modelled conditionally upon certain parameters, which themselves are given a probabilistic specification in terms of other parameters (known as hyperparameters). This kind of approach helps us to model complex multiparameter problems efficiently and can also facilitate computation for model fitting.

To give a concrete example, suppose that a researcher is interested in studying the relationship between health, as measured by a continuous variable, y, and a measure of individual socio-economic deprivation, x. Let us assume that the researcher has collected data on y and x in a simple random sample of n individuals, indexed by i. A classical linear regression would model:

$$y_i = \alpha + \beta x_i + \varepsilon_i, \text{ for individuals } i = 1, \ldots, n \quad (11.1)$$

where α is the intercept, β summarizes the change in y for a 1 unit change in x and ε is a normally distributed random error term with mean 0 and variance σ_ε^2. Now, assume that the researcher has collected data on a sample of 50 neighbourhoods (indexed by j), and within each neighbourhood, a random sample of individuals (indexed by i). It would be reasonable to assume that the health scores of individuals from the same neighbourhood might be more similar than those of individuals from different neighbourhoods, perhaps due to unmeasured environmental exposures that vary from neighbourhood to neighbourhood. If so, the outcomes observed in individuals from the same neighbourhood will be correlated, which violates a key assumption of the classical linear regression model.

A simple multilevel model for these data might be to assume instead that, at the level of the individual, the observed y for individual i in neighbourhood j depends on the observed value of x_{ij}, a neighbourhood-specific intercept, α_j, and an individual-level random error term ε_{ij}:

$$y_{ij} = \alpha_j + \beta x_{ij} + \varepsilon_{ij} \quad (11.2)$$

where $\varepsilon_{ij} \sim \text{Normal}(0,\sigma_\varepsilon^2)$. At the second level, a neighbourhood level model is specified for α_j, for example:

$$\alpha_j = \mu_\alpha + v_j \quad (11.3)$$

with $v_j \sim \text{Normal}(0,\sigma_v^2)$. In this simple example, one assumes that α_j comes from a distribution of neighbourhood intercepts that is normally distributed with mean μ_α and variance σ_v^2. Whereas in the classical linear regression model, the intercept (α) is treated as invariant over neighbourhoods, in the multilevel model, the intercept parameter is allowed to vary by neighbourhood and is given a probabilistic model. The relatively simple 2-level model just described is often referred to as a random intercept model. This second stage model could be further elaborated to incorporate additional neighbourhood level predictors.

The 2-level multilevel model could also be written in a single line as:

$$y_{ij} = \mu_\alpha + \beta x_{ij} + v_j + \varepsilon_{ij} \quad (11.4)$$

which highlights another way to think about this model. This is that one can also conceptualize the residual variation in y, conditional on the observed values of x, as having been partitioned into a between-neighbourhood component (v_j) and a within-neighbourhood component (ε_{ij}).

A key concept in hierarchical models is that of exchangeability (Gelman *et al.*, 2003). In a typical statistical analysis, the (often tacit) assumption is made that the outcomes y_i observed for n units of observation are exchangeable, meaning that their joint probability is invariant to permutation of the indexes. So one usually models outcomes from an exchangeable distribution as independently, identically distributed (i.i.d.) conditional on some unknown parameter vector θ (that may include the effects of known and observed explanatory variables). In a hierarchical model, one can speak of exchangeability at each level of units. So, in the simple example above, one treats individuals and their outcomes within each neighbourhood as exchangeable, and also treats the neighbourhoods as exchangeable (as reflected in the second stage model for α_j). In most analytic applications, one will want to make these assumptions of exchangeability at each level conditional on explanatory variables that are included as fixed effects in the model, e.g. in the above example, the assumption of exchangeability is conditional on the socio-economic deprivation variable x_{ij}.

An important consequence of exchangeability is that each parameter borrows strength from the other parameters at its level of the hierarchy, and as a result, estimates are 'shrunk' towards the population mean. This behaviour can be beneficial, especially when small numbers of individuals are observed in some of the units in the hierarchy. In these cases, the reduction in uncertainty for that unit can be quite large, because information from other groups or units with smaller variability is incorporated into the posterior estimates.

The goal in this chapter is to provide an introduction to the hierarchical modelling of spatial variation in health outcomes. In many health research applications, the georeferenced data of interest take the form of area-level aggregated counts, which are matched to population counts that are treated as known. Thus, I focus the discussion on multilevel Poisson regression models. An important consideration is specifying a reasonable model for the second stage parameters that appropriately captures the spatial variation in risk. I motivate the presentation by considering the setting in which one is interested in mapping smoothed estimates of disease rates and/or risks in order to reduce the statistical instability of small area estimates. I then consider two of the most popular approaches for accommodating local clustering of area level spatial variation in a hierarchical modelling framework: (i) a multilevel (nested) hierarchy of normally distributed random effects (Goldstein, 2011); and (ii) the popular intrinsic Gaussian conditionally autoregressive (CAR) approach by which local clustering is induced by a set of conditional autoregressions (Besag *et al.*, 1991).

The literature on hierarchical modelling approaches to spatially referenced health data is quite large, and excellent reviews and textbooks already exist that present the technical aspects in greater detail than can be accomplished here (Marshall, 1991; Clayton and Bernardinelli, 1992; Lawson *et al.*, 1999; Bithell, 2000; Wakefield *et al.*, 2000; Richardson, 2003; Banerjee *et al.*, 2004). Similarly, there is an extensive literature on multilevel models applied to problems in the social sciences and epidemiology (see, for example: Subramanian *et al.*, 2003; Gelman and Hill, 2007; Goldstein, 2011; Snidjers and Bosker, 2011). A particularly useful textbook that addresses the underlying theory and practical issues of implementation from both the disease mapping and multilevel perspectives is that of Lawson *et al.* (2003).

Here, it is useful to note a potential confusion in the nomenclature used to refer to these methods. Multilevel modelling grew out of work in the field of education in the 1980s (Aitkin *et al.*, 1981; Aitkin and Longford, 1986) where the units of analysis (e.g. students nested within classrooms within schools) could be organized into a nested hierarchy of levels. It makes sense that similar approaches could be applied to nested spatial data organized by geographical units (e.g. census tracts nested within counties or states) and even temporally organized data (repeated observations 'nested' within individuals in the longitudinal setting). In this way, the term 'multilevel' has become synonymous with hierarchically nested data structures (Blakely and Subramanian, 2006). However, while nested data clearly lend themselves to hierarchical modelling approaches, more complex, non-nested data structures do so as well. The observational units may no longer be neatly nested, but the models are still hierarchical in that the parameters that control the distribution of outcomes at the first level of the model may themselves be given a second stage model specified in terms of hyperparameters. In the multilevel modelling literature, these may be referred to as cross-classified structures. For clarity, I will use the word 'multilevel' to refer to models for nested data structures and use the word 'hierarchical' to refer to the broader class of modelling approaches.

Throughout, I make use of an illustrative data set of lung cancer deaths among the white non-Hispanic population observed in the 156 census tracts of the city of Boston, Massachusetts. The 156 census tracts are nested in 16 neighbourhoods, which potentially permits a three-level nested hierarchy of individuals nested in census tracts, nested in neighbourhoods. To obtain the data set, the 910 lung cancer deaths that occurred between 2000 and 2005 were geocoded to the census tract level and matched to age, race and gender-specific census tract population estimates from the US Census of 2000. These population estimates are multiplied by six (the number of years of data) to obtain person-time denominators.

11.1.1 Model implementation

Hierarchical model formulations have a particular affinity with the Bayesian inferential framework, as random effects naturally have a prior distribution (Gelman *et al.*, 2003). Thus, fully Bayesian and empirical Bayes (posterior approximation) methods are commonly used for fitting disease mapping models (Wakefield *et al.*, 2000; Best *et al.*, 2005). Suppose $\theta = (\theta_1, \ldots, \theta_p)$ is the vector of model parameters to be estimated and $y = (y_1, \ldots, y_n)$ is the observed data. In contrast to the usual frequentist approach that treats θ as a fixed parameter to be estimated, the Bayesian approach models the observed data and all unknown parameters as random. In addition to specifying the likelihood function, denoted by $f(y|\theta)$, a Bayesian model assumes that the vector θ is a random variable sampled from a prior distribution, $\pi(\theta|\lambda)$, where λ is a vector of hyperparameters that characterize this distribution. Sometimes, values of λ can be picked to reflect a strong prior belief about the values of θ. More often, however, one picks values so that θ can be free to vary across a very wide range — this is known as placing an 'uninformative prior' distribution on θ.

In the fully Bayesian approach, inference is based on the posterior distribution, $p(\theta|y)$, obtained using Markov Chain Monte Carlo (MCMC) methods. From the Bayesian viewpoint, all current knowledge about θ is summarized by the posterior distribution. Although the computation of the posterior distribution can often be difficult, subsequent Bayesian inferences are relatively straightforward once the posterior distribution has been obtained. For example, let us assume, for simplicity, that the parameter θ is univariate. Possible choices for a point estimate of θ are the mean, median or mode of the posterior distribution. The 95% credible set or Bayesian confidence interval for $\theta(q_L, q_U)$, can be determined empirically from the posterior distribution by choosing q_L and q_U as the 2.5th and 97.5th quantiles of the posterior distribution of θ. In addition, other useful summary quantities, perhaps involving combinations or manipulations of elements of θ, can be monitored at each iteration of the MCMC algorithm, and 95% credible intervals can be easily calculated. I give some examples of these in this chapter. Throughout, I take a Bayesian approach to model fitting using the popular WinBUGS (Bayesian inference Using Gibbs Sampling) software package (Lunn *et al.*, 2000). For each model, I ran two independent chains starting from different initial values. The first 10,000 iterations were discarded as a burn-in, and each chain was run for a further 40,000 iterations and thinned by eight (i.e. every 8th iteration was retained). Model convergence was evaluated by visual inspection of the time series plots of samples for each chain and by computing the Gelman–Rubin diagnostic (Gelman and Rubin, 1992). I report estimates and 95% credible intervals based on the mean and quantiles of the posterior samples.

To compare models, one can make use of the deviance information criterion (DIC), defined as the sum of the posterior mean of the deviance, $\bar{D}$ (–2 times the log likelihood), and an estimate of the 'effective' number of parameters, p_D (Spiegelhalter *et al.*, 2002, Best *et al.*, 2005). The latter can be thought of as a penalty term reflecting the model complexity or degrees of freedom, so that, broadly speaking, the DIC has a similar interpretation to Akaike's Information Criterion (AIC) in classical generalized linear models. Smaller values of the DIC reflect better model fit, and Spiegelhalter *et al.* (2002) suggests that models with DIC values >7 higher than that of the 'best' model are substantially inferior.

11.2 Disease Mapping

As a first step in addressing the question of 'How does the risk of this particular disease vary geographically?', consider the situation where one has geocoded records of deaths due to lung cancer, and wants to map these data to obtain a visual representation of where death due to lung cancer is more common and where it is less common. The map may be intended for simple descriptive purposes, to provide information on the health needs of the population, or to generate hypotheses about disease aetiology. As a first approach, one might be tempted to begin by mapping the locations of each case's geocoded address of residence, as I have done in Fig. 11.1 for (hypothetical) lung cancer deaths among white non-Hispanics in Boston in 2000–2005. While this gives a visual representation of where cases were recorded as living when they died of lung cancer, this does not provide a very satisfying summary of lung cancer mortality. First, there are likely to be confidentiality issues with plotting exact locations of cancer deaths (which is why I have only plotted hypothetical locations in Fig. 11.1). Secondly, and more importantly, the absolute number of deaths observed is sensitive to the population at risk, which varies across space. Thus, a more epidemiologically meaningful quantity to map is the mortality rate, defined as the number of deaths divided by the population (or person-time) at risk.

Even though the data set includes exact locations of deaths, population counts are only available aggregated over small areas (e.g. census block groups, census tracts, counties). Consequently, one has to aggregate the death counts to match the available units in the population data. This results in aggregated *count* data (also known as area or lattice data, as opposed to *point* data). That is, one observes y_i (the number of deaths in area i) and N_i (the population at risk in area i), from which one can estimate the crude mortality rate in area i as $\hat{r}_i = y_i/N_i$. In Fig. 11.2, I have mapped these using (real) data on lung cancer deaths among white non-Hispanics in Boston for 2000–2005. The resulting map allows one to visualize areas with low and high lung cancer mortality rates. However, it is still of limited use because it is well known that mortality rates are strongly related to age, and the age distribution may differ across areas.

A well-known way of dealing with this problem is to standardize the mortality rates by age using indirect standardization. If y_{ij} is the count of deaths in area i in age stratum j, then O_i is defined as the observed number of deaths in area i, summed up over the age strata, i.e.

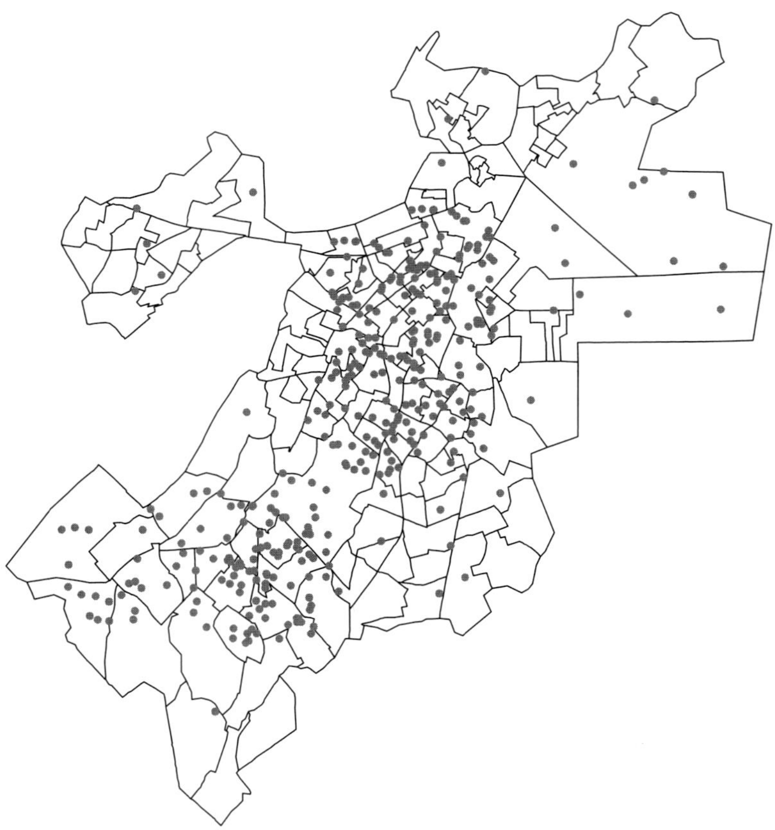

Fig. 11.1. A map of (hypothetical) residential addresses of lung cancer deaths among white non-Hispanics in Boston, Massachusetts.

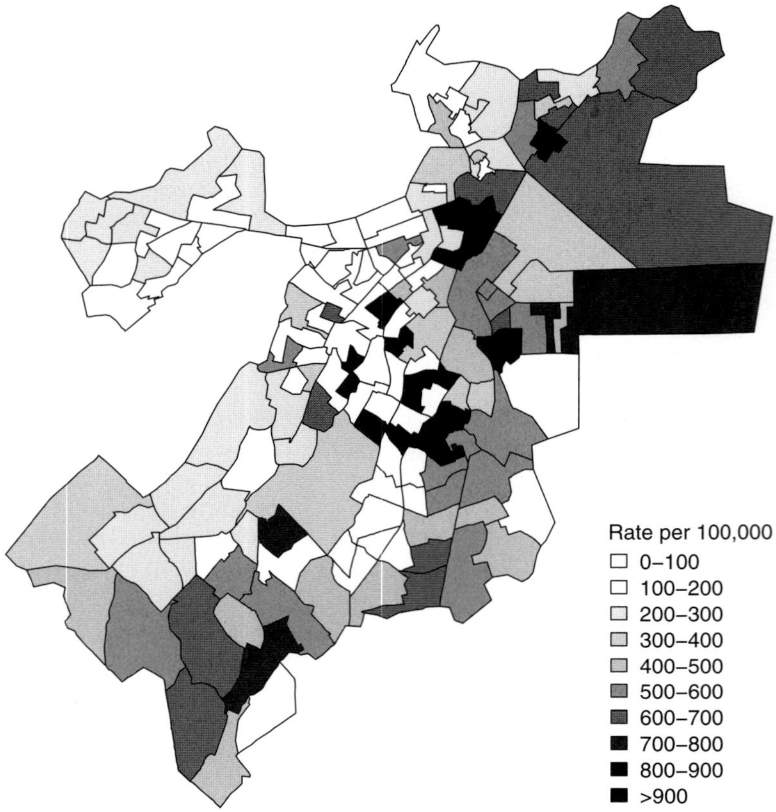

Fig. 11.2. Crude census tract lung cancer mortality rates for white non-Hispanics in Boston, 2000–2005.

$O_i = \Sigma_j\, y_{ij}$. The expected number of deaths, E_i, is computed by applying the age-specific mortality rates from a reference population to the age-specific population counts in each area:

$$E_i = \Sigma_j\, N_{ij} \times R_j \tag{11.5}$$

where N_{ij} is the person-time at risk in age group j in area i (computed by taking the population in age group j in area j × number of years), and R_j is the mortality rate age group j of a suitable reference population. The ratio O_i/E_i is known as the standardized incidence ratio (SIR), or, in the case of mortality outcomes, the standardized mortality ratio (SMR). This ratio is an estimate of the *relative risk* of mortality within each area, θ_i. For rare, non-communicable diseases, the standard statistical model for O_i is that of the Poisson distribution:

$$O_i \sim \text{Poisson}(\theta_i E_i) \tag{11.6}$$

The maximum likelihood estimator of θ_i is given by:

$$\hat{\theta} = \text{SMR}_i = O_i/E_i \tag{11.7}$$

with $\text{Var}(\text{SMR}_i) = \theta_i/E_i$, estimated by O_i/E_i^2. Note that $\text{Var}(\text{SMR}_i)$ is inversely proportional to E_i. To translate the relative risk into rates, one simply multiplies the SMR by the overall mortality rate from the reference population.

SMRs have been commonly used in disease maps, and are particularly useful when the age-specific counts of deaths are not available for each area. The method also produces rate estimates with a smaller asymptotic variance than the corresponding direct standardization method (Pickle and White, 1995). Because SMRs estimate the risk relative to the average risk over the entire study area, they are perhaps best visualized in colour with a divergent (or 'double-ended') colour gradient, which permits the identification of unusually high or unusually low SMRs; SMRs close to the null value of 1.0 are visualized with an unsaturated colour (Brewer, 2005). When maps are rendered in black and white, representation of the divergent scale is more difficult. In the print version of this chapter, maps of SMRs are presented using a sequential greyscale gradient. To see colour maps with a divergent colour gradient, with SMR < 1 represented in blues and SMR > 1 represented in reds, see www.albany.edu/~fboscoe/gisbook.

As summary measures, SMRs also have certain drawbacks. They are based on ratio estimators, and are thus sensitive to small changes in E_i. In particular, when E_i is close to zero, the SMR will be very large for any positive count. As the estimate of Var(SMR$_i$) is proportional to $1/E_i$, SMRs of zero do not distinguish variation in expected counts. Most importantly, the interpretability and comparability of SMRs based on indirectly age standardized data across areas depends on the assumption of independent area and age effects with respect to the standard population. This is known as the proportionality assumption, and assumes that $r_{ij} = \theta_i \times \alpha_j$, where α_j is an age effect that does not vary over areas.

Applying indirect age standardization to lung cancer mortality rates for white non-Hispanics in Boston (using age-specific lung cancer mortality reference rates from Massachusetts for the same period) yields the map in Fig. 11.3a. Here, the quantity mapped for each area is the ratio of the mortality rate in that particular area compared with the overall mean rate in the reference population. As Var(SMR$_i$) ≈ O_i/E_i^2, one can use this to calculate 95% confidence limits for the SMRs in the Boston example (Fig. 11.3b). Most of the confidence limits are wide and include the null value of 1. The resulting estimates are dominated by sampling variability, making comparison of mortality risks between areas difficult.

To overcome this variability, hierarchical models can be used to 'smooth' the raw rates. When faced with the problem of making inferences on many parameters $\{\theta_i\} = \theta_1, \ldots, \theta_n$, measured on n areas, one can imagine two possible extreme assumptions. At one extreme, one could assume that all of the $\{\theta_i\}$ are identical, in which case all the data can be pooled, and the individual units ignored. This is what one typically does when presenting summary rates and rate ratios over the whole area. At the other extreme, one could assume that all the $\{\theta_i\}$ are independent and entirely unrelated, in which case the results from each area would need to be analysed independently (no pooling). As we have seen in the SMR example above, this leads to statistical instability if the numbers are small. A third possible assumption lies somewhere between these two extremes. One could assume that the $\{\theta_i\}$ are 'similar' in

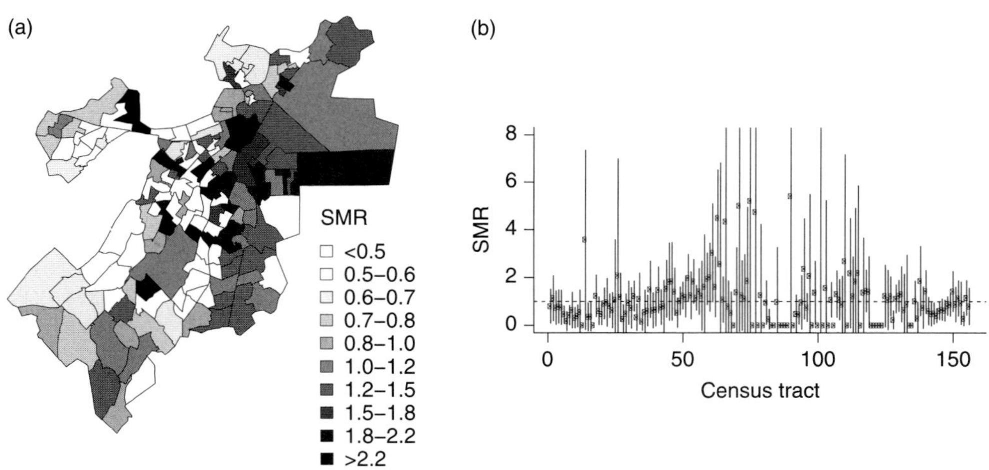

Fig. 11.3. Observed SMRs (standardized mortality ratios) for lung cancer mortality among white non-Hispanics in Boston, 2000–2005: (a) map, and (b) estimates and 95% confidence intervals.

the sense that the area labels convey no additional information. This is known as *exchangeability*, and is equivalent to assuming that the $\{\theta_i\}$ are drawn from a common prior distribution with unknown parameters.

11.3 A Poisson Gamma Model

A classic example of a hierarchical modelling approach building on exchangeability is presented by Clayton and Kaldor (1987), who developed a Bayesian analysis of a Poisson likelihood model. Their model is a useful introduction to the idea of hierarchical modelling of disease rates, because the second stage distribution for the area variability is analytically tractable. In the first stage of the hierarchy, one assumes that the observed death counts for each area are Poisson distributed, i.e. Eqn 11.6. In the second stage, a hierarchical prior is placed on θ_i:

$$O_i \sim \text{Poisson}(\theta_i E_i) \quad (11.8a)$$

$$\theta_i \sim \text{Gamma}(a, b) \quad (11.8b)$$

Recalling that the gamma distribution with parameters a and b has the mean a/b, this simply states that we expect the distribution of $\{\theta_i\}$ to follow a gamma distribution with mean a/b and variance a/b^2. As the gamma distribution is the conjugate prior of the Poisson, the posterior distribution of $p(\theta_i|O_i,E_i)$ also follows a gamma distribution:

$$\text{Gamma}(a + O_i, b + E_i) \quad (11.9)$$

with the mean given by

$$E(\theta_i \mid O_i, a, b) = \frac{a+O_i}{b+E_i}$$
$$= w_i \text{SMR}_i + (1-w_i)\frac{a}{b} \quad (11.10)$$

where

$$w_i = \frac{E_i}{b+E_i} \quad (11.11)$$

Thus, the posterior mean of the relative risk for the ith area is a weighted average of the SMR for the ith area and the average relative risk (a/b) in the overall map. The weight is inversely proportional to the variance of the SMR. Accordingly, when E_i is small (for rare diseases or small population counts), the variance is large, so the weight w_i is small. In this situation, the posterior mean is dominated by the prior mean, a/b. In areas with abundant data, the posterior mean is close to the observed SMR, O_i/E_i. This feature, whereby the amount of smoothing is proportional to the amount of information available for a particular area, is known as *precision weighting*. It has an intuitive appeal in that, when one does not observe a lot of information about an area (because the sample size is small and the risk estimate is unstable), one's 'best guess' concerning that area's mortality risk should be weighted towards what little is known from prior knowledge, i.e. that the risk is, on average, a/b. In contrast, if one observes a lot of information for an area (e.g. because the sample size is large), one is more likely to believe what the data say about mortality risk in that particular area, and so the 'best guess' would reasonably be weighted towards the observed SMR for that specific area.

In the fully Bayesian framework, one also treats the parameters of the gamma prior as unknown parameters to be estimated, and assigns prior distributions to a and b. This allows the data to inform the prior for the gamma distribution. If one selects relatively uninformative priors, such as:

$$a \sim \text{Exponential}(0.01) \quad (11.12a)$$

and

$$b \sim \text{Exponential}(0.01) \quad (11.12b)$$

then the choice of hyperparameters for these distributions does not heavily influence the lower level variation. In general, the posterior distribution of these parameters is not of closed form, but MCMC methods can be used to obtain posterior samples.

The resulting estimate of each θ_i 'borrows' strength from the likelihood contributions for all of the areas via their joint influence on the estimate of the unknown prior parameters a and b. This leads to global smoothing of the relative risks, as seen in Fig. 11.4, where the posterior estimates of the relative risks have been 'shrunk' towards the null value of 1. One obtains posterior distributions for each θ_i, and 95% credible intervals can be computed

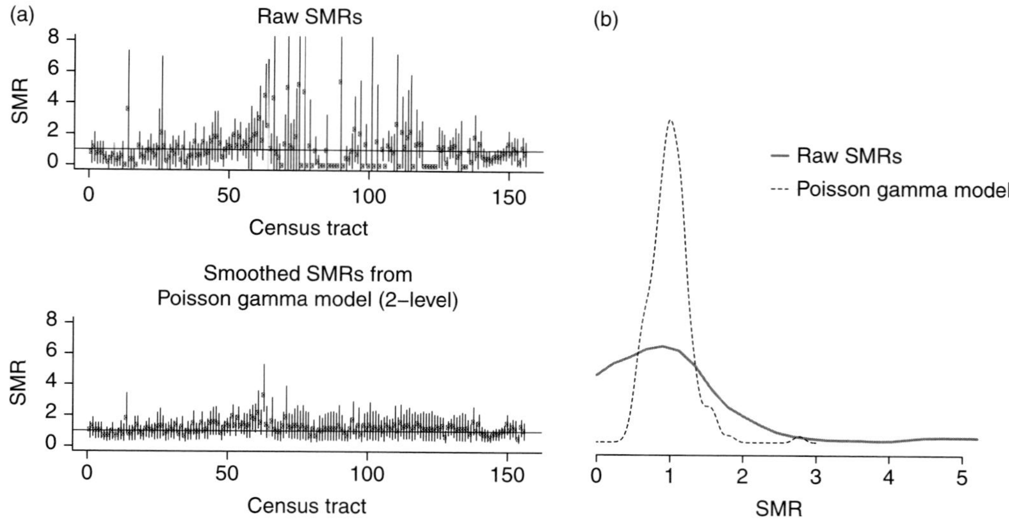

Fig. 11.4. Comparison of raw SMRs (standardized mortality ratios) and smoothed SMRs from the Poisson gamma model for lung cancer mortality among white non-Hispanics in Boston, 2000–2005: (a) raw SMRs and 95% confidence limits (top) and smoothed SMRS and 95% credible intervals (bottom); (b) distributions of raw SMRs and smoothed SMR estimates.

from quantiles of these distributions. The intervals that are computed show that the precision of the relative risk estimates is also improved by borrowing strength across areas. These estimates also reflect the uncertainty about the true values of *a* and *b*.

A comparison of the raw SMR map with the smoothed map from the Poisson gamma model (Fig. 11.5) also shows the substantial smoothing that has occurred. Most of the areas that appeared to have markedly higher or lower risk of lung cancer mortality in the raw SMR map (left) now appear to have fairly average risks, and only a few areas stand out as unusual in the second map (right).

11.4 A Poisson Log Normal Model

A gamma prior for $\{\theta_i\}$ is mathematically convenient, but may be restrictive. If the goal in hierarchical modelling is to be able to treat the units at each stage of the model as exchangeable, one is likely to want to adjust for observed covariates of disease risk. However, this is difficult in the Poisson gamma model. A normal prior for $\log(\theta_i)$ yields a more flexible model (Wakefield *et al.*, 2000; Lawson *et al.*, 2003):

$$O_i \sim \text{Poisson}(\theta_i E_i) \qquad (11.13a)$$

$$\log(\theta_i) = \alpha + v_i \qquad (11.13b)$$

$$v_i \sim \text{Normal}(0, \sigma_v^2) \qquad (11.13c)$$

where α is an intercept term representing the overall log relative risk of disease in the whole study region compared with the reference rate, and v_i is the residual log relative risk in area *i* compared with the average over the study region. Here, the $\{v_i\}$ are assumed to arise from a normal distribution with mean 0 and variance σ_v^2. This model is recognizable as a generalized linear mixed model, where 'mixed' refers to the fact that the model both contains 'random effects' (the $\{v_i\}$) and accommodates 'fixed' covariate effects, e.g.

$$\log(\theta_i) = \alpha + \beta_1 x_1 + \ldots + \beta_p x_p + v_i \qquad (11.14)$$

In this case the $\{v_i\}$ are interpretable as *residual* area-specific effects conditional on the *p* fixed covariates. Similarly, the βs are interpretable as covariate effects conditional on the area random effects.

It should be noted here that, as pointed out by Wolpert and Ickstadt (1998), the Poisson

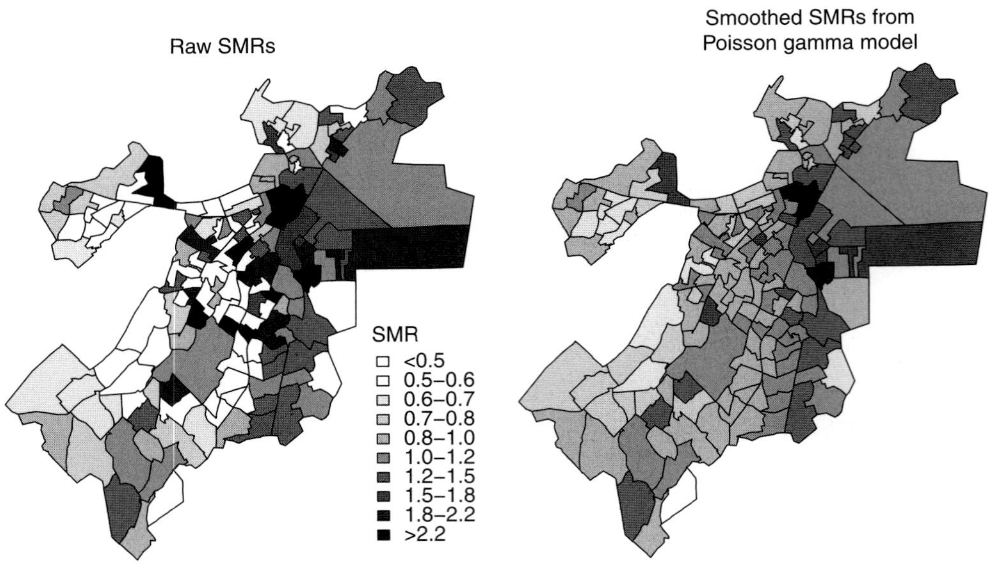

Fig. 11.5. Maps of relative risk estimates for lung cancer mortality (standardized mortality ratios, SMRs) among white non-Hispanics in Boston, 2000–2005: comparison of smoothed SMR estimates from the Poisson gamma model (right) with the raw SMRs (left).

log normal model does not aggregate consistently. That is, if one specifies a log normal distribution for each of the relative risks and then combines two areas and specifies a log normal distribution for the relative risk of the combined area, then these distributions are inconsistent (because the sum of log normal distributions is not log normal). This can be understood as a form of ecological bias whereby risk relationships do not remain constant across levels of aggregation (Wakefield *et al.*, 2000). Nevertheless, a normal second stage distribution has been observed empirically to provide a good model for log relative risks over a range of aggregations, and does present advantages with respect to model flexibility and ease of computation.

To complete the Bayesian specification, one needs to place hyperpriors on α and σ_v^2. For this example, I have specified a diffuse normal prior for $\alpha \sim$ Normal(0, 2000). Note that in WinBUGS, the normal distribution is specified in terms of the mean and the precision $\tau^2 = 1/\sigma^2$. Thus, the diffuse normal prior specified by dnorm(0, 0.0005) corresponds to a normal distribution with mean zero and variance of 2000. It is convenient in WinBUGS to specify a gamma prior for the precision of σ_v^2, e.g. $1/\sigma_v^2 \sim$ Gamma(0.5, 0.0005) (Kelsall and Wakefield, 1999; however, see Gelman, 2006, for a discussion about selecting appropriate prior distributions for the precision).

The estimate of the SMR for area *i* relative to the reference mortality rate (from the indirect age standardization) is $\exp(\alpha + v_i)$, while $\exp(v_i)$ is the residual relative risk for area *i* relative to the mean over the study area. Note that if an internal set of reference rates for indirect age standardization has been used, i.e. based on the observed rates over the whole study area itself, then α will generally be close to zero. The $\{v_i\}$ can also be thought of as latent variables that capture the effects of unknown or unmeasured area level covariates.

As shown in Fig. 11.6, the Poisson log normal model smooths the raw SMRs considerably, and yields a map similar to the one from the Poisson gamma model that was shown in Fig. 11.5. Similarly, in the density plot in Fig. 11.7, we see that the posterior distribution of the SMRs from the Poisson gamma and (2-level) Poisson log normal models are virtually the same, with both showing substantial smoothing compared with the raw SMRs.

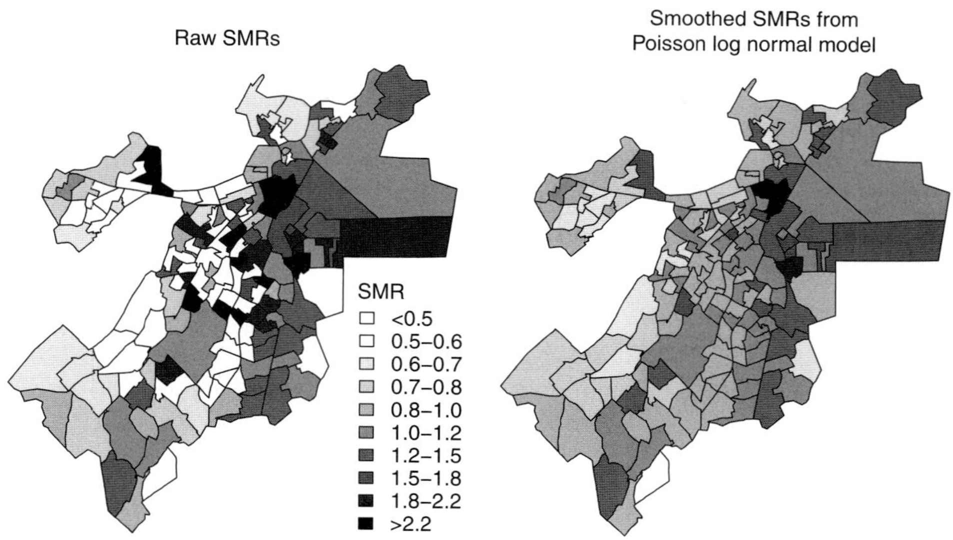

Fig. 11.6. Maps of relative risk estimates for lung cancer mortality (standardized mortality ratios, SMRs) among white non-Hispanics in Boston, 2000–2005: comparison of smoothed SMR estimates from the (2-level) Poisson log normal model (right) with raw SMRs (left).

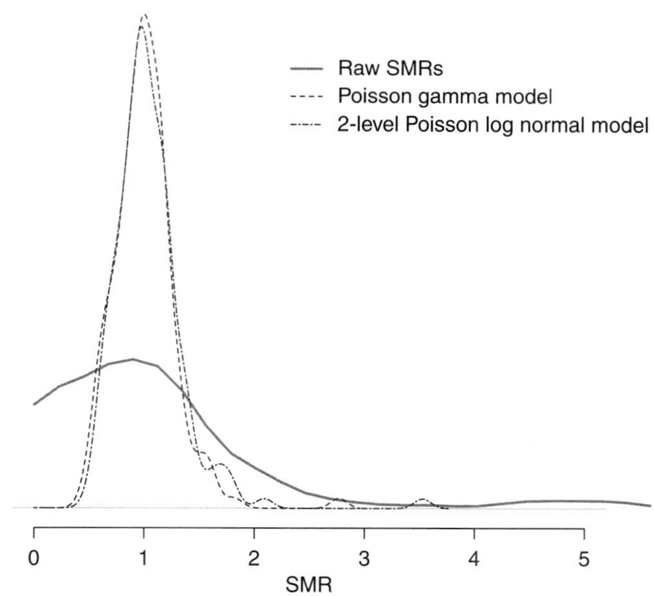

Fig. 11.7. Comparison of raw SMRs (standardized mortality ratios) and smoothed SMRs for lung cancer mortality among white non-Hispanics in Boston, 2000–2005: density plots of raw SMRs and posterior distributions from (2-level) Poisson log normal and gamma models.

Comparison of the DICs from the Poisson gamma model (DIC = 682.1) and the Poisson log normal model (DIC = 681.1) shows that both models are equally supported by the data and perform similarly in capturing the spatially varying risk surface.

The variance of the random effects (σ_v^2) reflects the amount of extra-Poisson variation in the data, but may be difficult to interpret on its own as it represents this variation on the log(SMR) scale. A useful alternative summary of the random effects variability is to look at the ratio of the quantiles of their empirical distribution (Gomez-Rubio *et al.*, 2010). For example, one can define $QR_{90} = \exp(q_{95\%} - q_{5\%})$, where $q_{5\%}$ is the log relative risk for the area ranked at the 5th percentile and $q_{95\%}$ is the log relative risk for the area ranked at the 95th percentile. QR_{90} is therefore interpretable as the relative risk between the top and bottom 5% of areas. Computing this based on the posterior samples of $\{v_i\}$ from the Poisson log normal model, one obtains an estimated QR_{90} of 3.80 (95% CI (credible interval) 2.90, 5.53). That is, there is an almost fourfold disparity in mortality when comparing the 5% of census tracts with the highest mortality rates with the 5% with the lowest mortality rates.

In both the Poisson gamma and Poisson log normal models, the smoothing is global: the random effects $\{v_i\}$ are treated as exchangeable and come from the same common distribution. As a result, all of the area-specific relative risks are shrunk to the same overall mean. This kind of global smoothing does not allow for spatial correlation between risks in nearby areas, as might be expected if there is local clustering in the spatial pattern of risks. Local clustering of risks may be due to risk factors that are shared within and across census tracts: individuals who share these spatially varying risk factors would be expected to have similar outcomes. If such local clustering exists, this is a violation of the assumption of exchangeability. If these risk factors are known and observed, the most straightforward solution would be to include them as covariates in the model. However, in most observational settings, one can rarely measure, or even know about, all of the relevant risk factors. If one suspects that these risk factors vary by area, it will be necessary to consider ways to allow for local clustering in models for $\{\theta_i\}$.

11.5 Multilevel Approaches to Clustering

If one has some a priori information about how census tracts are organized, one might consider modelling clustering by specifying an additional level in the multilevel hierarchy. For example, Boston has well defined neighbourhoods that are aggregations of census tracts (Fig. 11.8). The result is that Boston residents have a strong sense of neighbourhood identity. Additionally, neighbourhoods are used as administrative units, e.g. by the Boston Public Health Commission and Boston Housing Authority, so that there is good reason to believe that neighbourhood level policies might lead to clustering among census tracts (Chen *et al.*, 2006).

To adopt a multilevel (nested) approach to clustering, one can specify a 3-level Poisson log normal model with i indexing census tracts and j indexing neighbourhoods:

$$O_{ij} \sim \text{Poisson}(\theta_{ij}E_{ij}) \qquad (11.15a)$$

$$\log(\theta_{ij}) = \alpha + v_{ij} + z_j \qquad (11.15b)$$

$$v_{ij} \sim \text{Normal}(0, \sigma_v^2) \qquad (11.15c)$$

$$z_j \sim \text{Normal}(0, \sigma_z^2) \qquad (11.15d)$$

Here, the $\{v_{ij}\}$ are independently normally distributed *census tract* effects and the $\{z_j\}$ are independently normally distributed *neighbourhood* effects. Note that the census tracts and neighbourhood effects are conditionally independent. As with the 2-level Poisson log normal model described in the previous section Section 11.4), the model for $\log(\theta_i)$ could also include any number of fixed covariate effects, although for the moment I include just an intercept (α). Parameters of interest from this model include the census tract-specific SMRs ($SMR_i = \exp(\alpha + v_{ij} + z_j)$), the variance of the census tract random effects (σ_v^2), the variance of the neighbourhood random effects (σ_z^2), and the empirical ratio of the 95th to 5th percentiles of the SMRs (QR_{90}).

Figure 11.9 compares the resulting maps of the SMRs from the 2- and 3-level Poisson log normal models. The heavier lines in the second map (on the right) correspond to the neighbourhood boundaries. One can see that the 3-level model allows for local clustering of risk in certain neighbourhoods. The census tract level variance (σ_v^2) is 0.27 (95% CI 0.12, 0.39), the neighbourhood level variance (σ_z^2) is 0.29 (95% CI 0.17, 0.47) and the empirical ratio of the SMRs (QR_{90}) is 3.6 (95% CI 2.7, 4.9). Comparison of the DIC values for the 3-level Poisson log normal model (DIC = 672.3) and

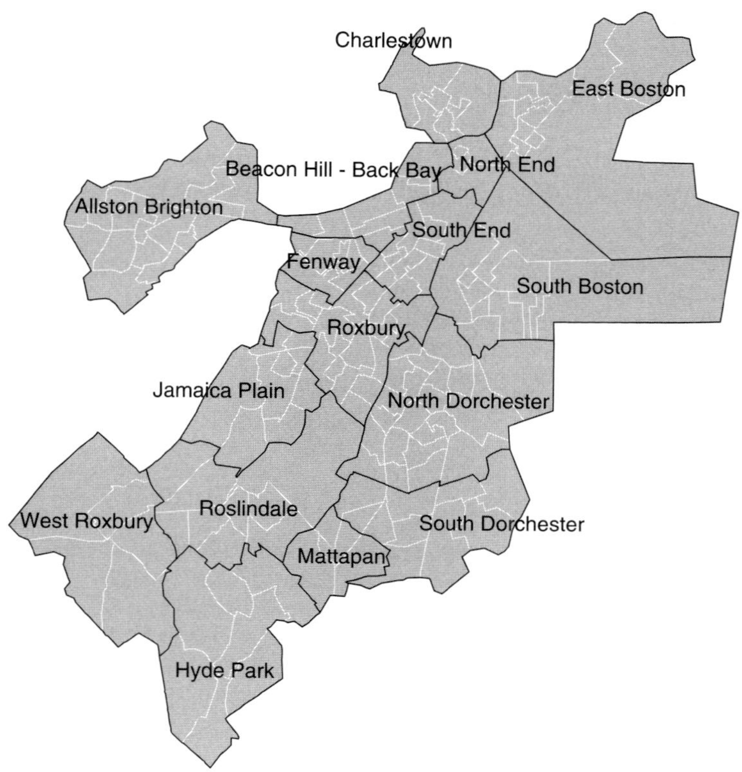

Fig. 11.8. Boston neighbourhoods defined by the Boston Public Health Commission of Massachusetts.

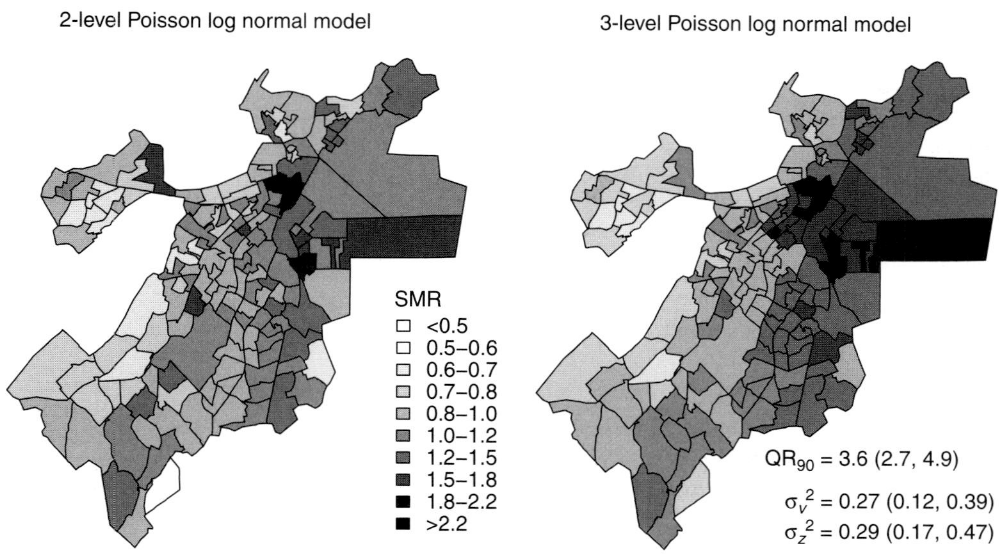

Fig. 11.9. Maps of relative risk estimates for lung cancer mortality (standardized mortality ratios, SMRs) among white non-Hispanics in Boston, 2000–2005: comparison of the mapped smoothed SMRs from the 2-level (left) and 3-level (right) Poisson log normal models. See text for explanations of QR_{90}, σ_v^2, σ_z^2.

the 2-level log normal model (DIC = 681.1) shows that the 3-level model offers a substantially better fit to the data. This is also evident in the density plots for the two models (Fig. 11.10).

11.6 Besag, York and Mollié Model

In the multilevel Poisson log normal model with independent census tracts and neighbourhoods, the neighbourhood units were specified a priori. In a sense, the neighbourhood boundaries are 'hard' boundaries, and crossing a boundary means that one's relative risk may jump by quite a lot. What if one wants to account for spatial correlation in a 'smoother' manner? One way to do this is to specify a multivariate normal prior distribution for all the area parameters with a spatially structured covariance matrix. Many different ways have been proposed to specify spatially structured multivariate normal distributions for $\log(\theta_i)$ (Wakefield *et al.*, 2000; Banerjee *et al.*, 2004).

One particular form of the multivariate normal distribution that is commonly used is the intrinsic Gaussian conditional autoregression (CAR) prior suggested by Clayton and Kaldor (1987) and developed by Besag *et al.* (1991). This is one of the most popular ways of dealing with spatial autocorrelation. The spatial structure is formulated through a set of conditional autoregressions, which uses the fact that if a vector of random variables has a multivariate normal distribution, then the distribution of each element of that vector conditional on all the other elements in the vector is also normal, with a mean and variance that depend on the original multivariate mean and covariance matrix.

As with the other models, the first stage model assumes that the observed counts are Poisson distributed, and that an additive model for $\log(\theta_i)$ can be specified for accommodating covariate effects:

$$O_i \sim \text{Poisson}(\theta_i E_i) \qquad (11.16a)$$

$$\log(\theta_i) = \alpha + u_i \qquad (11.16b)$$

where u_i is a spatially structured random effect. Then, instead of the independent normal prior for the distribution of the census tract effects, one models the effect for census tract i, u_i, as having a normal prior distribution conditional on the neighbours of i. That is,

$$u_i | u_{j,\, j\neq i} \sim \text{Normal}(\mu_i,\ \tau_u^2/m_i) \qquad (11.16c)$$

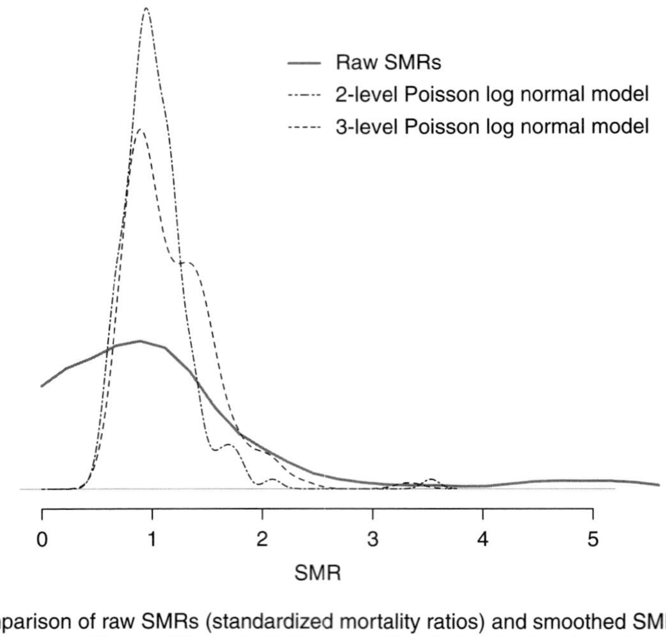

Fig. 11.10. Comparison of raw SMRs (standardized mortality ratios) and smoothed SMRs for lung cancer mortality among white non-Hispanics in Boston, 2000–2005: density plots of raw SMRs and posterior distributions from the 2-level and 3-level Poisson log normal models.

where u_i is the average of the census tract effects of the neighbouring census tracts, τ_u^2 is the conditional variance, m_i is the number of neighbours of census tract i.

To understand this, consider the highlighted census tract i in Fig. 11.11. If ∂_i is the set of areas adjacent to i, and one sets a weight w_{ij} to 1 for areas $j \in \partial_i$ and zero otherwise, then the prior distribution for u_i has conditional mean equal to the average of the neighbouring values $\{u_j\}$, i.e.

$$\mu_i = \frac{\Sigma_j w_{ij} u_j}{\Sigma_j w_{ij}} \qquad (11.17a)$$

where

$$w_{ij} = \begin{cases} 1 \text{ if } i, j \text{ are adjacent} \\ 0 \text{ if they are not} \end{cases} \qquad (11.17b)$$

Note that the conditional variance, τ_u^2, is scaled by:

$$\sum\nolimits_{j \in \partial_i} w_{ij} = m_i \qquad (11.17c)$$

i.e. the number of neighbours, to emphasize that it is only interpretable conditionally, and with variance (μ_i, τ_u^2/m_i) inversely proportional to the number of neighbours. Since the variance is scaled by the number of neighbours and only interpretable conditionally, I have changed the notation from σ_u^2 to τ_u^2.

Besag *et al.* (1991) recommended combining the CAR prior and the standard normal prior to allow for both spatially unstructured and spatially correlated random effects:

$$O_i \sim \text{Poisson}(\theta_i E_i) \qquad (11.18a)$$

$$\log(\theta_i) = \alpha + v_i + u_i \qquad (11.18b)$$

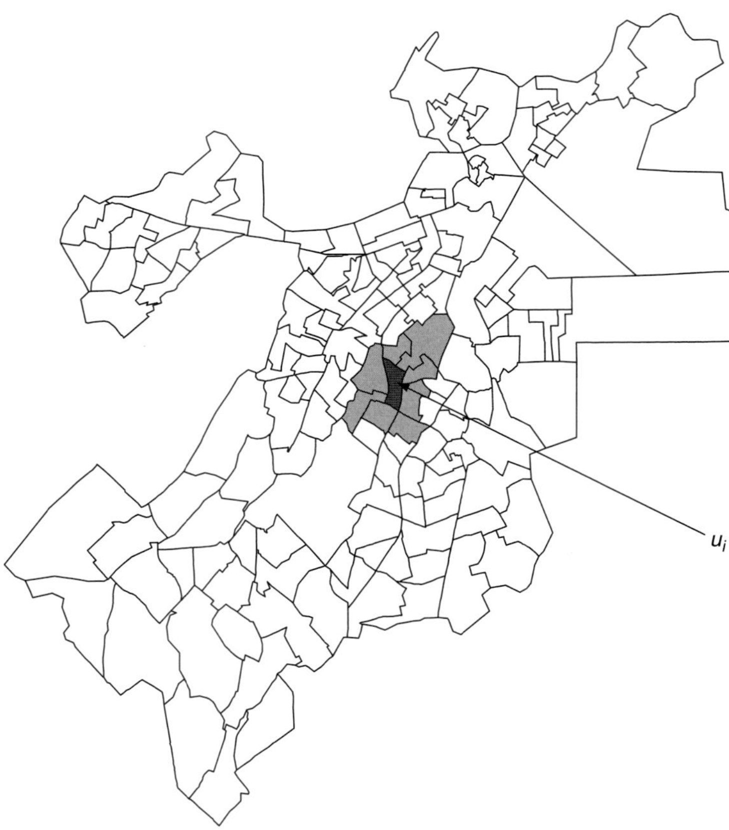

Fig. 11.11. An illustration of the CAR (Gaussian conditionally autoregressive) idea: u_i is smoothed towards the mean risk of the neighbouring areas.

$$v_i \sim \text{Normal}(0, \sigma_v^2) \qquad (11.18c)$$

$$u_i | u_{j,\ j \neq i} \sim \text{Normal}(\mu_i, \tau_u^2/m_i) \qquad (11.18d)$$

where v_i is a spatially unstructured random effect.

This model is often referred to as the convolution model, or the Besag, York and Mollié (BYM) model. The unstructured $\{v_i\}$ can be thought of as capturing unstructured heterogeneity, or correlation *within* areas. In contrast, the spatially structured $\{u_i\}$ capture spatial correlation *across* areas (Bernardinelli *et al.*, 1995). Note, however, that σ_v^2 (unstructured heterogeneity variance) and τ_u^2 (spatial variance) are not directly comparable: σ_v^2 reflects the marginal variability of the unstructured random effects between areas, while τ_u^2 is the conditional variance of the spatial effect in area *i*, conditional on values of neighbouring spatial effects. No closed-form expression is available for the marginal between-area variance of the spatial effects. However, in the Bayesian approach, the marginal spatial variance s_u^2 can be estimated empirically from the posterior samples of $\{u_i\}$:

$$s_u^2 = \Sigma_i (u_i - \bar{u})^2/(n-1) \qquad (11.19)$$

where $\bar{u}$ is the average of the $\{u_i\}$.

Technically, although the univariate conditional prior distributions for each u_i are well defined, the corresponding joint prior distribution for $\{u_i\}$ is now improper (undefined mean and infinite variance). It is necessary to impose a constraint to ensure that the model is identifiable. This is accomplished by constraining the $\{u_i\}$ to have a zero mean and specifying an improper uniform prior distribution for the intercept α.

With an estimate of the marginal between-area variance, one can also characterize the relative contribution of spatial versus unstructured heterogeneity:

$$\text{frac}_{\text{spatial}} = s_u^2/(s_u^2 + \sigma_v^2) \qquad (11.20)$$

When $\text{frac}_{\text{spatial}}$ is close to 1, spatial heterogeneity dominates. When $\text{frac}_{\text{spatial}}$ is close to 0, unstructured heterogeneity dominates (Best *et al.*, 2005).

Figure 11.12 compares the 3-level Poisson log normal model with the BYM model.

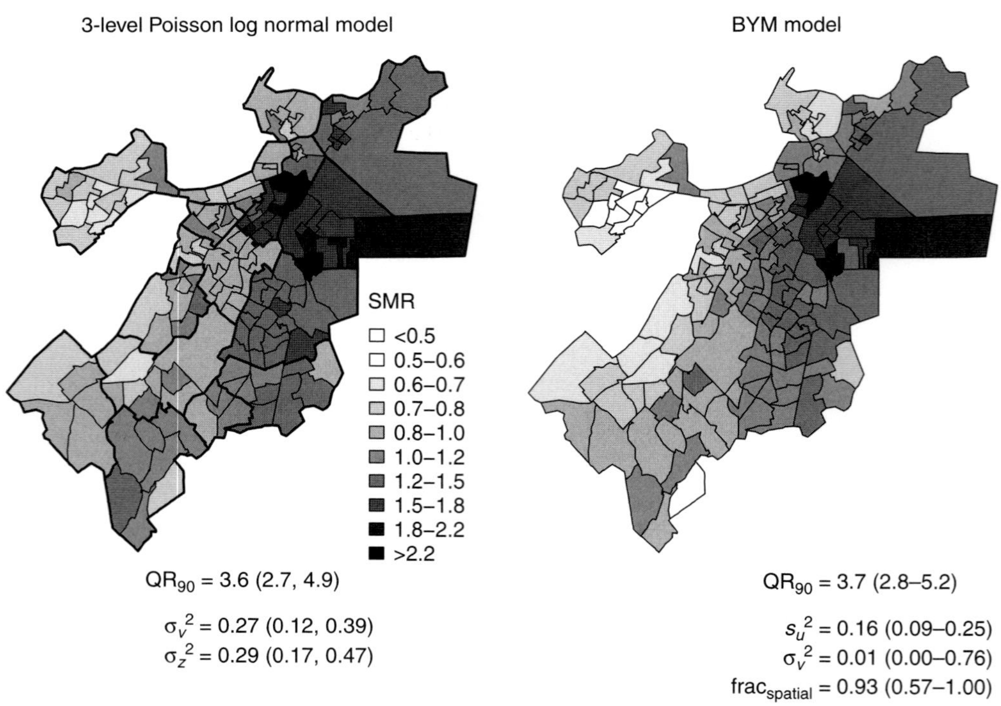

Fig. 11.12. Mapped smoothed SMRs (standardized mortality ratios) for lung cancer among white non-Hispanics in Boston, 2000–2005: comparison of BYM (Besag, York and Mollié) model (right) with 3-level Poisson log normal model (left). See text for explanations of QR_{90}, σ_v^2, σ_z^2, s_u^2.

Both models accommodate local clustering of census tract risks, compared with the 2-level Poisson log normal model (shown in Fig. 11.6, right, and Fig. 11.9, left), with some differences that are also reflected in the different distributions in Fig. 11.13. The marginal variance of the spatially structured effects, $s_u^2 = 0.16$ (95% CI 0.09, 0.25), is substantially larger than the variance of the unstructured effects, $\sigma_v^2 = 0.01$ (95% CI 0.00, 0.76), showing that the map is dominated by spatially structured heterogeneity ($frac_{spatial} = 0.93$, 95% CI 0.57, 1.00). Examination of the DICs suggests that the BYM model yields a better fit to the data (DIC = 665.9), compared with the 3-level Poisson log normal model (DIC = 672.3). One way to think about this is that, while the defined Boston neighbourhoods tend to reflect how the census tract level risks are clustered, the a priori defined neighbourhood structure does not compare this perfectly, while in the BYM model the clustering is informed by the data.

In the spatial modelling literature, the intrinsic CAR model based on adjacency weights has been a popular choice for modelling spatial variation in disease rates with local smoothing. However, the method entails making several assumptions about the weighting structure that should be acknowledged. First, there is the question of how to define adjacency, particularly for irregularly shaped areas. One basic choice involves deciding whether adjacent neighbours are to be defined based only on shared edges (rook neighbours) or on shared edges and vertices (queen neighbours; see Section 1.5). Secondly, while the intrinsic CAR model defines the conditional distributions using weights of 1 for adjacent areas and 0 for non-adjacent areas, other weighting schemes are possible for the general class of CAR models. For example, weights could be defined in a smoother manner as a decay function of distance, e.g. distance between population-weighted centroids of the areas. This function may be obtained empirically by fitting a correlogram to residuals from a model that does not include a spatially structured random effect, in order to determine the likely range of spatial autocorrelation (Cressie and Chan, 1989).

Published studies using various CAR approaches have rarely provided justification for the choice of the neighbourhood weight

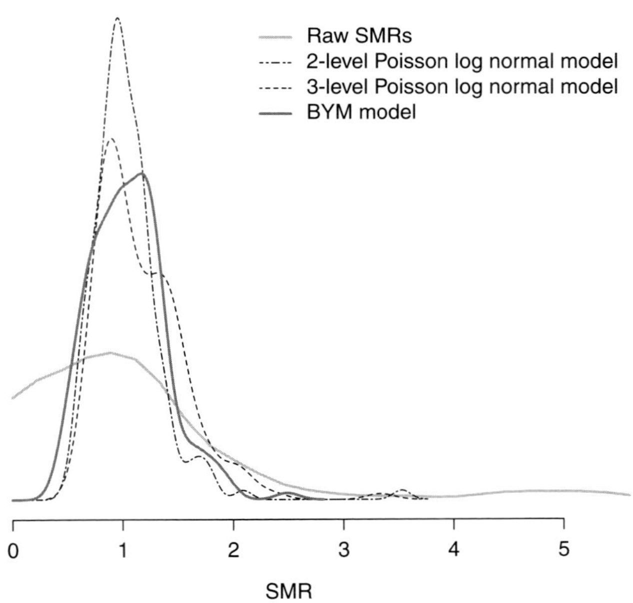

Fig. 11.13. Comparison of raw SMRs (standardized mortality ratios) and smoothed SMRs for lung cancer mortality among white non-Hispanics in Boston, 2000–2005: density plots of raw SMRs and posterior distributions from 2-level and 3-level Poisson log normal models and BYM (Besag, York and Mollié) model.

matrix structure. Best *et al.* (2001) investigated the relationship between benzene emissions and the incidence of childhood leukaemia in Greater London, and considered three alternative levels of data aggregation in their analysis. They examined adjacency versus distance-based neighbourhood spatial weights, and found, for both grid-level and ward-level analyses, that the adjacency based neighbourhood structure provided a better fit of the data, based on DIC comparisons. They also found a significant different in the estimates of the spatially structured random effects between the distance-based and adjacency-based neighbourhood structures for the ward-level analysis without any covariates. Earnest *et al.* (2007) explored a variety of adjacency- and distance-based weight matrices in a study of birth defects in New South Wales, Australia. They found that, in terms of agreement between observed and predicted relative risks, the distance-based matrices tended to perform better than those based on adjacency. They attributed this finding in part to the highly irregular shapes of the areas, and suggested that adjacency models would be expected to perform better with regular shaped areas such as grids. Thus, while the intrinsic CAR approach provides a convenient implementation of local smoothing, when possible, it is advisable to conduct an exploratory analysis of the neighbourhood weight matrix to guide the choice of a suitable weight scheme.

While the multilevel modelling framework is usually specified in terms of nested random normal effects, multilevel models can also accommodate spatial correlations via their extension to multiple membership models (Hill and Goldstein, 1998). Langford *et al.* (1999) showed how to use such models to fit spatial data, and Browne *et al.* (2001) present Bayesian extensions of this model as a member of the family of models called multiple-membership multiple-classification (MMMC) models.

11.7 CAR and Neighbourhood Effects

Given, on the one hand, an a priori belief in the importance of neighbourhoods and, on the other hand, an appreciation of the idea of smooth, spatially autocorrelated effects, one might be tempted to combine the CAR structure at the census tract level with independent neighbourhood effects by modelling:

$$O_{ij} \sim \text{Poisson}(\theta_{ij} E_{ij}) \qquad (11.21a)$$

$$\log(\theta_{ij}) = \alpha + v_{ij} + u_{ij} + z_j \qquad (11.21b)$$

$$v_i \sim \text{Normal}(0, \sigma_v^2) \qquad (11.21c)$$

$$u_i | u_{j,\, j \neq i} \sim \text{Normal}(\mu_i, \tau_u^2 / m_i) \qquad (11.21d)$$

$$z_j \sim \text{Normal}(0, \sigma_z^2) \qquad (11.21e)$$

This model includes spatially structured and unstructured effects at the census tract level along with neighbourhood level unstructured effects.

I compare this model – CAR + unstructured variability at the census tract level and unstructured neighbourhood variability – with the BYM model and the 3-level Poisson log normal model in Fig. 11.14. The map that the new more complex model generates is virtually indistinguishable from that obtained from the BYM model, but there is evidence that the more complex model is overspecified. The variance of the neighbourhood effects (σ_z^2) is close to zero and the DIC for this model (665.3) is not appreciably different from the DIC for the BYM model (665.9). Fig. 11.15 shows that the distribution of census tract effects is essentially the same as for the BYM model, leading one to conclude that the neighbourhood level effects do not add much beyond the clustering already captured by the conditionally autoregressive structure.

This exercise in model building suggests that, while one may have compelling conceptual reasons to specify a complex multilevel structure, care must be taken to ensure that the model is not overspecified and that the data support the proposed structure. In the Boston lung cancer mortality example, the conditionally autoregressive spatial structure captures most of the census tract level variability, including the local clustering, as evidenced by the high value for $\text{frac}_{\text{spatial}}$ and the fact that the neighbourhood level structure adds little to the model. Notably, the BYM model does support the notion of neighbourhood level variability in the sense of clustered census tracts that exhibit similarly elevated or depressed risks. However, the improved fit of the BYM model over the 3-level Poisson log normal

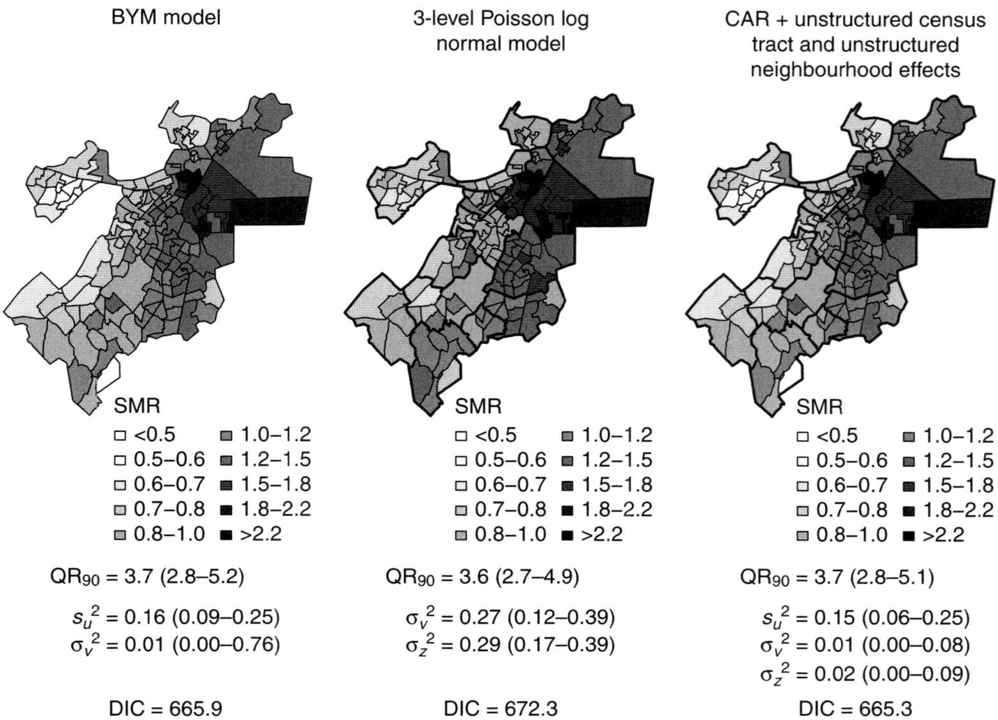

Fig. 11.14. Mapped smoothed SMRs (standardized mortality ratios) for lung cancer among white non-Hispanics in Boston, 2000–2005: comparison of BYM (Besag, York and Mollié) model, 3-level Poisson log normal model and a model with CAR (Gaussian conditionally autoregressive) + unstructured variability at the census tract level and unstructured neighbourhood variability. DIC, deviance information criterion. See text for explanations of QR_{90}, σ_v^2, σ_z^2, s_u^2.

model with predefined Boston neighbourhoods suggests that the official neighbourhood boundaries do not perfectly coincide with the actual pattern of spatial clustering of lung cancer mortality risks.

11.8 Covariate Effects

Having established that the BYM model best describes the census tract level variation in lung cancer mortality risk among white non-Hispanics, I now turn to fitting the BYM model with covariate effects. Documenting and monitoring socio-economic disparities in cancer outcomes is of great interest to social epidemiologists and public health policy makers, and a substantial literature has linked socio-economic deprivation to poorer cancer outcomes. To estimate socio-economic disparities in lung cancer mortality in white non-Hispanics in Boston, geocoded death records from 2000–2005 were linked to US Census 2000 estimates of the percentage of individuals living below the US defined poverty line at the census tract level. Figure 11.16 shows the geographic variation in census tract poverty in Boston, and indicates many areas where a substantial proportion of residents are living below the poverty line (≥20% below poverty). Census tract level poverty ranged from 2.3% to 57.4%, with a median of 17.4%. Over the whole city, 19.5% of Boston residents were living below the poverty line in 2000, compared with 9.3% of Massachusetts residents as a whole.

If this map is compared with the smoothed SMRs from the BYM model in Fig. 11.12, one sees that there are numerous areas where high poverty coincides with high lung cancer

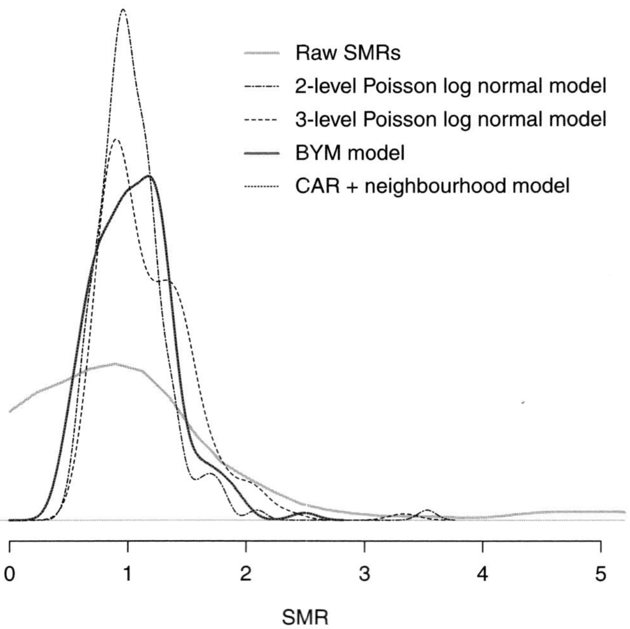

Fig. 11.15. Comparison of raw SMRs (standardized mortality ratios) and smoothed SMRs for lung cancer mortality among white non-Hispanics in Boston, 2000–2005: density plots of raw SMRs and posterior distributions from BYM (Besag, York and Mollié) and 3-level Poisson log normal models, and from a model with CAR (Gaussian conditionally autoregressive) + unstructured variability at the census tract level and unstructured neighbourhood variability.

mortality. However, there are also areas that do not follow this pattern, where high poverty coincides with more modest lung cancer mortality risk or where lower poverty coincides with higher lung cancer mortality risk.

To evaluate the overall association between census tract poverty across Boston census tracts, I fit the following model, which includes the census tract percentage below poverty measure as a continuous covariate:

$$O_{ij} \sim \text{Poisson}(\theta_{ij}E_{ij}) \quad (11.22a)$$

$$\log(\theta_{ij}) = \alpha + \beta^* \text{ poverty} + v_{ij} + u_{ij} \quad (11.22b)$$

$$v_i \sim \text{Normal}(0, \sigma_v^2) \quad (11.22c)$$

$$u_i|u_{j,j\neq i} \sim \text{Normal}(\mu_i, \tau_u^2/m_i) \quad (11.22d)$$

To fit the model in the fully Bayesian framework, I specify a diffuse normal prior for β (~ Normal(0, 10^4)). Table 11.1 presents the model results, including the estimated poverty gradient and summaries of area variation from the BYM model. I report the intercept and β for census tract poverty on the exponentiated scale so that these estimates are interpretable on the relative risk scale.

Recalling that the expected deaths in each census tract were computed using age-specific reference rates for Massachusetts as a whole, the intercept effect of exp(α) = 1.39 shows that white non-Hispanics in Boston experienced lung cancer mortality rates nearly 40% higher than the statewide lung cancer mortality rates. There was a strong socio-economic gradient in lung cancer mortality, with those living in more impoverished census tracts experiencing higher lung cancer mortality rates. As with the BYM model, the residual census tract variation in mortality was dominated by spatially structured heterogeneity ($\text{frac}_{\text{spatial}}$ = 0.96, 95% CI 0.70, 1.00).

Interestingly, while one observes a significant socio-economic gradient in lung cancer mortality by census tract poverty, adjusting for census tract poverty does not substantially reduce the census tract level variation. The empirical

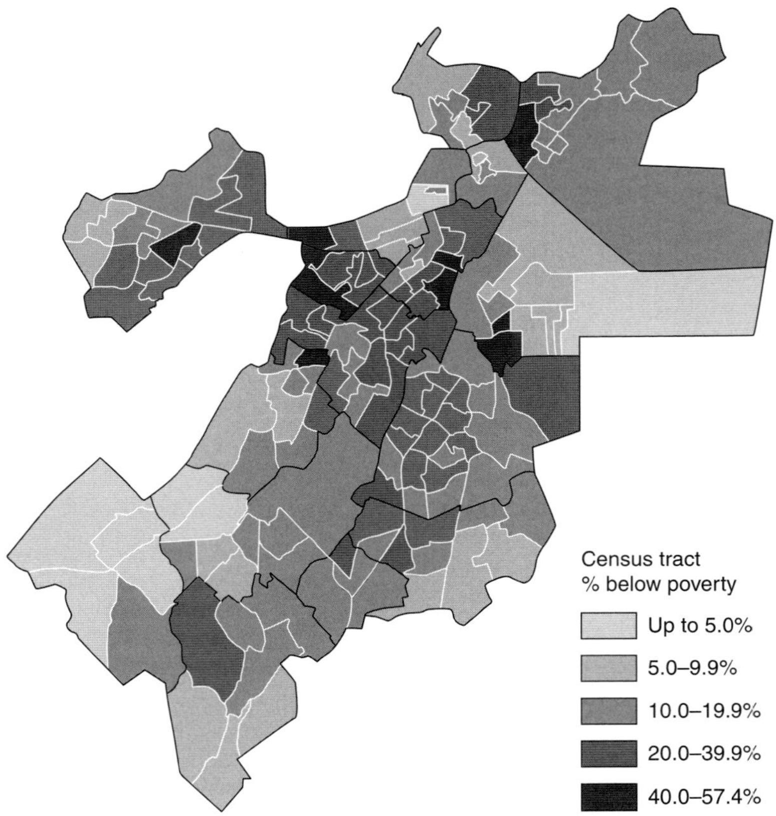

Fig. 11.16. Census tract percentages below poverty (US Census 2000 Summary File 3) in Boston, Massachusetts.

Table 11.1. Covariate effects and summaries of area variation from BYM (Besag, York and Mollié) model before and after adjustment for census tract poverty.

	Before	After
Covariate effects	**RR (95% CI)**[a]	**RR (95% CI)**
Intercept (e^{α})	1.13 (1.03, 1.24)	1.39 (1.26, 1.38)
Census tract % below poverty		3.54 (1.45, 8.66)
Other summary quantities	**Estimate (95% CI)**	**Estimate (95% CI)**
s_u^2	0.16 (0.09, 0.25)	0.16 (0.09, 0.24)
σ_v^2	0.01 (0.00, 0.08)	0.01 (0.00, 0.05)
$\text{frac}_{\text{spatial}}$	0.93 (0.57, 1.00)	0.96 (0.70, 1.00)
QR_{90}	3.73 (2.83, 5.17)	3.61 (2.73, 3.64)
DIC	665.9	662.6

[a]RR, relative risk, CI, confidence interval.

marginal variance of the CAR effects (s_u^2) was estimated as 0.16 in both this and the earlier BYM model. Similarly, in the model adjusting for census tract poverty, the DIC was 662.6, compared with 665.9 in the previous model. This leads one to the somewhat counterintuitive conclusion that census tract poverty is, on the one hand, a significant predictor of lung cancer mortality but, on the other hand, contributes only a small fraction to the overall census tract variation in lung cancer mortality risk.

As QR_{90} expresses the residual census tract variation in lung cancer mortality on the relative risk scale, one can gain a sense of what this variation means in terms of risk: the risk ratio comparing the 5% of census tracts with the highest mortality rates to the 5% with the lowest mortality rates is 3.61 (95% CI 2.73, 3.64). In contrast, based on the model estimate of the poverty gradient, comparing the census tract with the maximum census tract poverty level in Boston (54.7% below poverty) to census tracts with 0% poverty yields a risk ratio of around 2.0. Thus, the variation in lung cancer mortality risk across census tracts exceeds the variation due to poverty, and even after adjusting for census tract poverty, there remains a great deal of unexplained census tract level variation in mortality.

Figure 11.17 maps the posterior estimates of the census tract SMRs from the BYM model before and after adjusting for census tract poverty. As suggested by the model results on the lack of change in the variances of the structured and unstructured spatial heterogeneity, the maps show that adjustment for census tract poverty does little to change the observed pattern of lung cancer mortality risk, other than minor changes in the census tract SMRs for some of the census tracts. Of course, census tract poverty is but one area-based socio-economic variable, and there remain many potential risk factors, both individual and contextual, that may contribute to the area variation in lung cancer mortality rates. On a related note, because this socio-economic gradient is estimated on an area-based socio-economic measure, one must be cautious about making inferences about the relationship between an individual's socio-economic position and their risk of lung cancer death based on the observed ecological association. For an in-depth discussion of ecological bias, see Greenland (1992) and Elliott and Wakefield (1999). Similarly, while an area-based socio-economic variable can be conceptualized in its own right as reflecting 'contextual' socio-economic factors and not just as a proxy for individual-level socio-economic position, the estimated socio-economic effect from this model reflects both individual-level and contextual processes.

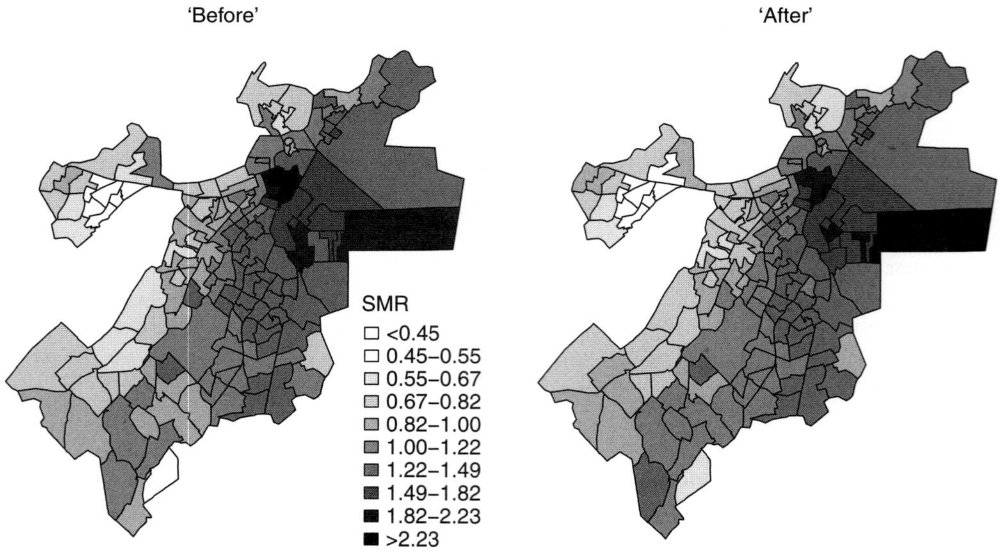

Fig. 11.17. Mapped smoothed SMRs (standardized mortality ratios) for lung cancer among white non-Hispanics in Boston, 2000–2005: comparison of census tract SMRs from the BYM (Besag, York and Mollié) model before and after adjustment for census tract poverty.

11.9 Conclusion

This chapter has presented an introduction to how health data in the form of georeferenced counts can be analysed using hierarchical models. These models are useful when one is interested in estimating, visualizing and comparing area-specific relative risks, particularly when the areas are small and the number of events in each area may be sparse. A key feature of this approach is that the unstable area-level parameters from the first stage of the model can be smoothed by specifying a second stage model that may, in turn, depend on a set of hyperparameters. This allows for more efficient estimation of regression parameters and also allows the standard errors of estimates to account appropriately for correlations between observations within areas and uncertainties in prediction and estimation.

I have compared several different modelling choices that allow for local clustering, including a multilevel approach based on nested independent normal effects at the census tract and neighbourhood levels, and the popular intrinsic Gaussian CAR model/BYM. Both models also allow for covariate adjustment and can be used to estimate the effect of fixed covariates conditional on the random effects structure. In our specific example focusing on the estimation and mapping of census tract level SMRs for lung cancer mortality among white non-Hispanics in Boston, the BYM model gave the best fit to the observed data.

In practice, however, the choice of modelling approach may depend on a priori beliefs about multilevel structure for a particular data set (e.g. the salience of administrative and policy relevant levels such as census tracts, counties, provinces or states) versus taking a more empirical approach to local smoothing. The inferential targets (i.e. estimates of the covariate effects versus posterior estimates of the area-specific effects) should also inform modelling choices. In particular, while hierarchical models are widely used in the spatial epidemiological literature, is important to note that estimates of the covariate effects from these hierarchical models are conditional on the correct specification of the random effects structure. If the model is not correctly specified, including if the random effects structure does not incorporate the relevant levels, this can potentially lead to bias. When interest focuses on the estimating covariate effects, and the correlation between observations from the same area is to be treated as a nuisance, an alternative strategy to modelling may be to use a generalized estimating equations (GEE) approach (Liang and Zeger, 1986). Parameter estimates from the GEE are consistent even when the covariance structure is mis-specified. Hubbard *et al.* (2010) argue that, when population averaged covariate effects are the primary interest, robustness to model mis-specification may be desirable.

Hierarchical models lend themselves to specification in the Bayesian framework and, as shown here, the posterior samples obtained from MCMC simulation can be used to obtain empirical estimates and credible intervals for several useful quantities (including, in these examples, QR_{90}, the marginal variance of CAR effects s_u^2 and $frac_{spatial}$). Caution must be used, however, as the Bayesian approach requires specifications of prior distributions of all model parameters, and model behaviour may be sensitive to these priors. While one typically tries to specify uninformative prior distributions so that the posterior likelihoods will be dominated by the data, in practice it is a good idea to try several different prior specifications in order to evaluate sensitivity. For example, in these models, I specified gamma(ε, ε) priors for the inverse of the variances of the random effects (i.e. σ_v^2, τ_u^2, σ_z^2), with ε very small (say 10^2 or 10^3) (Lawson *et al.*, 2003). However, Gelman (2006) and Kelsall and Wakefield (1999) point out that even small values of ε can be informative and that inferences become sensitive to ε. As an alternative, Gelman (2006) suggests using a half Cauchy prior for the precision of variance parameters.

While extremely flexible and able to deal with complex models, MCMC methods do involve computationally intensive simulations to obtain the posterior distribution for the parameters, and models for large data sets with many parameters may take a long time to fit. While multilevel Poisson models can also be fitted in a frequentist setting using a penalized quasi-likelihood algorithm (PQL), inference based on posterior samples is not available, and estimates of random effects may be biased in multilevel logistic models for binary response data. The Integrated Nested Laplace Approximation (INLA; Rue *et al.*, 2009) approach has been recently developed as a computationally efficient alternative to MCMC. INLA is designed for the broad class of latent Gaussian models, including (generalized) linear mixed, spatial and spatiotemporal models, and is gaining in popularity for spatial epidemiological applications.

While the BYM based on the intrinsic CAR prior is widely used in spatial epidemiological analyses, the development of hierarchical models for spatial and spatio-temporal data continues to be an active and vibrant research area. For example, some authors have argued that the parametric BYM model may result in oversmoothing of the risk surface, and have developed semiparametric spatial models that allow for discontinuities in the risk surface and make fewer distributional assumptions (Richardson *et al.*, 2004; Best *et al.*, 2005). The BYM model also requires a well defined set of areal boundaries in order to determine adjacency, and this can be complicated in the spatio-temporal setting if boundaries shift. Kelsall and Wakefield (1999) argue for the use of a smooth underlying surface based on a Gaussian random field prior to model areal data, with each areal observation related to the average of the surface over the defined area. Hund *et al.* (2012) build on this to develop a model for temporally misaligned data.

As a general framework for analysing disease risk across geographic areas, hierarchical modelling provides powerful and flexible tools for incorporating available information about how disease risk varies over populations in space. A multilevel statistical perspective can also encourage one to think creatively about causal processes that take place at multiple levels, and lead one to consider relevant exposures and covariates on multiple spatial scales. As methods and computational techniques for hierarchical models continue to evolve, and as rich georeferenced databases continue to proliferate, it is anticipated that these kinds of models will be used more and more widely by epidemiologists and health researchers.

References

Aitkin, M. and Longford, N. (1986) Statistical modelling in school effectiveness studies (with discussion). *Journal of the Royal Statistical Society, Series A (General)* 149, 1–43.

Aitkin, M., Anderson, D. and Hinde, J. (1981) Statistical modelling of data on teaching styles (with discussion). *Journal of the Royal Statistical Society, Series A (General)* 144, 148–161.

Banerjee, S., Carlin, B.P. and Gelfand, A.E. (2004) *Hierarchical Modeling and Analysis for Spatial Data*. Chapman and Hall/CRC, Boca Raton, Florida.

Bernardinelli, L., Clayton, D., Pascutto, C., Montomoli, C., Ghislandi, M. and Songini, M. (1995) Bayesian analysis of space–time variation in disease risk. *Statistics in Medicine* 14, 2433–2443.

Besag, J., York, J. and Mollié, A. (1991) Bayesian image restoration with two applications in spatial statistics. *Annals of the Institute of Statistical Mathematics* 43, 1–59.

Best, N., Cockings, S., Bennett, J., Wakefield, J. and Elliott, P. (2001) Ecological regression analysis of environmental benzene exposure and childhood leukaemia: sensitivity to data inaccuracies, geographical scale and ecological bias. *Journal of the Royal Statistical Society, Series A (Statistics in Society)* 164, 155–174.

Best, N., Richardson, S. and Thomson, A. (2005) A comparison of Bayesian spatial models for disease mapping. *Statistical Methods in Medical Research* 14, 35–49.

Bithell, J.F. (2000) A classification of disease mapping methods. *Statistics in Medicine* 19, 2203–2215.

Blakely, T. and Subramanian, S.V. (2006) Multilevel studies. In: Oakes, J.M. and Kaufman, J.S. (eds) *Methods in Social Epidemiology*. Jossey-Bass, San Francisco, California, pp. 316–340.

Brewer, C.A. (2005) *Designing Better Maps: A Guide for GIS Users*. Esri, Redlands, California.

Browne, W., Goldstein, H. and Rasbash, J. (2001) Multiple membership multiple classification (MMMC) models. *Statistical Modelling* 1, 103–124.

Chen, J.T., Rehkopf, D.H., Waterman, P.D., Subramanian, S.V., Coull, B.A., Cohen, B., Ostrem, M. and Krieger, N. (2006) Mapping and measuring social disparities in premature mortality: the impact of census tract poverty within and across Boston neighborhoods, 1999–2001. *Journal of Urban Health* 83, 1063–1084.

Clayton, D.G. and Bernardinelli, L. (1992) Bayesian methods for mapping disease risk. In: Elliott, P., Cuzick, J., English, D. and Stern, R. (eds) *Geographical and Environmental Epidemiology: Methods for Small-Area Studies*. Oxford University Press, Oxford, UK, pp. 205–220.

Clayton, D. and Kaldor, J. (1987) Empirical Bayes estimates of age-standardized relative risks for use in disease mapping. *Biometrics* 43, 671–681.

Cressie, N. and Chan, N.H. (1989) Spatial modelling of regional variables. *Journal of the American Statistical Association* 84, 393–401.

Earnest, A., Morgan, G., Mengersen, K., Ryan, L., Summerhayes, R. and Beard, J. (2007) Evaluating the effect of neighbourhood weight matrices on smoothing properties of Conditional Autoregressive (CAR) models. *International Journal of Health Geographics* 6, 54.

Elliott, P. and Wakefield, J.C. (1999) Bias and confounding in spatial epidemiology. In: Elliott, P., Wakefield, J.C., Best, N.G. and Briggs, D.J. (eds) *Spatial Epidemiology: Methods and Applications*. Oxford University Press, Oxford, UK, pp. 68–84.

Gelman, A. (2006) Prior distributions for variance parameters in hierarchical models. *Bayesian Analysis* 1, 515–533.

Gelman, A. and Hill, J. (2007) *Data Analysis Using Regression and Multilevel/Hierarchical Models*. Cambridge University Press, Cambridge, UK.

Gelman, A. and Rubin, D. (1992) Inference from iterative simulation using multiple sequences (with discussion). *Statistical Science* 7, 457–511.

Gelman, A., Carlin, J., Stern, H. and Rubin, D. (2003) *Bayesian Data Analysis*, 2nd edn. Chapman and Hall/CRC, Boca Raton, Florida.

Goldstein, H. (2011) *Multilevel Statistical Models*, 4th edn. Edward Arnold, London.

Gomez-Rubio, V., Best, N., Richardson, S., Li, G. and Clarke, P. (2010) Bayesian statistics small area estimation. Technical report. Imperial College, London. Available at http:// eprints. ncrm.ac. uk/1686/#sthash. KO306124.dpuf (accessed 30 June 2013).

Greenland, S. (1992) Divergent biases in ecologic and individual-level studies. *Statistics in Medicine* 11, 1209–1223.

Hill, P. and Goldstein, H. (1998) Multilevel modelling of educational data with cross-classifications and missing identification of units. *Journal of Educational and Behavioral Statistics* 23, 117–128.

Hubbard, A.E., Ahern, J., Fleischer, N.L., Van der Laan, M., Lippman, S.A., Jewell, N., Bruckner, T. and Satariano, W.A. (2010) To GEE or not to GEE: comparing population average and mixed models for estimating the associations between neighborhood risk factors and health. *Epidemiology* 21, 467–474.

Hund, L., Chen, J.T., Krieger, N. and Coull, B.A. (2012) A geostatistical approach to large-scale disease mapping with temporal misalignment. *Biometrics* 68, 849–858.

Kelsall, J.E. and Wakefield, J.C. (1999) Discussion of Bayesian models for spatially correlated disease and exposure data by N. Best, L. Waller, A. Thomas, E. Conlon and R. Arnold. In: Bernardo, J.M., Berger, J.O., Dawid, A.P. and Smith, A.F.M. (eds) *Bayesian Statistics 6: Sixth Valencia International Meeting on Bayesian Statistics, June 6–10, 1998*. Oxford University Press, Oxford, UK.

Langford, I., Leyland, A., Rasbash, J. and, Goldstein, H. (1999) Multilevel modelling of the geographical distribution of rare diseases. *Applied Statistics* 48, 253–268.

Lawson, A., Böhning, D., Biggeri, A., Lesaffe, E. and Viel, J.-F. (1999) Disease mapping and its uses. In: Lawson, A., Biggeri, A., Böhning, D., Lesaffe, E., Viel, J.-F. and Bertollini, R. (eds) *Disease Mapping and Risk Assessment for Public Health*. John Wiley, Chichester, UK, pp. 3–13.

Lawson, A., Browne, W.J. and Vidal Rodeiro, C.L. (2003) *Disease Mapping with WinBUGS and MLwiN*. John Wiley, Chichester, UK.

Liang, K.Y. and Zeger, S. (1986) Longitudinal data analysis using generalized linear models. *Biometrika* 73, 13–22.

Lunn, D.J., Thomas, A., Best, N. and Spiegelhalter, D. (2000) WinBUGS – a Bayesian modelling framework: concepts, structure, and extensibility. *Statistics and Computing* 10, 325–337.

Marshall, R. (1991) A review of methods for the statistical analysis of spatial patterns of disease. *Journal of the Royal Statistical Society, Series A (Statistics in Society)* 154, 421–441.

Pickle, L.W. and White, A.A. (1995) Effects of the choice of age-adjustment method on maps of death rates. *Statistics in Medicine* 14, 615–627.

Richardson, S. (2003) Spatial models in epidemiological applications. In: Green, P.J, Hjort, N.L. and Richardson, S. (eds) *Highly Structured Stochastic Systems*. Oxford University Press, Oxford, UK, pp. 237–259.

Richardson, S., Thomson, A., Best, N.G. and Elliott, P. (2004) Interpreting posterior relative risk estimates in disease-mapping studies. *Environmental Health Perspectives* 112, 1016–1025.

Rue, H., Martino, S. and Chopin, N. (2009) Approximate Bayesian inference for latent Gaussian models by using integrated nested Laplace approximations. *Journal of the Royal Statistical Society, Series B (Statistical Methodology)* 71, 1–35.

Snijders, T.A.B. and Bosker, R.J. (2011) *Multilevel Analysis: An Introduction to Basic and Advanced Multilevel Modeling*, 2nd edn. Sage, London.

Spiegelhalter, D.J, Best, N.G., Carlin, B.P. and van der Linde, A. (2002) Bayesian deviance, the effective number of parameters and the comparison of arbitrarily complex models (with discussion). *Journal of the Royal Statistical Society, Series B (Statistical Methodology)* 64, 583–640.

Subramanian, S., Jones, K. and Duncan, C. (2003) Multilevel methods for public health research. In: Kawachi, I. and Berkman, L. (eds) *Neighborhoods and Health*. Oxford University Press, New York, pp. 65–111.

Wakefield, J.C., Best, N.G. and Waller, L. (2000) Bayesian approaches to disease mapping. In: Elliott, P., Wakefield, J.C., Best, N.G. and Briggs, D.J. (eds) *Spatial Epidemiology: Methods and Applications*. Oxford University Press, Oxford, UK, pp. 104–127.

Wolpert, R.L. and Ickstadt, K. (1998) Poisson/gamma random field models for spatial statistics. *Biometrika* 85, 251–267.

Index

Page numbers in **bold** type refer to figures and tables